LECTURE NOTES ON

General Surgery

HAROLD ELLIS
CBE, DM, FRCS, FRCOG
Department of Anatomy
Guy's Hospital, London

SIR ROY Y. CALNE
MS, FRCS, FRS
Department of Surgery
Addenbrooke's Hospital, Cambridge

CHRISTOPHER J.E. WATSON
MD, FRCS
The Nuffield Department of Surgery
The John Radcliffe Hospital
Oxford

Ninth edition

b

Blackwell
Science

© 1965, 1968, 1970, 1972, 1977, 1983,
1987, 1993, 1998 by
Blackwell Science Ltd
Editorial Offices:
Osney Mead, Oxford OX2 0EL
25 John Street, London WC1N 2BL
23 Ainslie Place, Edinburgh EH3 6AJ
350 Main Street, Malden
  MA 02148 5018, USA
54 University Street, Carlton
  Victoria 3053, Australia
10, rue Casimir Delavigne
  75006 Paris, France

Other Editorial Offices:
Blackwell Wissenschafts-Verlag GmbH
Kurfürstendamm 57
10707 Berlin, Germany

Blackwell Science KK
MG Kodenmacho Building
7-10 Kodenmacho Nihombashi
Chuo-ku, Tokyo 104, Japan

The right of the Authors to be
identified as the Author of this Work
has been asserted in accordance
with the Copyright, Designs and
Patents Act 1988.

Set by Excel Typesetters, Co.,
  Hong Kong
Printed and bound in the United Kingdom
at the University Press, Cambridge

First published 1965
Revised edition 1966
Second edition 1968
Greek edition 1968
Third edition 1970
Fourth edition 1972
Reprinted 1974
Revised reprint 1976
Fifth edition 1977
Portuguese edition 1979
Reprinted 1979, 1980
Sixth edition 1983,
Reprinted 1984, 1985, 1986
Seventh edition 1987
Reprinted 1989 (twice)
Eighth edition 1993
Reprinted 1994. 1996
Ninth edition 1998
Reprinted 1999

A catalogue record for this title
is available from the British Library

ISBN 0-86542-768-2

Library of Congress
Cataloging-in-publication Data

Ellis, Harold, 1926–
    Lecture notes on general
surgery/Harold Ellis, Sir Roy Calne,
C. Watson.—9th ed.
        p.   cm.
    Includes index.
    ISBN 0-86542-768-2
    1. Surgery — Handbooks,
manuals, etc
    I. Calne, Roy Yorke.
    II. Watson, Christopher J. E.
Christopher John Edward)
    III. Title
    [DNLM: 1. Surgery.   WO 100
    E47L 1998]
RD37.E44   1998
617–dc21
DNLM/DLC
for Library of Congress   97-42474
                                        CIP

DISTRIBUTORS

Marston Book Services Ltd
PO Box 269
Abingdon Oxon OX14 4YN
(Orders: Tel: 01235 465500
        Fax: 01235 465555)

USA
Blackwell Science, Inc.
Commerce Place
350 Main Street
Malden, MA 02148 5018
(Orders: Tel: 800 759 6102
                781 388 8250
        Fax: 781 388 8255)

Canada
Login Brothers Book Company
324 Saulteaux Crescent
Winnipeg, Manitoba R3J 3T2
(Orders: Tel: 204 837-2987)

Australia
Blackwell Science Pty Ltd
54 University Street
Carlton, Victoria 3053
(Orders: Tel: 3 9347 0300
        Fax: 3 9347 5001)

For further information on
Blackwell Science, visit our website:
www.blackwell-science.com

Contents

Introduction

The ideal medical student at the end of the clinical course will have written his or her own textbook—a digest of the lectures and tutorials assiduously attended and of the textbooks meticulously read. Unfortunately, few students are perfect, and most approach the qualifying examinations depressed by the thought of the thousands of pages of excellent and exhaustive textbooks wherein lies the wisdom required of them by the examiners.

We believe that there is a serious need in these days of widening knowledge and expanding syllabus for a book that will set out briefly the important facts in general surgery that are classified, analysed and as far as possible rationalized for the revision student. These lecture notes represent our own final-year teaching; they are in no way a substitute for the standard textbooks but are our attempts to draw together in some sort of logical way the fundamentals of general surgery.

Because this book is written at student level, principles of treatment only are presented, not details of surgical technique.

We recommend the companion volume *Spot Diagnosis in General Surgery* (1993, Blackwell Science), which provides colour illustrations and questions and answers based on the text of *Lecture Notes on General Surgery*.

In the Ninth Edition, the two senior authors, having been involved for more than three decades in successive revisions, are fortunate in being joined by Mr Christopher Watson. He brings with him the fresh approach of the new generation of surgical teachers and has carefully reviewed every paragraph of the text. The numerous important advances in surgery that have been made in recent years have inevitably resulted in some increase in the amount of text, which we have partly controlled by judicious excisions of out-of-date material. Space has also been saved by the use of summary boxes. We are confident that this volume will continue to serve the needs of medical students into the next millenium.

H. E.
R. Y. C.
C. J. E. W.

Acknowledgements

We are grateful to our colleagues—registrars, housemen and students — who have read and criticized this text during its production, and to many readers and reviewers for their constructve criticisms. Mr R. Macfarlane, Mr P. Hall, Dr M. Lindop and Dr J. Firth at Addenbrooke's Hospital gave valuable advice.

Finally, we would like to acknowledge the continued help given by the staff at Blackwell Science, in particular Dr Michael Stein.

CHAPTER 1

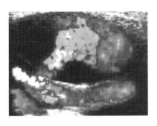

Fluid and Electrolyte Management

The management of a patient's fluid status is vital to a successful outcome in surgery. This requires pre-operative assessment, with resuscitation if required, and post-operative replacement of normal and abnormal losses until the patient can resume a normal diet. This chapter will review the normal state and the mechanisms that maintain homeostasis, and will then discuss the aberrations and their management.

Body fluid compartments
(Fig. 1.1)

In the average person, water contributes 60% to the total body weight. Forty per cent of the body weight is intracellular fluid, the remaining 20% extracellular. This extracellular fluid can be subdivided into intravascular (5%) and extravascular, or interstitial (15%). Fluid may cross from compartment to compartment by osmosis, which depends on a solute gradient, and filtration, which is the result of a hydrostatic pressure gradient.

The electrolyte composition of each compartment differs. Intracellular fluid has a low sodium and a high potassium concentration. In contrast, extracellular fluid (intravascular and interstitial) has a high sodium and low potassium concentration. Only 2% of the total body potassium is in the extracellular fluid. There is also difference in protein con-centration within the extracellular compartment, with the interstitial fluid having a very low concentration compared with the high protein concentration of the intravascular compartment.

Knowledge of fluid compartments and their composition becomes very important when considering fluid replacement. In order rapidly to fill the intravascular compartment, a plasma substitute or blood is the fluid of choice. Such fluids, with high colloid osmotic potential, remain within the intravascular space, in contrast to a saline solution, which rapidly distributes over the entire extravas-cular compartment, which is four times as large as the intravascular compartment alone. Thus, of the original litre of saline, only 250 ml would remain in the intravascular compart-ment. Five per cent dextrose, which is water with a small amount of dextrose added to render it isotonic, will redistribute across both intracellular and extracellular spaces.

Fluid and electrolyte losses

In order to calculate daily fluid and electrolyte requirements, the daily losses should be measured or estimated. Fluid is lost from four routes: the kidney, the gastrointestinal tract, the skin and the respiratory tract. Losses from the latter two routes are termed insensible losses.

1

FLUID AND ELECTROLYTE DISTRIBUTION

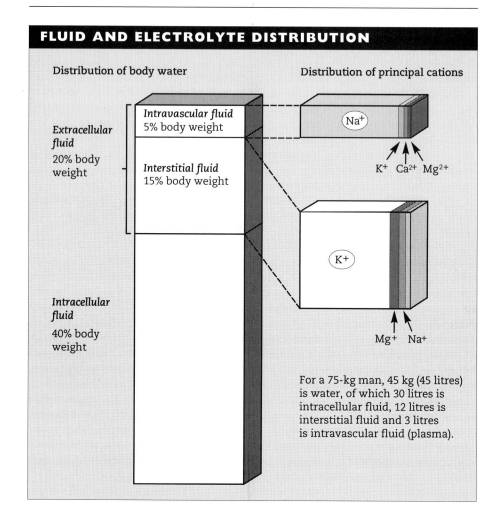

Distribution of body water

Extracellular fluid
20% body weight

Intravascular fluid
5% body weight

Interstitial fluid
15% body weight

Intracellular fluid
40% body weight

Distribution of principal cations

Na⁺

K⁺ Ca²⁺ Mg²⁺

K⁺

Mg⁺ Na⁺

For a 75-kg man, 45 kg (45 litres) is water, of which 30 litres is intracellular fluid, 12 litres is interstitial fluid and 3 litres is intravascular fluid (plasma).

Fig. 1.1 Distribution of fluid and electrolytes within the body.

Normal fluid losses (Table 1.1)
The kidney
In the absence of intrinsic renal disease, fluid losses from the kidney are regulated by aldosterone and antidiuretic hormone (ADH). These two hormone systems regulate the circulating volume and its osmolarity, and are thus crucial to homeostasis. Aldosterone responds to a fall in glomerular perfusion by salt retention. ADH responds to the increased solute concentration by retaining water in the renal tubules. Normal urinary losses are around 1500–2000 ml/day.

The gastrointestinal tract
The stomach, liver and pancreas secrete a large amount of electrolyte-rich fluid into the gut. After digestion and absorption, the waste material enters the colon, where the remaining water is resorbed. Approximately 300 ml is lost into the faeces each day.

Insensible losses
Inspired air is humidified in its passage to the alveoli, and much of this water is lost with

NORMAL FLUID LOSSES

Fluid loss	Volume (ml)	Na+ (mmol)	K+ (mmol)
Urine	2000	80–130	60
Faeces	300		
Insensible	400		
Total	2700		

Table 1.1 Normal fluid losses.

expiration. Fluid is also lost from the skin, and the total of these insensible losses is around 700 ml/day. This may be balanced by insensible production of fluid, with around 300 ml of 'metabolic' water being produced endogenously.

Abnormal fluid losses
The kidney
Impaired tubular function may cause increased losses. Resolving acute tubular necrosis (p. 330), diabetes insipidus and head injury may result in loss of several litres of dilute urine. In contrast, production of ADH by tumours (the syndrome of inappropriate ADH, or SIADH) causes water retention and haemodilution.

The gastrointestinal tract
Loss of water by the gastrointestinal tract is increased in diarrhoea and in the presence of an ileostomy, where colonic water resorption is absent.

Vomiting, naso-gastric aspiration and fistulous losses result in loss of electrolyte-rich fluid. Disturbance of the acid–base balance may also occur if predominantly acid or alkali fluid is lost, as occurs with pyloric stenosis and with a pancreatic fistula, respectively.

Large occult losses occur in paralytic ileus and intestinal obstruction. Several litres of fluid may be sequestered in the gut contributing to the hypovolaemia. Resolution of an ileus is marked by absorption of the fluid

and the resultant hypervolaemia produces a diuresis.

Insensible losses
Hyperventilation, as may happen with pain or chest infection, increases respiratory losses. Losses from the skin are increased by pyrexia and sweating, with up to a litre of sweat per hour in extreme cases. Sweat contains a large amount of salt.

Effects of surgery

ADH is released in response to surgery, conserving water. Hypovolaemia will cause aldosterone secretion and salt retention by the kidney. Potassium is released by damaged tissues, and the potassium level may be further increased by blood transfusion, each unit containing in excess of 20 mmol. If renal perfusion is poor, and urine output sparse, this potassium will not be excreted and accumulates, causing life-threatening arrhythmias. This is the basis of the recommendation that supplementary potassium is not necessary in the first 48 hours following surgery or trauma.

Prescribing fluids for the surgical patient
The majority of patients require fluid replacement for only a brief period post-operatively until they resume a normal diet. Some require resuscitation pre-operatively, and others require replacement of specific losses such as those from a fistula. In severely ill patients, and those with impaired gastrointestinal function, long-term nutritional support is necessary.

The amount of fluid required = Normal losses (insensible and urinary)

+ Abnormal losses (e.g. fistula, surgical drain)

+ Initial fluid deficit (estimated)

Replacement of normal losses

Table 1.1 shows the normal daily fluid losses. Replacement of this lost fluid (Table 1.2) is achieved by the administration of 3 litres of fluid, which may comprise 1 litre of normal saline (150 mmol of NaCl) together with 2 litres of water (as 5% dextrose). Potassium may be added to each litre bag (20 mmol/L). Adjustments to this regimen should be based on regular examination, measurement of losses (e.g. urine output) and regular blood samples for electrolyte determination. For example, if the patient is anuric, 1 L/day of hypertonic dextrose without potassium may suffice, which has the added advantage or reducing catabolism with the breakdown of protein and accumulation of urea. Daily weighing of the patient will give an estimate of changes in the total amount of body fluid.

Replacement of special losses

Special losses include naso-gastric aspirates, losses from fistulae, diarrhoea and stomas, and covert losses as occur with an ileus. Loss of plasma in burns is considered elsewhere (Chapter 6). All fluid losses should be measured carefully where possible, and this volume added to the normal daily requirements. The composition of these special losses varies (Table 1.3), but as a rough guide replacement with an equal volume of normal saline should suffice. Extra potassium supplements may be required where losses are high, such as in diarrhoea. Analysis of the electrolyte content of fistula drainage may be useful.

Resuscitation

Estimation of the fluid deficit in patients is particularly important when they first present

Table 1.2 Electrolyte content of intravenous fluids.

INTRAVENOUS FLUIDS

Intravenous infusion	Na$^+$ (mmol/L)	Cl$^-$ (mmol/L)	K$^+$ (mmol/L)	HCO$_3^-$ (mmol/L)	Ca^{2+} (mmol/L)
Normal saline (0.9% saline)	150	150	—	—	—
4% dextrose 0.18% saline	30	30	—	—	—
Hartmann's (compound sodium lactate)	131	111	5	29	2
Normal plasma values	140	103	4.5	26	2.5

Table 1.3 Daily volume and composition of gastrointestinal fluids.

GASTROINTESTINAL FLUIDS

Fluid	Volume (ml)	Na$^+$ (mmol/L)	K$^+$ (mmol/L)	Cl$^-$ (mmol/L)	H$^+$/HCO$_3^-$ (mmol/L)	
Gastric	2500	30–80	5–20	100–150	H$^+$	40–60
Bile	500	130	10	100	HCO$_3^-$	30–50
Pancreatic	1000	130	10	75	HCO$_3^-$	70–110
Small bowel	5000	130	10	90–130	HCO$_3^-$	20–40

in order to enable accurate replacement. Dry mucous membranes, loss of skin turgor, tachycardia and postural hypotension, together with a low jugular venous pressure suggest a loss of between 5 and 15% of total body water. Fluid losses of under 5% body water are difficult to detect clinically; over 15% there is marked circulatory collapse.

As an example, consider a 70-kg man presenting with a perforated peptic ulcer. On examination he is noted to have dry mucous membranes, a tachycardia and slight postural fall in arterial blood pressure. If the loss is estimated at 10% of the total body water, itself 60% of body weight, the volume deficit is 10% $\times$ 60% of 70 kg, or 10% of 42 litres = 4.2 litres. As this loss is largely isotonic (gastric juices and the peritoneal inflammatory response), infusion of isotonic saline (normal saline) is appropriate. A general rule of thumb is to replace half of the estimated loss quickly, and then reassess before replacement of the rest. The best guide to the success of resuscitation is the resumption of normal urine output, therefore hourly urine output should be measured. Placement of a central venous catheter once initial resuscitation has begun will also help in the adjustment of rate of infusion.

Nutrition

Many patients undergoing elective and emergency surgery are reasonably well nourished and do not require special supplementation pre- or post-operatively. Recovery from surgery is usually swift, and the patient resumes a normal diet before he or she has become seriously malnourished. There are, however, certain categories of patients where nutrition prior to surgery is poor and may be a critical factor in determining the outcome of an operation, lowering their resistance to infection and impairing wound healing. Such patients include those with chronic intestinal fistulae, malabsorption, chronic liver disease, neoplasia, starvation, and after chemo- and radiotherapy. Wherever possible, nutritional support should be instituted before surgery, as post-operative recovery will be much quicker.

Enteral feeding

If the gastrointestinal tract is functioning satisfactorily, oral intake can be supplemented by a basic diet introduced through a fine naso-gastric tube directly into the stomach. The constituents of the diet are designed to be readily absorbable protein, fat and carbohydrate. Such a diet can provide 8400 kJ with 70 g protein in a volume of 2 litres. The commonest complication is diarrhoea, which is usually self-limiting.

If a prolonged post-operative recovery is anticipated, or a large pre-operative nutritional deficit needs to be corrected, consideration should be given to insertion of a feeding jejunostomy at the time of surgery. This has the advantage of avoiding a naso-gastric tube.

Parenteral feeding

For patients with intestinal fistulae, prolonged ileus or malabsorption, nutrition cannot be supplemented through the gastrointestinal tract and therefore parenteral feeding is necessary. This is usually administered via a catheter in a central vein because of the high osmolarity of the solutions used; there is a high risk of phlebitis in smaller veins with lower blood flow. However, peripheral parenteral nutrition with less hyperosmolar solutions such as Vitlipid can be used for short-term feeding. The exact management is best directed by an expert in nutrition, but in principle is to provide the patient with protein in the form of amino acids, carbohydrate in the form of glucose, and fat emulsions such as Intralipid. Energy is derived from the carbohydrate and fat (30–50% fat), which must be given when amino acids are given, usually in a ratio of 1000 kJ/g protein nitrogen. Trace elements, such as zinc, magnesium and copper, as well as vitamins such as vitamin B_{12} and ascorbic acid, and the lipid-soluble vitamins A, D, E and K, are usually added to the fluid, which is infused as a 2.5-litre volume over 24 hours. Daily weights as well as biochemical estimations of electrolytes and albumin are useful guides to continued requirements.

The ability of a patient to benefit from intravenous feeding depends on the general state of metabolism and residual liver function. Nutritional support should be continued in the post-operative period until gastrointestinal function returns and the patient is restored to positive nitrogen balance from the perioperative catabolic state. Restoration of a positive nitrogen balance is often apparent to the nurses and doctors as a sudden occurrence, when the patient starts smiling and asks for food. Occasionally in chronic malnutrition with intestinal fistulae or in patients who have lost most of the small bowel, parenteral feeding may be necessary on a long-term basis.

Complications of total parenteral nutrition (TPN) include sepsis, thrombosis, hyponatraemia, hyperglycaemia and liver damage. To minimize sepsis, the central venous catheter is tunnelled with a subcutaneous Dacron cuff at the exit site to reduce the risk of line infection. Thrombosis may occur on any indwelling venous catheter, and in patients requiring long-term TPN this is a major cause of morbidity. Hyperglycaemia is common, particularly following pancreatitis, and may necessitate infusion of insulin.

CHAPTER 2

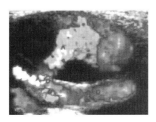

Shock

Shock is characterized by inadequate perfusion of vital organs, principally the heart and brain.

Aetiology

Tissue perfusion requires an adequate blood pressure, which is dependent upon the systemic vascular resistance and cardiac output; the cardiac output is a function of the heart rate and the stroke volume. These may be expressed in mathematical terms:

$$CO = HR \times SV$$
$$BP = CO \times SVR$$

where CO is cardiac output, SV is stroke volume, HR is heart rate, BP is arterial blood pressure and SVR is systemic vascular resistance.

Normal regulation of tissue perfusion

The autonomic nervous system is able to alter heart rate and peripheral vascular resistance in response to changes in blood pressure detected by the carotid sinus and aortic arch baroreceptors; changes in systemic vascular resistance may alter venous return by changing the amount of fluid circulating in the cutaneous and splanchnic vascular beds. Venous return determines stroke volume; increasing venous return causes an increase in stroke volume, the heart acting as a permissive pump (Starling's law*: the output depends on the degree of stretch of the heart muscle in diastole). Volume regulation is achieved by the kidney, in particular by the regulation of sodium loss by the renin–angiotensin–aldosterone system (p. 68) and antidiuretic hormone (ADH) produced by the posterior pituitary; in addition, a fall in circulating volume prompts the sensation of thirst, stimulating increased fluid intake.

Abnormal regulation of tissue perfusion

Inadequate tissue perfusion (shock) may result from factors related to the pump (the heart) and factors relating to the systemic circulation. The causes of shock may be classified accordingly, as follows.

1 *Cardiogenic shock.* A primary failure of cardiac output in which the heart is unable to maintain adequate stroke volume in spite of satisfactory filling. Compensation involves an increase in heart rate and systemic vascular resistance, manifested clinically by a tachycardia, sweating (due to sympathetic nervous system outflow), pallor and coldness (due to cutaneous vasoconstriction). Causes include:

---

*E. H. Starling (1866–1927), Professor of Physiology, University College, London. Described capillary flow events and discovered secretin with Bayliss.

(a) massive myocardial infarction;
(b) pulmonary embolism;
(c) acute ventricular–septal defect;
(d) mitral or aortic valve rupture;
(e) acute cardiac tamponade.

2 *Fluid loss.* Reduction in circulating volume results in a reduction in stroke volume and cardiac output. Blood pressure is initially maintained as in cardiogenic shock, with increased sympathetic activity raising the peripheral vascular resistance leading to the clinical picture of a cold, clammy patient with a tachycardia. As volume losses increase, the blood pressure falls. In severe cases the patient is confused or semi-conscious. Causes include:

(a) haemorrhage, overt or covert;
(b) burns, with massive loss of plasma and electrolytes;
(c) severe diarrhoea or vomiting, with fluid and electrolyte loss, particularly in colitis or pyloric stenosis;
(d) bowel obstruction, where large amounts of fluid are sequestered into the gut, in addition to the losses due to vomiting;
(e) peritonitis, with large fluid losses into the abdomen as a consequence of infection or chemical irritation;
(f) gastrointestinal fistulae with fluid and electrolyte loss;
(g) urinary losses, e.g. the osmotic diuresis of diabetic ketoacidosis, or polyuria in resolving acute tubular necrosis (p. 330).

3 *Reduction in systemic vascular resistance.* Reduction in systemic vascular resistance increases the size of the systemic vascular bed, producing a relative hypovolaemia, reduced diastolic filling, reduced stroke volume and thus a fall in blood pressure. Unlike the previous two causes, vasodilatation occurs as part of the pathogenesis, so the patient appears warm ('hot shock'), not cold and peripherally shut down. The heart compensates with a tachycardia. The principal causes are:

(a) anaphylaxis;
(b) sepsis;
(c) spinal shock.

4 *Confounding factors: β-blockers for hypertension.* Pre-existing medical conditions and medications may confuse the clinical picture. Consider a patient with hypertension and taking β-blockers such as atenolol. For that patient a systolic blood pressure of 110 mmHg may be very low, while the atenolol prevents a tachycardia response.

Special causes of shock

Adreno-cortical failure
Loss of the hormones produced by the cortex of the suprarenal gland may follow bilateral suprarenal haemorrhage, adrenalectomy, Addison's disease or lack of corticosteroid replacement in patients who have been on long-term glucocorticoids.

Loss of aldosterone results in volume depletion and glucocorticoid deficiency, which impairs autonomic responses. The ability to respond to minor stress is severely compromised and may provoke an Addisonian crisis characterized by bradycardia and postural hypotension, which is responsive to corticosteroid replacement. No patient should die from unexplained hypotension without first receiving a bolus of hydrocortisone.

Sympathetic interruption
This reduces the effective blood volume by widespread vasodilatation. It follows transection of the spinal cord (spinal shock), but may also occur after a high spinal anaesthetic.

The vasovagal syndrome (faint)
The vasovagal syndrome is produced by severe pain or emotional disturbance. It is due to reflex vasodilatation together with cardiac slowing due to vagal activity. Hypotension is due to a fall in cardiac output due both to bradycardia and reduced venous return, the latter due to peripheral vasodilatation. Clinically, it is recognized by the presence of a bradycardia and responds to the simple measure of lying the patient flat with elevation of the legs.

Septic shock
Shock may be produced as the result of severe infection from either Gram-positive or, more

commonly, Gram-negative organisms. The latter is particularly seen after colonic, biliary and urological surgery, and with infected severe burns. The principal effect of endotoxins is to cause vasodilatation of the peripheral circulation together with increased capillary permeability. The effects are partly direct, and partly due to activation of normal tissue inflammatory responses such as the complement system and mediators such as tumour necrosis factor.

Activation of the clotting cascade results in *disseminated intravascular coagulation* (DIC), and blockage of the arterial microcirculation by microemboli may ensue. Fibrin and platelets are consumed excessively, with resultant haemorrhages into the skin, the gastrointestinal tract, the lungs, mouth and nose.

Sequelae of shock

A continued low blood pressure produces a series of irreversible changes, so that the patient may die in spite of treatment. The oxygen lack affects all the vital organs.
- *Cerebral hypoperfusion* results in confusion or coma.
- *Renal hypoperfusion* results in reduced glomerular filtration, with oliguria or anuria. As renal ischaemia progresses, tubular necrosis may occur, and profound ischaemia may lead to cortical necrosis (p. 330).
- *The heart* may fail due to inadequate coronary perfusion.
- *Pulmonary capillaries* may reflect the changes in the systemic circulation with transudation of fluid resulting in pulmonary oedema, hampering oxygen transfer and causing further arterial hypoxaemia and thus tissue hypoxia. Pulmonary capillary function may also be impaired following multiple blood transfusions and contusions resulting from chest trauma, a picture known as acute lung injury (previously termed 'shock lung').
- *DIC* precipitated by sepsis may be further aggravated by hypothermia unless active rewarming is undertaken.

Principles in the management of patients in shock

Immediate measures
The immediate treatment of patients in shock vary according to cause. Two causes merit mention for immediate treatment: bleeding and anaphylaxis.

Bleeding
Direct pressure should be applied to a bleeding wound. Immediate surgical exploration is indicated where continued bleeding is likely, such as is caused by peptic ulcer haemorrhage, ruptured spleen, ruptured aortic aneurysm or ruptured ectopic pregnancy. In these cases, resuscitation cannot overcome the losses until the rate of blood loss is curtailed.

Anaphylaxis
In a surgical practice, this may arise as an allergic reaction to an antibiotic or radiological contrast medium. In addition to hypotension (due to vasodilatation), bronchospasm and laryngeal oedema may be present and warrant immediate therapy. The immediate treatment for anaphylaxis is the administration of adrenaline (0.5 ml of 1 : 1000 adrenaline) intramuscularly or subcutaneously, repeated every 10–30 minutes as required. Subsequently hydrocortisone and antihistamine agents may be given (e.g. chlorpheniramine).

For milder reactions, aliquots of 1 ml of 1 : 10 000 adrenaline are given and titrated to effect.

Monitoring and subsequent management
The severely shocked patient should be admitted to an intensive care ward where continuous supervision by specially trained nursing staff is available. As well as careful clinical surveillance, the following need to be monitored.
- Core temperature, pulse, respiration rate and blood pressure.
- Hourly urine output (via a urinary catheter).
- Central venous pressure.

- Pulse oximetry. Oxygen is administered to ensure adequate oxygenation. Mechanical ventilation may be required.
- Electrocardiogram (ECG).
- Serum electrolytes, haemoglobin and white blood cell count.
- Arterial Po_2, Pco_2, pH.
- The cardiac output, left atrial and pulmonary arterial pressures using a Swan–Ganz catheter (see below).

The frequency of these measurements depends on the patient's condition and response to treatment. It is particularly important that doctors remember that, in this environment of recording machinery and scientific nursing, the patient remains a human being, who deserves to be treated with dignity and tenderness. If the patient is conscious, he or she may well be terrified, in pain and acutely aware of all that is going on. Proper explanations and appropriate analgesia must be provided.

Swan–Ganz catheter*

The Swan–Ganz catheter is a multiple-lumen catheter, which is passed via a central vein (internal jugular or subclavian) into the right atrium. At this stage, a small balloon on the end of the catheter is inflated. The inflated balloon then 'floats' with the blood returning to the heart across the tricuspid and pulmonary valves into the pulmonary artery. Once in the pulmonary artery, the catheter is advanced until it wedges itself in a small branch of a pulmonary artery. The balloon is then deflated. During insertion, the position of the catheter can be monitored by the changing pressure waveform recorded by a transducer connected to the lumen. The catheter also has a temperature probe near its tip, which facilitates the measurement of cardiac output.

Cardiac output is calculated by the Fick principle after injecting a bolus of cold saline through the catheter and monitoring the change in temperature. Importantly, the

*H. J. C. Swan, Cardiologist, Cedars of Lebanon Hospital, Los Angeles, USA. W. Ganz, Engineer, Cedars of Lebanon Hospital, Los Angeles, USA.

catheter also allows calculation of the systemic and pulmonary vascular resistances.

When the balloon is inflated no flow comes past the tip. The catheter is wedged and the pressure that is recorded, referred to as the wedge pressure, is an approximation of the left atrial pressure.

Fluid management
See Chapter 1.

Prevention of hypothermia
Patients may cool down due to neglect, infusion of cold fluids particularly unwarmed blood, and extracorporeal circulations such as haemodialysis or haemofiltration circuits. Allowing a patient to cool down to subnormal temperatures (35°C and below) impairs the normal coagulation mechanisms and promotes fibrinolysis, possibly resulting in DIC.

To prevent this, all infusions should be prewarmed, and the patient actively rewarmed using warm air blankets.

Pharmacological agents
The shocked patient may require significant pharmacological support. The principal drugs used are catecholamines or their derivatives, in addition to drugs to treat specific causes such as antimicrobial therapy for septicaemia. Patients in cardiogenic shock benefit from positive inotropic agents, while patients with low systemic vascular resistance due to sepsis require agents to increase vascular resistance. The drugs used in this context are sympathomimetics, with differing degrees of α (peripheral vasoconstriction), β_1 (inotropic and chronotropic) and β_2 (peripheral vasodilatation) effects. Examples of such drugs include the following.

Dopamine
Dopamine has three separate actions according to dose.

1 At low doses (2 µg/kg/min) dopaminergic actions dominate, causing increased renal perfusion. This is the commonest indication for the use of dopamine.

2 *At moderate doses* (5 μg/kg/min), β_1 effects predominate with positive inotropic activity (increasing myocardial contractility and rate).
3 *At higher doses* (over 5 μg/kg/min), α effects predominate with vasoconstriction.

Dobutamine
Dobutamine has predominantly β_1 actions increasing myocardial contractility and rate. It is used principally in cardiogenic shock.

Noradrenaline
Noradrenaline has predominantly α effects, but with modest β activity. It is used to increase systemic vascular resistance through its vasoconstrictor α effects.

Adrenaline
Adrenaline has strong α and β actions, and may be used to increase peripheral resistance while also increasing cardiac output. The powerful vasoconstrictor actions of both adrenaline and noradrenaline may result in ischaemia and infarction of peripheral tissues, most commonly fingers, toes, and the tips of the nose and ears.

CHAPTER 3

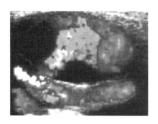

Post-operative Complications

Classification

Any operation carries with it the risk of complications. These should be considered as:

• *Local*—involving the operation site itself.

• *General*— affecting any of the other systems of the body, e.g. respiratory, urological or cardiovascular complications.

In addition, post-operative complications should be classified into:

• *Immediate*—within the first 24 hours.

• *Early*—within the first 4 weeks.

• *Late* — any subsequent period, often long after the patient has left hospital.

A useful table of post-operative complications following abdominal surgery is presented in Table 3.1. This scheme can be modified for operations concerning any other system.

Wound infection

The incidence of wound infection after surgical operations is still in the region of 10%. It is especially high where pre-operative sepsis already exists. In pre-antibiotic days it was particularly the haemolytic *Streptococcus* that was feared, but now, as this is still usually penicillin sensitive, the principal causes of wound infection are the penicillin-resistant *Staphylococcus aureus*, together with *Streptococcus faecalis*, *Pseudomonas*, coliform bacilli and other bowel bacteria including bacteroides. With continued use of antibiotics, more resistant strains of the organisms are appearing, such as the methicillin-resistant *Staphylococcus aureus* (MRSA) and the vancomycin-resistant *Enterococcus* (VRE).

Aetiology

In considering the aetiology of any post-operative complication the following classification should be used:

• *pre-operative*—factors already existing before the operation is carried out;

• *operative*—factors that come into play during the operation itself;

• *post-operative* — factors introduced after the patient's return to the ward.

Pre-operative factors

There may be pre-existing infection, e.g. a perforated appendix or an infected compound fracture. The patient may be a nasal carrier of staphylococci or have a skin infection, e.g. a crop of boils.

Operative factors

These are lapses in theatre technique, e.g. failure of adequate sterilization of instruments, the surgeon's hands or dressings. There may be nasal or skin carriers of staphylococci among the nursing and surgical staff. Wound infections are especially common when the alimentary, biliary or urinary tract is opened during surgery, allowing bacterial contamination to occur. Wounds placed in poorly

ABDOMINAL SURGERY COMPLICATIONS

Time	Local	General
0 hours to 24 hours	Reactionary haemorrhage	Asphyxia ⟨ Obstructed airway / Inhaled vomit
2nd day to 3 weeks	Paralytic ileus	Pulmonary ⟨ Collapse / Broncho-pneumonia / Embolus
	Infection ⟨ Wound / Peritonitis / Pelvic / Subphrenic	Urinary ⟨ Retention / Suppression of production (tubular necrosis)
	Secondary haemorrhage	
	Dehiscence ⟨ Wound / Anastomosis	Deep venous thrombosis Enterocolitis Bed sores
	Obstruction due to fibrinous adhesions	
Late	Obstruction due to fibrous adhesions Incisional hernia Persistent sinus Recurrence of original lesion (e.g. stomal ulcer or malignancy)	*After extensive resections or gastrectomy* Anaemia Vitamin deficiency Steatorrhoea and/or diarrhoea Osteoporosis Dumping syndrome

Table 3.1 Post-operative complications following abdominal surgery.

vascularized tissue, such as an amputation stump, are also prone to infection, as necrotic tissue is a good medium for bacterial growth, and a good blood supply is necessary to provide access for the inflammatory cells.

Post-operative factors
Cross-infection may occur from infected cases in the ward during dressing changes or wound inspection, or there may be contamination of the wound from the nose or hands of the surgical or nursing staff.

Clinical features
The onset of wound infection is usually a few days after operation; this may be delayed still further, even up to weeks, if antimicrobial chemotherapy has been employed. The patient complains of pain and swelling in the wound, of the general effects of infection (malaise, anorexia, vomiting) and runs a swinging pyrexia. The wound is red, swollen, hot and tender. Removal of sutures or probing of the wound releases the contained pus.

Treatment
Prophylaxis comprises scrupulous theatre and dressing technique, the isolation of infected cases and the elimination of carriers with colds or septic lesions among the medical and nursing staff.

Established infection is treated by drainage; antibiotics are given if there is, in addition, a spreading cellulitis.

Antimicrobial prophylaxis
Prophylactic antimicrobial chemotherapy (or prophylactic antibiotics as they are more usually known), was, in the early days of its use,

believed to herald the end of wound infections. Unfortunately, this soon proved to be a false hope, and the widespread use of these drugs simply saw the emergence of resistant strains of bacteria and of many examples of diarrhoea, skin rashes and other unpleasant side-effects.

There are instances where prophylactic antibiotics are indicated, as follows, and the antibiotics chosen are those specific to the likely bacterial flora encountered. The principle of prophylaxis is to treat before contamination occurs, and this is particularly important with antibiotics, where an adequate antibiotic concentration needs to be present in the blood at the time of exposure to infection.

• *Valvular heart disease.* In patients with valvular heart disease, commonly rheumatic mitral valve disease, prophylaxis is given against haematogenous bacterial colonization of the valve resulting in infective endocarditis.

• *Implantation or presence of a foreign body.* Where a foreign body such as a prosthetic heart valve or prosthetic joint is implanted, antibiotics are used to prevent infection of the prosthesis at the time of surgery. The commonest infecting agent is *Staphylococcus aureus*, therefore the antibiotic spectrum should cover this organism. Haematogenous spread of an organism during other procedures should also be borne in mind, occurring in a similar manner to infective endocarditis.

• *Vascular surgery and organ transplant surgery,* especially where prosthetic material is used and where immunosuppression or ischaemia exists.

• *Amputation of an ischaemic limb.* Here the risk of gas gangrene is high, particularly above the knee where contamination by perineal and faecal organisms may occur: penicillin is the antibiotic of choice.

• *Penetrating wounds and compound fractures.* Again principally as prophylaxis against clostridial infections.

• *Where there is a high risk of bacterial contamination,* such as in operations that involve opening the biliary or alimentary tract (especially the large bowel), prophylactic systemic or local broad-spectrum antibiotics are indicated.

In colonic surgery, cover against anaerobic organisms is particularly important and is afforded by metronidazole.

Antibiotic-associated enterocolitis

Broad-spectrum antibiotics result in the destruction of the normal commensal gut organisms, selecting out resistant forms, such as the toxin-producing strains of *Clostridium difficile*. The patient experiences severe watery diarrhoea due to extensive enterocolitis, and the bowel shows mucosal inflammation with pseudo-membrane formation — pseudo-membranous colitis.

When first described, there was a strong association with preceding lincomycin or clindamycin therapy; today, cephalosporins and co-amoxiclav are the commonest culprits, reflecting their widespread use in clinical practice.

Clinical features

Antibiotic-associated enterocolitis usually occurs in the first post-operative week in patients who have received broad-spectrum antibiotics. The condition is particularly likely to occur after large-bowel surgery. Mild cases present simply with watery diarrhoea. Severe cases have a cholera-like picture with a sudden onset of profuse, watery diarrhoea with excess mucus, abdominal distension and shock due to the profound fluid loss. Occasionally, *Clostridium difficile* infection may present with a toxic dilatation of the colon.

Sigmoidoscopy reveals a red, friable mucosa with whitish yellow plaques, which may coalesce to form a pseudo-membrane.

Treatment

Intravenous fluid and electrolyte replacement is essential. Other antibiotics are stopped and oral metronidazole, or vancomycin (which is not absorbed from the gut and which rapidly eliminates *Clostridium difficile*), is prescribed.

Pulmonary collapse and infection

Some degree of pulmonary collapse occurs after almost every abdominal or trans-thoracic procedure. Mucus is retained in the bronchial tree, blocking the smaller bronchi; the alveolar air is then absorbed, with collapse of the supplied lung segments (usually the basal lobes). The collapsed lung continues to be perfused and acts as a shunt, which reduces oxygenation. The lung segment may become secondarily infected by inhaled or aspirated organisms, and rarely abscess formation may occur.

Aetiology
Pre-operative factors
• *Pre-existing acute or chronic pulmonary infection* increases the amount of bronchial secretion and adds the extra factor of pathogenic bacteria.
• *Smokers* are at particular risk, with increased secretions and ineffective cilia.
• *Chronic pulmonary disease*, e.g. emphysema.
• *Chest wall disease*, e.g. ankylosing spondylitis, which makes coughing difficult.

Operative factors
• *Anaesthetic drugs* increase mucus secretion and depress the action of the bronchial cilia.
• *Atropine* in addition increases the viscosity of the mucus.

Post-operative factors
• *Pain*. The pain of the thoracic or abdominal incision, which inhibits expectoration of the accumulated bronchial secretions, is the most important cause of mucus retention.

Clinical features
Pulmonary collapse occurs within the first post-operative 48 hours. The patient is dyspnoeic with a rapid pulse and elevated temperature. There may be cyanosis. The patient attempts to cough, but this is painful and unless encouraged, he or she may fail to expectorate.

The sputum is at first frothy and clear, but later may become purulent.

Examination reveals that the patient is distressed with a typical painful 'fruity cough'. This results from the sound of the bronchial secretions rattling within the chest and a good clinician should be able to make the diagnosis while still several yards away from the patient. The chest movements are diminished, particularly on the affected side; there is basal dullness and air entry is depressed with the addition of coarse crackles.

Pulse oximetry indicates a reduced saturation, and chest X-ray may reveal an opacity of the involved segment (usually basal or midzone), together with mediastinal shift to the affected side.

Treatment
Pre-operatively, breathing exercises are given, smoking is forbidden and antibiotics prescribed if any chronic respiratory infection is present. Surgery should be postponed when possible until all pre-existing chest infection has resolved. Post-operatively, the patient is encouraged to cough, and breathing exercises are instituted, usually under the supervision of a physiotherapist. Small repeated doses of opiates diminish the pain of coughing but are insufficient to dull the cough reflex. Epidural anaesthesia and intercostal nerve blocks may help reduce the inhibitory pain of an abdominal or thoracic incision, without affecting the respiratory drive. Antibiotics are only prescribed if the sputum is infected; their selection is based on the sensitivity of the cultured organisms.

Deep vein thrombosis in the lower limb

In the post-operative period, the patient has an increased predisposition to venous thrombosis in the veins of the calf muscles, the main deep venous channels of the leg and in pelvic veins. This predisposition has three main components.

1 *Increased thrombotic tendency.* Increase in platelets and their stickiness and increase in fibrinogen. Following blood loss and platelet consumption intra-operatively, more platelets are produced, numbers peaking around day 10. The new platelets have an increased tendency to aggregate. Fibrinogen levels also increase.

2 *Changes in blood flow.* Increased stagnation within the veins occurs as a result of im-mobilization on the operating table and post-operatively in bed, and with depression of respiration.

3 *Damage to the vein wall* prompts thrombus formation on the damaged endothelium. The damage may be due to an inflammatory process in the pelvis, or may be produced by pressure of the mattress against the calf or direct damage at operation (particularly the pelvic veins during pelvic procedures) or by disease (e.g. pelvic sepsis).

Platelets deposit on the damaged endothe-lium, the vein is occluded by thrombus and a propagated fibrin clot then develops, which may detach and form a pulmonary embolus (see below).

This complication is particularly likely to occur in elderly patients, the obese, those with malignant disease, patients who have varicose veins or a history of previous deep vein throm-bosis, those undergoing abdominal, pelvic and particularly hip surgery, and women who are taking oestrogen-containing oral con-traceptives and hormone-replacement tablets. In addition, some patients may be predisposed to thrombosis due to reduced levels of the endogenous anticoagulants protein C, protein S, antithrombin III, or due to possession of the Leiden mutation of the coagulation Factor V.

Clinical features

Deep vein thrombosis can be 'silent', but typi-cally symptoms and signs usually occur during the second post-operative week, although they may be earlier or later. Earlier thrombosis particularly occurs when the patient has already been in hospital for some time pre-operatively. Studies using radio-iodine-labelled fibrinogen, which is deposited as fibrin in the developing thrombus and which can be detected by scanning the leg, suggest that the thrombotic process usually commences at, or soon after, the operation.

The patient complains of pain in the calf, and on examination there is tenderness of the calf and swelling of the foot, often with oedema, raised skin temperature and dilatation of the superficial veins of the leg. This is accom-panied by a mild pyrexia. If the pelvic veins or the femoral vein are affected, there is massive swelling of the whole lower limb.

Special investigations

• *Venography.* This is the definitive investiga-tion but cannot be repeated frequently nor employed for routine screening.

• *Duplex scanning.* The course of the iliac and femoral veins can be scanned and filling defects due to thrombi detected. In skilled hands, duplex scanning can detect thrombi in all the major veins at and above the knee, but is unre-liable below this. It has the advantage that it is simple and non-invasive.

• *^{125}I-labelled fibrinogen.* A highly sensitive test that enables the legs to be scanned at daily intervals. It demonstrates the presence of deep vein thrombosis in approximately one-third of all post-operative patients, with a particularly high incidence in the high-risk groups listed above. Only half of the thrombi picked up on scanning can be detected on careful clinical examination. Due to scatter from the radio-active iodine excreted in the urine and held in the bladder, the test is unreliable in the pelvic and thigh region and is only significant from the knee downwards.

Management
Prophylaxis

• *Treat avoidable risk factors.* Elective surgery on anyone with a treatable risk factor should be avoided. For example, elective surgery on a patient taking the contraceptive pill should be delayed for several weeks after stopping the pill.

• *Active mobilization.* Stimulation of blood flow by encouraging early mobilzation reduces the risks, and this may be extended to the intraoperative period by the application of inter-mittent calf compression using inflatable bags, which have been shown to reduce the inci-dence of thrombosis.

• *Graded compression stockings* and *elevation of the legs* to increase venous return are simple and effective.

• *Subcutaneous heparin injections*, particularly low-molecular-weight heparins such as enoxa-parin, should be started pre-operatively and continued while the patient remains at risk. Controlled trials have shown reduction in the incidence of venous thrombosis with a less certain reduction in pulmonary embolism in the treated groups.

Treatment

In the established case, anticoagulant therapy with intravenous heparin is commenced to prevent further propagation of the clot, and to increase fibrinolysis; this is usually given by continuous pump infusion. Once anticoagu-lated, the patient can be mobilized with the lower limbs supported in elastic stockings to prevent oedema, and intravenous anticoagul-ation replaced with oral anticoagulation with warfarin.

The decision to anticoagulate a patient is particularly difficult if thrombosis occurs in the immediate post-operative period, as antico-agulation carries a serious risk of haemorrhage at the operation site. If bleeding occurs, the heparin is immediately discontinued and protamine sulphate may be given to reverse its effect.

If pulmonary embolism occurs in spite of anticoagulation, percutaneous insertion of an umbrella-like filter into the inferior vena cava such as the Greenfield filter may be indicated to prevent recurrent episodes of pulmonary embolization.

Pulmonary embolus

This occurs when a clot from a vein, originating in the femoral vein or the pelvis (and occasion-ally in the calf muscles), detaches and becomes lodged in the pulmonary arterial tree.

Clinical features

The clinical features of pulmonary embolus may vary from dyspnoea or mild pleuritic chest pain, to sudden death due to an ob-structed pulmonary artery trunk. Minor symp-toms include pleuritic chest pain, dyspnoea and haemoptysis. Severe dyspnoea may occur with cyanosis and shock, and larger emboli may prompt acute right-heart failure and death.

The dyspnoea may be sudden in onset, or progressive as further showers of emboli dis-lodge. The chest pain is pleuritic, and where basal lung segments are affected diaphragma-tic irritation may occur and result in shoulder tip pain. In elderly patients, confusion due to hypoxia may be the presenting symptom. Pulmonary emboli classically occur around the 10th post-operative day. They often occur while straining at stool, as the increased intra-abdominal pressure dislodges a pelvic venous thrombus.

Examination

On examination, the patient is tachypnoeic, often with a spike of fever. There is a tachycar-dia and a raised jugular venous pressure (JVP) reflecting the pulmonary hypertension. There may be tenderness in the calves at the site of a deep-vein thrombosis, but this is not common. Cyanosis may be present if the embolus is large, and a pleural rub may be audible in small and peripherally located emboli.

If the patient survives the embolus, com-plete clearing of the clot occurs quite rapidly. Infarction of the lung is uncommon because the lungs themselves are perfused via the bronchial arteries. It may occur in those patients with cardiac failure where there is pre-existing pul-monary congestion.

Diagnosis of an embolus is often difficult. The main differential diagnosis of a major em-bolus is a myocardial infarction, while small emboli may be confused with a chest infection.

Special investigations

• *Chest X-ray* in the early stages is often normal, although within a few hours patchy shadowing of the affected segment takes place.

• *Electrocardiogram (ECG)* may help in differentiating pulmonary embolus from myocardial infarction. In the case of an embolus there may be rhythm changes (atrial fibrillation, heart block) or features of right-heart strain (ST segment depression in leads V1 to V3, III and AVF, with right-axis deviation), as the heart pumps against the obstructed pulmonary arterial tree. The characteristic 'S1 Q3 T3' pattern (S wave in lead I, with a Q wave and an inverted T wave in lead III) is seldom present.

• *Arterial blood gasses* may confirm the hypoxia. Hypocapnia (low CO_2) may also be present secondary to tachypnoea.

• *Ventilation–perfusion scintigraphy (V/Q scan).* This is a radionuclide technique in which a radiolabelled inert gas such as xenon (^{133}Xe) or krypton (^{81}Kr) is inhaled and its distribution throughout the lung measured. This is followed by intravenous injection of technetium (^{99}Tc)-labelled human albumin particles. The albumin particles are trapped in the lung capillaries and their distribution reflects lung perfusion. In a pulmonary embolus, the perfusion scan will show uneven circulation through the lungs, with multiple perfusion defects, but a simultaneous ventilation scan is normal in the absence of pre-existing pulmonary disease.

• *Pulmonary angiography* gives the definitive diagnosis demonstrating a filling defect in the pulmonary artery. This may be indicated in the critically ill patient if the diagnosis is in doubt and is also performed if pulmonary embolectomy is planned.

It is important to appreciate that pulmonary embolus may occur without any preceding warning signs of thrombosis in the leg. Indeed, once there are obvious clinical features of deep vein thrombosis, detachment of an organized and adherent clot from this limb is rather unlikely, especially if anticoagulant therapy has been commenced so that fresh clot formation is inhibited. The great majority of fatal pulmonary emboli are unheralded.

Treatment
Opiate analgesia is given for pain, oxygen administered and heparin commenced if the patient is not already on anticoagulants. Lysis of a massive embolus may be effected with an intravenous infusion of streptokinase, especially if delivered via a pulmonary catheter at the time of pulmonary angiography. Recent surgery is a relative contraindication to thrombolysis. In the critically ill patient, pulmonary embolectomy carried out with cardiopulmonary bypass may be successful.

Burst abdomen

Aetiology
Dehiscence of the abdominal wound may result from a number of factors.

Pre-operative
Uraemia, cachexia with protein deficiency, vitamin C deficiency, jaundice, obesity, steroids, distension and chronic cough (the latter two because of the strain put upon the abdominal incision).

Operative
Poor technique in closing the abdominal wound or the use of suture material of low tensile strength, which ruptures post-operatively. Badly tied knots may come undone and sutures too near the edge of the incision may cut through the tissues like a cheese wire through cheese, especially if these tissues are weakened by infection.

Post-operative
Cough or abdominal distension, which puts a strain on the suture line; infection or haematoma of the wound, which weakens it.

Clinical features
The abdomen usually dehisces on about the 10th day. There may be a warning of this if pink fluid discharges through the abdominal incision. This represents the serous effusion (which is always present during the first week or two within the abdominal cavity after operation), which is tinged with blood and which seeps through the breaking-down wound. If

this 'pink fluid sign' is ignored the patient finds a loop of intestine or the omentum protruding through the wound, usually after a cough or strain — a most alarming finding both for the patient and staff.

Sometimes, the deep layer of the abdominal incision gives way but the skin sutures hold; such cases result in a massive incisional hernia.

Treatment

The patient with a burst abdomen is usually in mortal fear. The patient should be reassured and the reassurance supplemented by an injection of morphine. The abdominal contents are covered with sterile towels soaked in saline and the patient prepared for operation. The abdominal wound is resutured under a general anaesthetic using strong nylon stitches passed through all the layers of the abdominal wall including the skin. The prognosis after this procedure is good unless the patient succumbs to the underlying disease. The wound usually heals rapidly, but there is a high incidence of subsequent incisional herniation.

Post-operative fistula

Definition

A fistula is defined as an abnormal connection between two epithelial surfaces.

Aetiology

The development of a fistula involving the alimentary canal or its biliary or pancreatic adnexae following abdominal surgery is a serious complication. A fistula may result from general or local factors.

General factors

The patient's general condition may be poor due to uraemia, anaemia, jaundice, protein deficiency or cachexia from malignant disease.

Local factors

• Poor surgical technique.

• Poor blood supply at the anastomotic line, particularly in operations on the oesophagus and rectum.
• Sepsis incurred before or during the operation leading to suture line breakdown. (Sepsis is, of course, inevitable once leakage has occurred.)
• Presence of distal obstruction. Thus, a biliary fistula is likely to occur if stones are left behind in the common bile duct after cholecystectomy.
• Local malignant or inflammatory disease, e.g. Crohn's disease.

Clinical features

Diagnosis is usually all too obvious, with the escape of bowel contents or bile through the wound or drainage site. If there is any doubt, methylene blue given by mouth will appear in the effluent of an alimentary fistula, and the fluid can be tested for bile to diagnose a biliary leak, creatinine for a urinary tract leak while the fluid from a pancreatic leak is rich in amylase. An injection of radio-opaque fluid will outline the fistulous tract and provide valuable information about its size and whether or not distal obstruction exists.

The enzyme-rich fluid of the upper alimentary tract and of a pancreatic fistula produces rapid excoriation of the surrounding skin. This is much less marked in a faecal fistula, as the contents of the colon are relatively poor in proteolytic enzymes. The patient is toxic and passes into a severe catabolic state compounded by infection and starvation due to loss of intestinal fluid. Rapid wasting occurs from fluid loss and protein depletion.

Treatment

The early management has three aims.
1 *To protect the skin around the fistula from ulceration.* The edges of the wound are covered by Stomadhesive (which adheres even to moist surfaces), or aluminum paint or silicone barrier cream. It may be possible to collect the effluent by means of a colostomy appliance and thus reduce skin soilage. If the mouth of the fistula is large, continuous suction may be necessary.

2 *To replace the loss of fluid, electrolytes, nutrients and vitamins.* In a high alimentary fistula, this will require intravenous feeding via a central line. Calories are given in the form of glucose and fat emulsion and protein depletion is countered by amino acids. Vitamins and electrolytes are also required. Such prolonged intravenous feeding must be carefully monitored by serial biochemical studies. If the fistula is low in the alimentary tract, an elemental diet can be given by mouth. This is rapidly absorbed in the upper intestine and is thus not lost through the fistula.

3 *To reduce sepsis.* This is achieved by judicious drainage of pus collections and by antibiotic therapy.

On this conservative regimen, a side-fistula without distal obstruction may well heal spontaneously. However, if the fistula is large or complete, or there is a distal obstruction, or the fistula is malignant in origin or it is at the site of an inflammatory disease such as Crohn's disease, subsequent surgery is required to close the leak and to deal with the obstruction. This can only be successful if carried out at the stage when the patient's condition has improved and when a positive nitrogen balance has been achieved.

Post-operative pyrexia

There are many causes of a pyrexia following surgery, and diagnosis requires a methodical approach. A mild pyrexia is a common post-operative feature immediately following surgery and is a normal response to tissue injury. The following procedure is valuable in elucidating the cause of such a fever.

1 *Inspect the wound*: superficial wound infection or haematoma.

2 *Inspect venous cannula sites*: thrombophlebitis is common when a cannula has remained *in situ* for a few days, or through which irritant infusions have passed.

3 *Examine the chest clinically* and if necessary order a chest X-ray and ultrasound: exclude pulmonary collapse, infection, infarction and subphrenic abscess.

4 *Examine the legs*: deep vein thrombosis.

5 *Rectal examination*: pelvic abscess.

6 *Urine culture*: urinary infection.

7 *Stool culture*: for *Clostridium difficile* toxin to exclude enterocolitis.

8 Finally, consider the possibility of *drug sensitivity*.

CHAPTER 4

Acute Infections

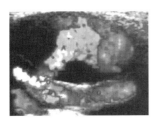

There is an important general principle in treating acute infection anywhere in the body: antibiotics are invaluable when the infection is spreading through the tissues (e.g. cellulitis, peritonitis, pneumonia), but drainage is essential when abscess formation has occurred.

Cellulitis

Cellulitis is a spreading inflammation of connective tissues. It is generally subcutaneous, but the term may also be applied to pelvic, perinephric, pharyngeal and other connective tissue infections. The common causative agent is the β-haemolytic *Streptococcus*. The invasiveness of this organism is due to the production of hyaluronidase and streptokinase, which respectively dissolve the intercellular matrix and the fibrin inflammatory barrier.

Characteristically, the skin is dark red with local oedema and heat; it blanches on pressure. There may be vesicles and, in severe cases, cutaneous gangrene. Cellulitis is often accompanied by lymphangitis and lymphadenitis, and there may be an associated septicaemia.

Treatment

Immobilization, elevation and antibiotics. If a local abscess forms, this must be drained.

Abscess

An abscess is a localized collection of pus, usually, but not invariably, produced by pyogenic organisms. Occasionally, a sterile abscess results from the injection of irritants into soft tissues (e.g. thiopentone).

An abscess commences as a hard, red, painful swelling, which then softens and becomes fluctuant. If not drained, it may discharge spontaneously onto the surface or into an adjacent viscus or body cavity. There are the associated features of bacterial infection, namely a swinging fever, malaise, anorexia and sweating with a polymorph leucocytosis.

Treatment

An established abscess in any situation requires drainage. Antimicrobial agents cannot diffuse in sufficient quantity to sterilize an abscess completely. Pus left undrained continues to act as a source of toxaemia and becomes surrounded by dense, fibrous tissue.

The technique of abscess drainage depends on the site. The classical method, which is applicable to a superficial abscess, is to wait until there is fluctuation and to insert the tip of a scalpel blade at this point. The track is widened by means of sinus forceps, which can be inserted without fear of damaging adjacent structures. If there is room, the surgeon's finger can be used to explore the abscess cavity and break down undrained loculi. Drainage is

21

then maintained until the abscess cavity heals from below upwards, otherwise the superficial layers can close over, with recurrence of the abscess. The cavity is therefore kept open by means of a gauze wick, a corrugated drain or a tube; the drain is gradually withdrawn until complete healing is achieved.

Deep abscesses can be localized and drained using ultrasound or computed tomography (CT) guidance.

Boil

A boil (furuncle) is an abscess, usually due to the pyogenic *Staphylococcus*, which involves a hair follicle and its associated glands. It is therefore not found on the hairless palm or sole, but is usually encountered where the skin is hairy, injured by friction, or dirty and macerated by sweat; thus, it occurs particularly on the neck, axilla and the perianal region. Occasionally, a furuncle may be the primary source of a staphylococcal septicaemia and be responsible for osteomyelitis, perinephric abscess or empyema, particularly in debilitated patients. A boil on the face may be complicated by a pyelophlebitis spreading along the facial veins resulting in thrombosis of the cavernous sinus.

Differential diagnosis

Multiple infected foci in the axillae or groins due to infection of the apocrine sweat glands of these regions (*hydradenitis suppurativa*) are usually misdiagnosed as boils. They do not respond to antibiotic therapy and can only be treated effectively by excision of the affected skin area; if this is extensive, the defect may require grafting.

Treatment

When pus is visible, the boil should be incised. Recurrent crops of boils should be treated by improving the general hygiene of the patient, and by the use of ultraviolet light and hexa-chlorophene baths, but systemic antibiotic therapy is not indicated.

Carbuncle

A carbuncle is an area of subcutaneous necrosis that discharges onto the surface through multiple sinuses. It is usually staphylococcal in origin. The subcutaneous tissues become honeycombed by small abscesses separated by fibrous strands. The condition is often associated with general debility and particularly with diabetes. The urine should always be tested for sugar in this or any other septic condition.

Treatment

Surgery is rarely indicated initially. Antibiotic therapy is given and the carbuncle merely protected with sterile dressings. Occasionally, a large sloughing area eventually requires excision and a skin graft. Diabetes, if present, should be controlled.

Specific infections

Tetanus

Tetanus is now a rare disease in the Western world, thanks to a comprehensive immunization policy. In the developing world it remains prevalent with a mortality of up to 60%.

Pathology

Tetanus is caused by *Clostridium tetani*, an anaerobic, exotoxin-secreting, Gram-positive bacillus. It is characterized by formation of a terminal spore ('drumstick'), and is a normal inhabitant of soil and faeces. The bacillus remains at the site of inoculation and produces a powerful exotoxin. This toxin causes increase in muscle tone and excitability by effects both at the motor end-plate and in the anterior horn cells of the spinal cord.

Tetanus follows the implantation of spores into a deep, devitalized wound where anaerobic conditions occur. Infection is related less to the severity of the wound than to its nature; thus, an extensive injury that has received early and adequate wound toilet is far less at risk than a contaminated puncture wound that has been neglected.

Clinical features

The incubation time is 24 hours to 24 days, the initial injury often being trivial and forgotten. Muscle spasm first develops at the site of inoculation and then involves the facial muscles and the muscles of the neck and spine. As a rule, it is the trismus of the facial spasm (producing the typical 'risus sardonicus') that is the first reliable indication of developing tetanus. This may be so severe that it becomes impossible for the patient to open his or her mouth ('lock-jaw'). The period of spasm is followed, except in mild cases, by violent and extremely painful convulsions, which occur within 24–72 hours of the onset of symptoms and may be precipitated by some trivial stimulus, such as a sudden noise. The convulsions, like the muscle spasm, affect the muscles of the neck, face and trunk. Characteristically, the muscles remain in spasm between the convulsions. The temperature is a little elevated but the pulse is rapid and weak.

In favourable cases, the convulsions, if present at all, become less frequent and then cease and the tonic spasm gradually lessens. It may, however, be some weeks before muscle tone returns to normal and the risus sardonicus disappears. In fatal cases, paroxysms become more severe and frequent; death occurs from asphyxia due to involvement of the respiratory muscles or from exhaustion, inhalation of vomit or pneumonia.

Poor prognostic features are a short incubation period from the time of injury to the onset of spasm (under 5 days) and the occurrence of convulsions within 48 hours of the onset of muscle spasm.

Differential diagnosis

• *Tetany*: characteristically affects the limbs, producing carpopedal spasm.
• *Strychnine poisoning*: flaccidity occurs between convulsions whereas in tetanus the spasm persists.
• *Meningitis*: because of the neck stiffness.

• *Epilepsy*.
• *Hysteria*.

Treatment
Prophylaxis
Active immunization. Comprises two initial injections of tetanus toxoid (formalin-treated exotoxin) at an interval of 6 weeks. Booster doses are given at intervals of 10 years, or at the time of any injury. Toxoid should be given to any population at risk of injury, particularly the elderly in whom cover may have lapsed.

Wound toilet. The risk of tetanus can be reduced almost to zero if penetrating and contaminated wounds are adequately excised to remove all dead tissue, and a course of prophylactic penicillin (or erythromycin for sensitive patients) is given. Antibiotic therapy is no substitute for thorough wound debridement.

Passive immunization. Patients who have previously received toxoid should be given a booster dose. If toxoid has not been given in the past, human tetanus immunoglobulin (HTIG), prepared from fully immunized subjects, should be given if the wound is heavily contaminated or a puncture wound, and more than 6 hours have elapsed before treatment is received. HTIG is insufficient to confer long-term immunity, and a course of toxoid should also be given.

Curative treatment
Control convulsions. The patient is nursed in isolation, quiet and darkness and is heavily sedated with phenobarbitone or chlorpromazine. In severe cases, paralysis with tracheostomy and intermittent positive-pressure mechanical ventilation is required and this may have to be continued for up to 4 weeks. It is terminated when the spasms and rigidity are absent during a trial period without muscle relaxants. These serious cases are best transferred to a special respiratory unit.

Control the local infection. Excision and drainage of any wound is carried out under a general anaesthetic. High-dose penicillin (or erythromycin for sensitive patients) is administered.

Nutrition. Feed the patient by fine-bore naso-gastric tube to maintain the general condition and electrolyte balance.

Administer tetanus toxoid. Human tetanus immunoglobulin does not confer immunity and therefore, if the patient has not previously been immunized, the first dose of tetanus toxoid should be given. If previous active immunization has been carried out, a booster dose of toxoid is administered.

Gas gangrene
Pathology
Results from infection by *Clostridium perfringens* (*welchii*) and other *Clostridium* species. The organism, a Gram-positive, spore-forming bacillus like *Clostridium tetani*, also produces powerful exotoxins. The toxins have various activities, including phospholipase, collagenase, proteinase and hyaluronidase, which facilitate aggressive local spread of infection along tissue planes, with liberation of CO_2, H_2S and NH_3 by protein destruction. The organisms are found in soil and in faeces.

Typically, gas gangrene is an infection of deep penetrating wounds, particularly of war, but sometimes involvement of the abdominal wall or cavity may follow operations upon the alimentary system. Occasionally, gas gangrene complicates amputation of an ischaemic lower limb, or follows abortion or puerperal infection.

Clinical features
The incubation period is about 24 hours. Toxaemia is severe with tachycardia, shock and vomiting. The temperature is first elevated and then becomes subnormal. The affected tissues are swollen, and crepitus is palpable due to gas. The skin becomes gangrenous and the infection spreads along the muscle planes, produc-ing at first dark-red swollen muscle and then frank gangrene.

Treatment
Prophylaxis
This consists of adequate excision of wounds, which removes both the organisms and the dead tissues that are essential for their anaerobic growth. Seriously contused wounds (such as those produced by a gunshot wound) or contaminated wounds are *left open* and lightly packed with gauze. Delayed primary suture can then safely be performed after 5 or 6 days, by which time the wound is usually healthy and granulating. Penicillin is given in all heavily contaminated wounds and to patients undergoing amputation of an ischaemic leg.

Curative
In the established case, all involved tissue must be excised. Implication of all muscle groups in a limb is an indication for amputation, which in the lower limb may mean a disarticulation at the hip. High-dose penicillin is given, and other supportive measures as required. Hyperbaric oxygen therapy, to eliminate the anaerobic environment, is theoretically sound but as it is combined with all the other modalities of treatment its efficacy cannot be judged. If a hyperbaric chamber is available, it should certainly be employed.

The value of anti-gas gangrene serum, both as a prophylactic and curative measure, is not established.

Synergistic gangrene
Pathology
Synergistic gangrene, also known as progressive bacterial gangrene and Meleny's gangrene, is caused by the synergistic action of two or more organisms, commonly aerobic haemolytic *Staphylococcus* and micro-aerophilic non-haemolytic *Streptococcus*. It is more common in diabetics and is often related to recent trauma or infection. Where it affects the scrotum and perineum it has been termed Fournier's gangrene.

Clinical features

There may be no precipitating factor, but most follow infections or recent surgery (previously termed progressive post-operative gangrene). Around the wound an area of cellulitis appears, which spreads rapidly. The area is exquisitely tender, and as gangrene evolves it liberates an offensive odour. The patient becomes profoundly septic and unwell.

Treatment

High-dose, broad-spectrum antibiotics should be commenced immediately, but the mainstay of treatment is a radical debridement of all the affected area. Following the initial debridement, the wound should be inspected twice daily at least for evidence of spread, and further debridement performed until all the affected area is cleared.

CHAPTER 5

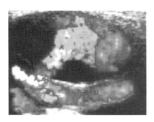

Tumours

A medical student was asked on a ward round 'What would you think of if a patient had central abdominal pain, vomited and then the pain shifted to the right iliac fossa?' He replied 'Cancer, Sir.' In this answer there existed a grain of truth. New growths are so common and widespread that their consideration must at least pass through the mind in most clinical situations. It therefore behoves the student, both for examinations and, still more important, for future practical doctoring, to have a standard scheme with which to tabulate the pathology, diagnosis, treatment and prognosis of neoplastic disease.

Pathology

When considering the tumours affecting any organ this simple classification should be used:
1 Benign.
2 Malignant:
  (a) primary;
  (b) secondary.
It is surprising how often failure to remember this basic scheme leads one to omit such an elementary fact that common tumours of brain and bone are secondary deposits.

For each particular tumour, the following headings should be used.
• Incidence.
• Age distribution.
• Sex distribution.
• Geographical distribution (where relevant).
• Predisposing factors.
• Macroscopic appearances.

• Microscopic appearances.
• Pathways of spread of the tumour.
• Prognosis.

Clinical features and diagnosis

A malignant tumour may manifest itself in four ways.
1 The effects of the primary tumour itself.
2 The effects produced by secondary deposits.
3 The general effects of malignant disease.
4 Paraneoplastic syndromes. These are remote effects caused by hormone or other tumour-cell products, which are most common in carcinoma of the lung, particularly small-cell tumours. For example, ectopic adrenocor-ticotrophic hormone (ACTH) production may present like Cushing's syndrome, and ectopic parathormone (PTH) production may present with hypercalcaemia and its symptoms.
(The only common exceptions are primary tumours of the central nervous system (CNS), which seldom produce secondary deposits.)

Diagnosis is always made by history, clinical examination and, where necessary, special investigations. Let us now, as an example, apply this scheme to carcinoma of the lung — the commonest lethal cancer in the UK.

History
• *The primary tumour* may present with cough, haemoptysis, dyspnoea, pneumonia (sometimes recurrent pneumonia due to partial bronchial obstruction).

- *Secondary deposits* in bone may produce pathological fracture or bone pains; cerebral metastases may produce headaches or drowsiness; liver deposits may result in jaundice.
- *Paraneoplastic syndromes*, such as ectopic hormone production, myasthenia-like syndrome (Eaton–Lambert syndrome*), hypertrophic pulmonary osteoarthropathy (HPOA) and finger clubbing.
- *General effects of malignant disease*: the patient may present with malaise, lassitude or loss of weight.

Examination
- *The primary tumour* may produce signs in the chest.
- *Secondary deposits* may produce cervical lymph-node enlargement, hepatomegaly or obvious bony deposits.
- *The general effects of malignancy* may be suggested by pallor or weight loss.

Special investigations
- *The primary tumour*: chest X-ray, computed tomography (CT), bronchoscopy, cytology of sputum and needle biopsy.
- *Secondary deposits*: isotope bone scan, bone X-ray and ultrasound of liver.
- *Paraneoplastic hormone production*: hormone assay.
- *General manifestation of malignancy*: a blood count may reveal anaemia. The erythrocyte sedimentation rate (ESR) may be raised.
- *Tumour markers*: these are blood chemicals (often fetal proteins) produced by the malignant cells. Some tumours have a characteristic marker associated with them, such as α-fetoprotein (AFP) in hepatoma and teratoma, prostate-specific antigen (PSA) in carcinoma of the prostate (Table 5.1). Tumour markers may indicate malignant change in a benign condition, and are useful in post-operative monitoring. If a marker was raised pre-treatment, it

*L. M. Eaton (1905–58), Professor of Neurology, Mayo Clinic, USA. E. H. Lambert (1915–?), Neurophysiologist at Mayo Clinic, Professor of Physiology, University of Minnesota, USA.

should fall when the disease is controlled, but will rise again if recurrence occurs. Some tumours produce excess amounts of the appropriate hormone, such as medullary carcinoma of the thyroid and calcitonin, in which case hormone assay may be used to detect tumour activity.

This simple scheme applied to any of the principal malignant tumours will enable the student to present a very full clinical picture of the disease with little mental effort.

Treatment
The treatment of malignant disease should be considered under two headings.

1 *Curative*: an attempt is made to ablate the disease completely.

2 *Palliative*: although the disease is incurable or has recurred after treatment, measures can still be taken to ease the symptoms of the patient.

In this section we shall summarize the possible lines of treatment for malignant disease in general; in subsequent chapters, the management of specific tumours will be considered in more detail.

Curative treatment
1 *Surgery*.

2 *Radiotherapy* alone (e.g. tumours of the mouth and pharynx).

3 *A combination* of surgery and radiotherapy (e.g. carcinoma of cervix).

4 *Cytotoxic therapy* where the tumour is particularly sensitive to particular agents, such as teratoma of the testis to platinum compounds. Like radiotherapy, this may be combined with surgery.

Palliative treatment
1 *Surgery*. The palliative excision of a primary lesion may be indicated, although secondary deposits may be present. For example, a carcinoma of the rectum may be excised to prevent pain, bleeding and mucus discharge, although secondary deposits may already be present in the liver. Irremovable obstructing growths in the bowel may be bypassed. Inoper-

TUMOUR MARKERS

Marker	Nature of marker	Malignant marker
α-Fetoprotein (AFP)	Protein secreted by fetal liver	Hepatoma and testicular teratoma
Ca 12.5	Monoclonal antibody to high-molecular-weight mucinous protein cell product	Ovarian and some colo-rectal tumours
Ca 19.9	Monoclonal antibody to high-molecular-weight mucinous glycoprotein cell product	Colo-rectal (advanced disease), gastric, pancreatic and hepatocellular tumours
Carcinoembryonic antigen (CEA)	Protein secreted by fetal gut	Advanced colo-rectal carcinoma
Prostatic acid phosphatase (PAP)	Prostatic isoenzyme of acid phosphatase	Advanced prostatic carcinoma (extracapsular spread)
Prostate-specific antigen (PSA)		Prostatic tumours

Table 5.1 Tumour markers. Some tumour markers are also present in some benign diseases.

able obstructing tumours of the oesophagus or cardia of the stomach may be intubated by means of a plastic tube so that dysphagia can be relieved. Surgery may also be used for pain relief by interrupting nerve pathways, e.g. cordotomy in which the contralateral spino-thalamic tract within the spinal cord is divided.

2 *Radiotherapy*: palliative treatment may be given to localized secondary deposits in bone, irremovable breast tumours, inoperable lymph-node deposits, etc. It is particularly indicated for localized irremovable disease.

3 *Hormone therapy*: applicable in carcinoma of the breast and prostate.

4 *Cytotoxic therapy*: a wide range of drugs have anti-cancer action but this is not specific and all of them also damage normal dividing cells, especially those of the bone marrow, the gut, the skin and the gonads. They may be classified into:

(a) alkylating agents (e.g. cyclophosphamide, chlorambucil);

(b) anti-metabolites (e.g. 5-fluorouracil, methotrexate);

(c) plant alkaloids (e.g. vincristine);

(d) anti-tumour antibiotics (e.g. adriamycin, bleomycin);

(e) platinum compounds (e.g. cisplatin and carboplatin);

(f) epipodophyllotoxins (e.g. etoposide).

Multiple drugs are frequently used (combination chemotherapy) where their modes of action and toxicity profiles are different.

A balance must be made between the chances of regression of the tumour in relatively fit patients with tumours likely to be sensitive (e.g. breast, ovary, testis), and the toxic effects of the drug regimen.

5 *Drugs* for pain relief (non-steroidal analgesics, opiates), hypnotics, tranquillizers and anti-emetics (e.g. chlorpromazine).

6 *Nerve blocks* with phenol or alcohol for relief of pain.

7 *Maintenance of morale* by cheerful and kindly attitude of medical and nursing staff.

Prognosis

The prognosis of any tumour depends on four main features:

1 the extent of spread;
2 microscopic appearance;
3 anatomical situation;
4 general condition of the patient.

The extent of spread (staging)

The extent of the tumour (its *staging*) on clinical examination, at operation or on studying the excised surgical specimen, is of great prognostic importance. Obviously, the clinical findings of palpable distant secondaries or gross fixation of the primary tumour are serious. Similarly, the local invasiveness of the tumour at operation or evidence of distant spread are of great significance. Finally, histological study may reveal involvement of the nodes, which had not been detected clinically, or microscopic extension of the growth to the edges of the resected specimen with consequent worsening of the outlook for the patient.

The *TNM classification* is an international system for tumour staging. Tumours are staged by scoring them according to the **t**umour characteristics (size, degree of invasion, etc.), the extent of lymph-**n**ode involvement and the presence of **m**etastases. Some tumours have additional classifications, which predate the TNM classification, and which are more useful to the clinician. Examples of such are Dukes' staging of rectal carcinoma (p. 220), and the Manchester staging of breast carcinoma (p. 287).

Microscopic appearance (histological differentiation)

As a general principle, the prognosis of a tumour is related to its degree of histological differentiation (its *grading*) on the spectrum between well differentiated and anaplastic.

The spread of the tumour and its histological differentiation should be considered in conjunction with each other. A small tumour with no apparent spread at the time of operation may still have poor prognosis if it is highly anaplastic, whereas an extensive tumour is not incompatible with long survival of the patient after operation if the microscopic examination reveals a high degree of differentiation.

Anatomical situation

The site of the tumour may preclude its adequate removal and thus seriously affect the prognosis. For example, a tumour at the lower end of the oesophagus may be easily removable whereas an exactly similar tumour situated behind the arch of the aorta may be technically inoperable; a brain tumour located in the frontal lobe may be resected whereas a similar tumour in the brain stem will be a desperate surgical proposition.

General condition of the patient

A patient apparently curable from the point of view of the local condition may be inoperable because of poor general health. For example, gross congestive cardiac failure may convert what is technically an operable carcinoma of the rectum into a hopeless anaesthetic risk.

Screening

Screening is the process of testing individuals for a specific condition. It is commonly performed in the context of tumours, but may be used in other contexts such as abdominal aortic aneurysm and hypertension. Effective screening for a given condition using a particular test has several prerequisites.

• The condition, if untreated, is sufficiently serious to warrant its prevention.
• The condition has a recognizable early stage.
• Treatment at an early stage can improve the prognosis.
• Effective treatment is available.
• The screening test is simple, and acceptable to the patient.
• The screening test should have minimal false-positive and false-negative outcomes. Incorrect diagnosis has serious consequences.

In reality, cost-effective screening requires restricting the testing to those groups at highest risk of a condition. This may involve large-scale population screening or screening families where a genetic predisposition exists.

Population screening

Examples of population screening include breast cancer screening by mammography, which is restricted to older women (over 50 years) and cervical cancer screening for women over 20 years. In cervical cancer, for example, a distinct progression exists from dysplasia to carcinoma-*in-situ*, and this may take 10 years. Hence, screening the population every 3–5 years by cervical smear cytology is adequate and cost-effective.

Screening for high-risk individuals

A number of cancer syndromes exist in which there is an inherited predisposition (e.g. familial adenomatous polyposis (FAP)), or a familial risk (e.g. breast and ovarian cancer).

Inherited cancer syndromes. Like FAP, most inherited cancers are autosomal dominantly inherited. In at-risk families, early identification may be possible either through genetic mapping of the cancer or early recognition of a component of the syndrome. In FAP, early colonoscopy may identify villous adenomas (polyps) while they are still dysplastic, before they become malignant, at which stage prophylactic colectomy is indicated. Alternatively, identification of the gene (located on chromosome 5q21) will also signify carriage.

Familial clustering. Many of the familial cancers are now being associated with specific genes. Incomplete expression of the gene may account for the sporadic incidence of the tumour. For breast cancer, two genes have been identified, *BrCa*1 (chromosome 17q21) and *BrCa*2 (chromosome 13q12). Presence of either gene confers an 80% risk of breast cancer by the age of 70 years, together with an increased risk of ovarian cancer. Screening tests based on the detection of these genes differ from the other screening tests mentioned above, as they identify a tendency to malignancy and not premalignant change or early curable malignancy. There is no consensus as to the best management of such patients.

CHAPTER 6

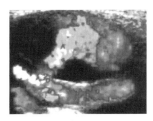

Burns

Pathology

The commonest cause of a burn is a thermal injury to the skin, although electrical and chemical injuries may also result in burns. Burns may be classified into partial thickness and full thickness, depending on whether or not the germinal epithelial layer of the skin is intact or destroyed (Fig. 6.1; Table 6.1).

A *partial thickness* burn may be quite superficial, with erythema due to capillary dilatation and with or without areas of blistering produced by exudation of plasma beneath coagulated epidermis. The underlying germinal layer is intact, and complete healing takes place within a few days. Deeper partial thickness burns extend down to the germinal layer and may partially destroy it. There is intense blistering followed by the formation of a slough. This separates after about 10 days, leaving healthy, newly formed, pink epithelium beneath.

Full-thickness burns completely destroy the skin. There may be initial blistering but this is soon replaced by a coagulum or slough; more often this is present from the onset in an intense deep burn. Unlike the more superficial burns, this slough separates only slowly over 3 or 4 weeks, leaving an underlying surface of granulation tissue. Very small deep burns may heal from an ingrowth of epithelium from adjacent healthy skin; more extensive burns, unless grafted, heal by dense scar tissue with consequent contracture and deformity.

Clinical features

Pain

This is due to the stimulation of numerous nerve endings in the damaged skin. It is more severe in superficial burns and, indeed, deep burns may be relatively painless, due to extensive destruction of nerve endings.

Plasma loss

Loss of the epidermis, together with the intense exudation of plasma through the damaged capillaries, which is especially marked in the first 24 hours after burning, results in an enormous loss of plasma. By the time a coagulum has formed (about 48 hours) this plasma loss ceases. The amount of this loss is proportional to the area of the burn and not its depth.

Hypovolaemic shock

Shock is a direct result of plasma loss. The intravascular volume is rapidly depleted as plasma is lost from the surface of the burn.

Anaemia

This results partly from destruction of red cells within involved skin capillaries and partly from toxic inhibition of the bone marrow if infection of the burnt area occurs.

Airway

Smoke inhalation or thermal injury of the respiratory tract may rapidly result in respira-

BURN CLASSIFICATION

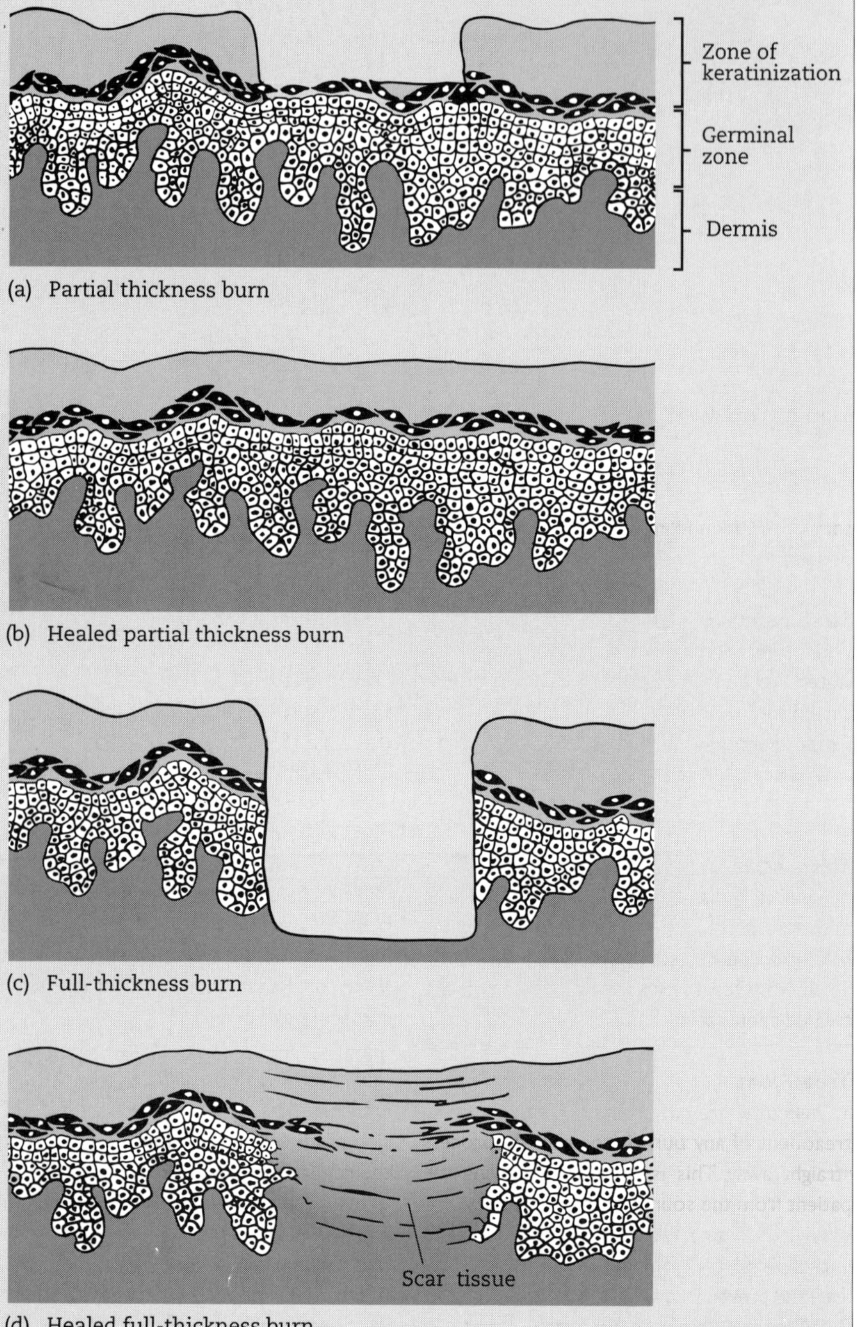

Zone of keratinization

Germinal zone

Dermis

(a) Partial thickness burn

(b) Healed partial thickness burn

(c) Full-thickness burn

Scar tissue

(d) Healed full-thickness burn

Fig. 6.1 A partial thickness burn (a) leaves part or the whole of the germinal epithelium intact. Complete healing takes place (b). A full-thickness burn (c) destroys the germinal layer and, unless very small, can only heal by dense scar tissue (d).

BURN COMPARISON		
	Partial thickness	Full thickness
Depth	Superficial	Deep
Underlying germinal layer	Intact	Destroyed
Sensation	Present	Absent
Healing	Complete	Scarring and contracture
Blistering	Prominent, followed by slough	Slight, slough dominates

Table 6.1 Comparison of superficial and deep burns.

tory obstruction from pharyngeal or laryngeal oedema.

Stress reaction

The adreno-cortical response of sodium and water retention, potassium loss and protein catabolism occurs as in any severe injury. Peptic ulceration (Curling's ulcers*) may occur as a reaction to the stress.

Toxaemia

This is a combination of factors, which include biochemical disturbances, plasma loss and infection. It has also been postulated that a toxin may be produced by the burnt tissues. Toxaemia is less often seen now that burns are treated adequately.

Treatment

1 *Immediate first-aid treatment.* The immediate treatment of any burn is to stop the process straight away. This is done by removing the patient from the source of the burn, removing overlying clothing, which may contain the heat, and applying cold running water to cool the area and prevent continued damage.

2 *Subsequent treatment.* Thereafter the principles of the treatment of burns are:

*Thomas Blizzard Curling (1811–88), Surgeon, The London Hospital, London.

(a) management of the local condition — prevent infection and promote healing;

(b) general treatment — mitigate the effects of burns listed above.

Local treatment

Partial thickness burns affecting a small area (less than 15% in adults, 10% in children) can be managed by cleaning the wound and covering it with a non-adherent dressing such as paraffin gauze or with silver sulphadiazine (Flamazine) cream. Hands, which are commonly burned, may be liberally covered with silver sulphadiazine and placed in polythene bags. The wounds will re-epithelialize in 2–3 weeks. Extensive burns on hands should be treated by early surgery and grafting.

Full-thickness burns are best treated by immediate excision and split-skin grafting. Excision of the burned skin (burn eschar) removes the culture medium for bacteria such as *Streptococcus pyogenes* and *Pseudomonas aeruginosa*. Immediate grafting reduces the risk of sepsis further. However, where a large surface area is burned there may be insufficient skin left from which a donor skin graft may be taken. Under these circumstances, donor skin may be used from a relative or skin bank (allograft), or pig (xenograft). More recently, skin produced by tissue culture has been used. While these grafts may later be lost, they tide the patient over the critical period to a time when a second graft may be taken from what donor sites there are, or alternative means of skin closure may be used.

Electrical burns are full-thickness burns, and are usually far more extensive than is initially suspected. The severity of an electrical burn is proportional to the electrical current, rather than the voltage. The current passes through the body from its source to an earth, and produces entry and exit site burns. In between, the tissues conducting the current sustain varying degrees of injury.

Circumferential full-thickness burns affecting the chest or limb contract and may restrict breathing and impair blood flow to the limbs. Such contractions must be incised acutely to save the limb (escharotomy).

Inhalational burns are indicated by burnt skin and soot around the face particularly the mouth and nostrils. Burns to the airway produce oedema, particularly laryngeal oedema, which may necessitate intubation or tracheostomy. Evidence of hypoxia and pulmonary oedema should be treated by ventilation with humidified oxygen and antibiotics. The presence of carboxyhaemoglobin in the blood is further evidence suggesting inhalational burns.

Priority areas for skin grafting. Skin grafting is carried out immediately if the eyelids are involved in order to prevent ectropion with the risk of corneal ulceration. The face, hands and the joint flexures are next in priority for skin grafting procedures, as scarring at these sites will obviously produce considerable deformity and disability.

General treatment
Pain. Relieve pain with intravenous opiates (e.g. morphine).

Hypovolaemic shock. Rapid fluid loss occurs, the rate of loss being quickest in the first 12 hours. Aggressive replacement of this fluid as soon as possible is essential. There are two underlying principles in this replacement: first the correct *amount* of fluid should be replaced, and secondly the correct *type* of fluid is important.

1 *Amount of fluid replacement.* This depends upon the total *area* burnt. As a guide the 'rule of nine' is helpful. The body is divided into zones of percentage of surface area as follows (Fig. 6.2):

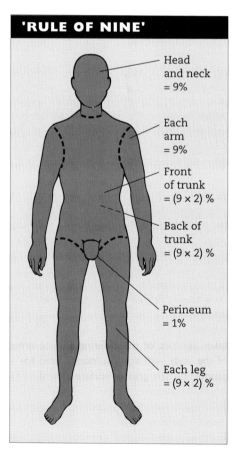

'RULE OF NINE'

Head and neck = 9%

Each arm = 9%

Front of trunk = (9 × 2) %

Back of trunk = (9 × 2) %

Perineum = 1%

Each leg = (9 × 2) %

Fig. 6.2 The 'rule of nine'—a useful guide to the estimation of the area of a burned surface. (Note also that a patient's hand represents 1% of the body surface area.)

MOUNT VERNON FORMULA

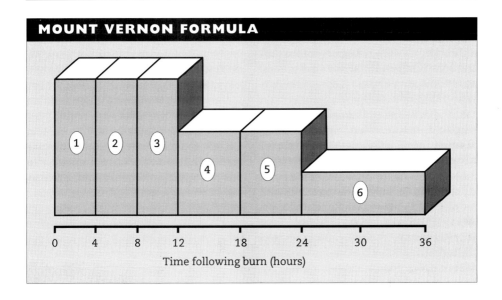

Time following burn (hours)

Fig. 6.3 The Mount Vernon formula for fluid replacement, where each period is represented by a box. One period of volume replacement = weight (kg) × % burn / 2. Fluid replacement is calculated from the time the burn occurred.

	Per cent surface area
Head and neck	9
Each arm	9
Each leg	2 × 9 = 18
Front of the trunk	2 × 9 = 18
Back of the trunk	2 × 9 = 18
Perineum	1

As a rough rule, the patient's hand is approximately 1% of the body surface area. An alternative is the Lund and Browder chart, which takes account of the differing surface areas of the body with age. An infant's head has a proportionately greater surface area than an adult's, for example.

The rate of fluid replacement must take into account that most fluid is lost in the first few hours after the burn, before a coagulum forms. As a rule, burns greater than 10% in children and 15% in adults require intravenous fluid replacement. Less extensive burns can be managed by oral replacement. The Mount Vernon Burns Unit* formula gives a good guide to the amount and rate of fluid replacement required in the first 36 hours, based on the estimated losses:

Fluid replacement (ml) per period =

$$\frac{\text{Weight (kg)} \times \text{\% burn area}}{2}$$

For example, a 70-kg patient with a 40% burn would, on this formula, give a figure of 70 × 40 / 2 = 1400 ml per period. Starting from the time of the burn, the calculated volume of fluid is given every 4 hours for the first 12 hours, every 6 hours for the next 12 hours and then 12-hourly for the next 12 hours. Hence, six volumes of fluid are given over the first 36 hours (Fig. 6.3), decreasing the rate with time. This is in addition to the patient's normal daily fluid requirement (3 litres of crystalloid in an adult).

During the resuscitation phase, careful clinical assessment of the patient should include monitoring hourly urinary output, general condition of shock (pulse, blood pressure), central venous pressure monitoring and

*Mount Vernon Hospital, Northwood, Middlesex, UK.

core temperature, together with regular haematocrit estimations.

2 *Type of fluid used for replacement.* The exudate across the burn is plasma and it should be replaced with plasma or a plasma substitute (e.g. 4.5% human albumin solution). If the burns are full thickness, approximately 50% of the fluid replacement should be given as blood in order to replace the extensive red-cell destruction that occurs within the affected area.

Antimicrobial chemotherapy. Topical agents are used in preference to systemic prophylactic antimicrobial therapy. Secondary infection of the burns may also require local application of antibiotics, and silver sulphadiazine is the commonest used. Invasive infection does require systemic administration of broad-spectrum antibiotics. Where necrotic tissue is present, antibiotics will not eliminate infection, and there is the risk that resistant organisms will eventually proliferate. The best protection against infection is to excise the eschar and obtain skin cover.

Nutrition. The patient's nutrition should be maintained especially where burns are extensive. If enteral nutrition is not possible, parenteral feeding should be instituted early (within 24 hours of the injury). Patients rapidly become catabolic, and adequate calorie and protein replacement are necessary to avoid a negative nitrogen balance.

Complications
Local
• Wound sepsis, usually *Streptococcus pyogenes* or *Pseudomonas aeruginosa.*
• Scarring (full thickness).
• Wound contractures.

General
• *Sepsis*, particularly chest infection in inhalational injury, urinary tract infection resulting from catheterization, and septicaemia directly from wound invasion.
• *Acute peptic ulceration* (Curling's ulcer).
• *Seizures* in children, due to electrolyte imbalance.
• *Renal failure* resulting from the initial hypovolaemia due to plasma loss, precipitation of haemoglobin or myoglobin, or due to nephrotoxic antimicrobial agents.
• *Psychological disturbance.*

Prognosis
Prognosis depends on the extent and depth of the burns, and whether or not infection occurs. Young infants and the elderly carry a higher mortality than young adults. No matter which methods of treatment are used, few patients survive more than a 70% body area full-thickness burn. As a very rough guide, if the patient's age + percentage body area of full-thickness burn exceeds 100, the chances of survival are low.

CHAPTER 7

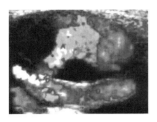

The Skin and its Adnexae

Sebaceous cyst

A sebaceous cyst (epidermoid cyst or wen) is a retention cyst produced by obstruction to the mouth of a sebaceous gland. Sebaceous cysts may therefore occur wherever sebaceous glands exist and are not found on the gland-free palms and soles. They are especially common on the scalp, face, scrotum and vulva and on the lobe of the ear. The cyst is fluctuant and cannot be moved separately from the overlying skin. There may be a typical central punctum and the contents are cheesy with an unpleasant smell. The lining membrane consists of squamous epithelium.

Complications
- Infection.
- Ulceration, which may then resemble a fungating carcinoma ('Cock's peculiar tumour'*).
- Calcification, producing a hard subcutaneous tumour misnamed a 'benign calcifying epithelioma'.
- Horn formation.
- Malignant change—very rare.

*Edward Cock (1805–92), Surgeon, Guy's Hospital, London.

Treatment
The uninfected sebaceous cyst should be removed to prevent possible complications. A small elliptical skin incision is made around the punctum of the cyst under local anaesthetic; the capsule is identified and the cyst removed intact. Failure to remove the cyst in its entirety may lead to recurrence.

If acutely inflamed, drainage will be required, followed later by excision of the capsule wall.

Dermoid cyst

There are two types of dermoid cyst: implantation dermoids and sequestration dermoids.

Implantation dermoid
This is a painless, subcutaneous, cystic swelling commonly found on the pulps of the fingers, neither attached to the skin nor to the deeper structures. It usually follows a puncture injury (e.g. a rose thorn) with consequent implantation of epithelial cells into the subcutaneous tissues. The cyst typically contains a white, greasy material, which results from degeneration of the desquamated cells. An old healed scar over the cyst may help confirm the diagnosis.

Sequestration dermoid

This is a subcutaneous cystic swelling resulting from an embryological rest of epithelial cells along a line of fusion. The common sites are over the external angular process of the frontal bone (the upper outer margin of the orbit — the external angular dermoid), the root of the nose (internal angular dermoid) and in the midline. When in relation to the skull, the underlying bone is usually hollowed out around it. The possibility of communication with an intracranial dermoid or the meninges should be excluded by skull radiography or computed tomography (CT) scan prior to excision.

Verruca vulgaris (wart)

This is the familiar well-localized horny projection that is common on the fingers, hands, feet and knees, particularly of children and young adults. Crops of warts may occur on the genitalia and perianal region, in many cases spread by sexual contact. The lesion is often multiple and is due to a papilloma virus.

Microscopically, there is a local hyperplasia of the prickle cell layer of the skin (acanthosis) with marked surface cornification.

Treatment

Untreated, warts usually vanish spontaneously within 2 years, hence the apparent efficacy of folklore 'wart cures'. Often reassurance that these lesions will disappear is all that is required, but if treatment is demanded they can be burnt down by the application of a silver nitrate stick or podophyllin, frozen with liquid nitrogen, or curetted under local or general anaesthesia.

Plantar warts

These are verrucas that occur on the weight-bearing areas of the foot. Pressure forces the wart into the deeper tissues, producing intense local pain on walking. They may occur in epidemics in schools etc., where the hygiene of the communal bath or changing room is not of a high standard.

They should be treated by podophyllin or curettage.

Keratoacanthoma (molluscum sebaceum)

This is a lesion that occurs most commonly on the face and nose (75%) but may also be found on the fingers, hands and elsewhere on the skin in patients of the 50–60 year age group. It appears as a rapidly growing nodule, which may reach 3 cm or more in diameter in a few weeks with a characteristic central crater filled by a keratin plug. It closely resembles a squamous carcinoma or rodent ulcer in appearance, and it is only the history of very rapid growth that helps differentiate it from the latter.

Histologically, it consists of a central crater filled with keratin surrounded by hypertrophied squamous stratified epithelium. There is no invasion of the surrounding tissues.

If left untreated, the lesion disappears over a period of 4 or 5 months, leaving a faint white scar. Its aetiology is unknown, but it does not appear to be a virus infection; attempts to transfer it by means of tissue extract have failed. Its solitary situation and occurrence in mainly elderly patients also indicate that it does not have a viral origin.

Treatment

It is safest to remove the lesion to establish histological proof of the diagnosis.

Ganglion

Ganglia present as cystic, subcutaneous, pea-sized lumps, which occur especially around the wrist and the dorsum of the foot (joint-capsule origin), or along the flexor aspect of the fingers and on the peroneal tendons (tendon-sheath origin). Although ganglia are amongst the commonest of surgical lumps, their origin is uncertain. They may represent a benign myxoma of joint capsule or tendon sheath, a hamartoma or a myxomatous degeneration due to trauma.

They are unilocular, thin-walled cysts with a synovial lining, which contain mucoid fluid having the microscopic appearances of Wharton's jelly. Histologically, they are indistinguishable from cysts of the lateral cartilage of the knee and semi-membranosus bursae.

Treatment

The patient may complain of discomfort or of the cosmetic appearance; if so the cyst should be excised under a general anaesthetic using a bloodless field produced by a tourniquet. The old-fashioned treatment of hitting the ganglion with the family Bible ruptures the cyst, but recurrence usually occurs after some time. Recurrence is unfortunately also common after surgical excision if even a fragment of the ganglion wall is left behind.

Pilonidal sinus

The majority of pilonidal sinuses occur in the skin of the natal cleft. They may be solitary or appear as a row in the midline. Frequently tufts of hair are found lying free within the sinus (Latin *pilus* = hair, *nidus* = nest).

Usually, young adults are affected, males more than females, and more often in dark-haired individuals; the sinuses are rarely seen in children and do not present until adolescence. They may also occur in the clefts between the fingers as an occupational disease of barbers and are occasionally found in the axilla, at the umbilicus, the perineum and the sole of the foot as well as on amputation stumps.

Aetiology

The occurrence of pilonidal sinuses remote from the natal cleft, and the occurrence of such sinuses on the hands and feet of people working with cattle, where the contained hair is clearly of animal origin, suggests the hypothesis that these sinuses occur by implantation of hair into the skin; these set up a foreign-body reaction and produce a chronic infected sinus. It may be that in some cases post-anal pits act as traps for loose hairs, thus combining both

the congenital and acquired theories of origin. The hair enters the skin follicles from its distal end and works its way in due to tapered lateral hair extensions angled proximally.

Clinical features

The pilonidal sinus is symptomless until it becomes infected; there is then a typical history of recurrent abscesses, which either require drainage or discharge spontaneously.

Treatment

If an acute abscess is present, this must be drained in the usual way. In the quiescent phase, the track is excised or simply laid open and allowed to heal by granulation. Recurrence is diminished by keeping the surrounding skin free from hair by rubbing with fine sandpaper, shaving or the use of depilatory creams.

The nails

The nails are the site of some common and important surgical conditions.

Paronychia

Paronychia denotes infection of the nail fold, usually of the finger, but it may complicate an ingrowing toenail (see below).

Diagnosis of acute paronychia is obvious; the nail fold is red, swollen and tender, and pus may be visible beneath the skin.

Treatment

If seen before pus has formed, at the cellulitic stage, infection may be aborted by a course of flucloxacillin or other appropriate anti-staphylococcal antibiotic together with immobilization by a splint to the finger and a sling to the arm. If pus is present, drainage is performed through an incision carried proximally through the nail fold, combined with removal of the base of the nail if pus has tracked beneath it.

Chronic paronychia is seen in those whose occupation requires constant soaking of the hands in water, but it may also occur as a result of fungus infection (*Candida*) of the nails and where the peripheral circulation is deficient, e.g. Raynaud's phenomenon (see p. 81).

Ingrowing toenail

This is nearly always confined to the hallux and is usually due to a combination of tight shoes (particularly trainers) and the habit of paring the nail downwards into the nail fold, rather than transversely; the sharp edge of the nail then grows into the side of the nail bed, producing ulceration and infection.

Treatment

If seen before infection has occurred, advice is given on correct cutting of the nails; nylon socks and trainers are vetoed. A pledget of cotton wool tucked daily into the side of the nail bed, after preliminary soaking of the feet in hot water to soften the nails, enables the nail to grow up out of the fold.

If an acute paronychia is present, drainage will be required by means of removal of the side of the nail or avulsion of the whole nail. For recurrent cases when the infection has settled, the affected side may be excised together with the nail root (wedge excision), or the entire nail may be obliterated completely by excision of the nail root (Zadik's operation*) or by treating the nail bed with aqueous phenol.

Onychogryphosis

This condition of an intensely coiled 'ram's horn' deformity of the nail may affect any of the toes, although the hallux is the commonest site. It may follow trauma to the nail bed and is usually found in elderly subjects.

Treatment

Relatively mild examples can be kept under control by trimming the nail with bone-cutting forceps. Merely avulsing the nail is invariably followed by recurrence, and the only adequate treatment is excision of the nail root.

Lesions of the nail bed

It is convenient to list a number of relatively common conditions that affect the nail bed.

Haematoma

As a result of crush injury to the terminal phalanx, with or without fracture of the underlying bone, a tense, painful haematoma may develop beneath the nail. Relief is afforded by evacuating the clot through a hole made either by a dental drill or by a red-hot needle; both procedures are painless. Occasionally, a small haematoma may develop after a trivial or forgotten injury and clinically may closely simulate a subungual melanoma.

Subungual exostosis

This is nearly always confined to the hallux and is especially found in adolescents and young adults. It appears as a reddish brown area under the nail, which is tender on pressure. The exostosis may ulcerate through the overlying nail, producing an infected granulating mass. The diagnosis is confirmed by X-ray of the toe, and treatment is to remove the nail and excise the underlying exostosis.

Melanoma

The nail bed is a common site for malignant melanoma (see p. 44), with a long history of slow growth; often there is a misleading history of trauma. The lesion should be confirmed by excision biopsy followed by amputation of the digit. If the regional lymph nodes are involved, block dissection is performed.

Glomus tumour

The nail bed of the fingers and toes is a common site of this extremely painful lesion, which is a benign tumour arising in a subcutaneous glomus body (highly innervated arterio-venous anastomosis). It is considered on page 47.

*Frank Raphael Zadik (contemporary), Orthopaedic Surgeon, Sheffield, UK.

Tumours of the skin and subcutaneous tissues

Classification
1 Epidermal.
   (a) Benign: papilloma, senile keratosis, seborrhoeic keratosis.
   (b) Malignant: Bowen's disease, squamous cell carcinoma, basal cell carcinoma, secondary deposits (e.g. from carcinoma of breast and lung, leukaemia, Hodgkin's disease).
2 Benign and malignant melanomas.
3 Tumours of sebaceous and sweat glands.
4 Dermal tumours from blood vessels, lymphatics, nerves, fibrous tissue or fat.

Epidermal tumours
Papilloma
This is a common, benign, pedunculated tumour, often pigmented with melanin. Microscopically, it comprises a keratinized papillary tumour of squamous epithelium.

Seborrhoeic keratosis (basal cell papilloma)
This is a common tumour occurring after the age of 40 years. It appears as a yellowish or brown raised lesion on the face, arms or trunk and is often multiple. It often appears greasy, and its surface is characterized by a network of crypts.

Microscopically, there is hyperkeratosis, proliferation of the basal cell layer and melanin pigmentation.

The lesion is quite benign, but differential diagnosis from a melanoma can only be made with certainty by excising the lump and submitting it to histological examination.

Senile (solar or actinic) keratosis
This is a small, hard, brown, scaly tumour on sun-exposed areas of skin (e.g. the forehead, ears and backs of hands) of the elderly. Keratoses are more common in individuals with fair skin, and after prolonged exposure to ultraviolet light.

Microscopically, hyperkeratosis is present, often with atypical dividing cells in the prickle cell layer.

The lesions may be treated with liquid nitrogen cryotherapy, or curettage; large areas may require topical chemotherapy (e.g. 5-fluorouracil).

The importance of this lesion is that it may undergo change into a squamous cell carcinoma.

Bowen's disease*
This appears as a very slowly growing, red, scaly plaque, and represents 'carcinoma-in-situ'. It may be mistaken for a psoriatic plaque, but has a different distribution.

Microscopically, there is marked mitotic activity in the prickle cell layer with the presence of giant cells and large, clear Paget cells.

Treatment is adequate excision; if left untreated, eventually a squamous cell carcinoma will supervene.

Squamous cell carcinoma (epithelioma)
Occurs usually in the elderly male, especially in skin areas exposed to sunshine, e.g. face and backs of the hands. Like solar keratoses, it is relatively common in white subjects who live in the tropics.

Predisposing factors
These include:
• solar keratosis;
• Bowen's disease;
• exposure to sunshine or ultraviolet irradiation;
• carcinogens, e.g. pitch, tar, soot, mineral oils;
• chronic ulceration, particularly in burns scars (Marjolin's ulcer—see below);
• lupus vulgaris (cutaneous tuberculosis);
• immunosuppressive drugs.

Pathology
Macroscopically, it presents as a typical carci-

*John Templeton Bowen (1857–1941), Dermatologist, Harvard Medical School, Boston, USA.

nomatous ulcer with raised everted edges and a central scab. Microscopically, there are solid columns of epithelial cells growing into the dermis with epithelial pearls of central keratin surrounded by prickle cells. Occasionally, anaplastic tumours are seen in which these pearls are absent.

Spread occurs by local infiltration and then by lymphatics. Blood spread occurs only in very advanced cases.

Treatment

Treatment consists of either wide excision or radiotherapy, depending on the site of the lesion. If the regional lymph nodes are involved, block dissection is indicated.

Marjolin's ulcer*

The name applied to malignant change in a scar, ulcer or sinus, e.g. a chronic venous ulcer, an unhealed burn or the sinus of chronic osteomyelitis. It has the following characteristics:
• slow growth, because the lesion is relatively avascular;
• painless, because the scar tissue does not contain cutaneous nerve fibres;
• lymphatic spread is late, because the scar tissue produces lymphatic obliteration.

Once the tumour reaches the normal tissues beyond the diseased area, rapid growth, pain and lymphatic involvement take place.

Basal cell carcinoma (rodent ulcer)

This is the most common form of skin cancer in white people. It occurs usually in elderly subjects, males twice as commonly as females. Ninety per cent are found on the face above a line joining the angle of the mouth to the external auditory meatus, particularly around the eye, the naso-labial folds and the hair line of the scalp. The tumour may, however, arise on any part of the skin and this includes the anal margin. Predisposing factors are exposure to sunlight or irradiation.

*Jean Nicholas Marjolin (1780–1850), Surgeon, Hôpital Sainte-Eugénie, Paris, France.

Pathology

Macroscopically, the tumour has raised, rolled, but not everted edges. It consists of pearly nodules over which fine blood vessels can be seen to course (telangiectasia). Starting as a small nodule, the tumour very slowly grows over the years with central ulceration and scabbing.

Microscopically, solid sheets of uniform, darkly staining cells arising from the basal layer of the skin are seen. Prickle cells and epithelial pearls are both absent.

Spread is by infiltration with slow but steady destruction of surrounding tissues; in advanced cases, the underlying skull may be eroded or the face, nose and eye may be destroyed, hence the name 'rodent'. Lymphatic and blood spread occur with extreme rarity.

Treatment

Treatment is by excision, where this can be done with an adequate margin and without cosmetic deformity. It is also indicated in late cases where the tumour has recurred after irradiation or has invaded underlying bone or cartilage. In the majority of cases, however, superficial radiotherapy gives excellent results. Where the tumour occurs on or near the eyelid, the conjunctiva must be protected by means of a lead shield during irradiation therapy.

Melanoma
Aetiology

Melanomas develop from melanocytes, which are situated in the basal layer of the epidermis and which originate from the neuro-ectoderm of the embryonic neural crest. Some melanocytes contain no visible pigment, but all are characterized by a positive dihydroxyphenylalanine (DOPA) reaction—they can all convert DOPA into melanin.

Classification

Melanomas may be classified into:
• intradermal melanoma or naevus (the common mole);
• junctional melanoma or naevus;
• compound melanoma or naevus;

- juvenile melanoma;
- malignant melanoma.

Nearly everyone possesses one or more moles; some have hundreds, although they may not become apparent until after puberty. Those moles that are entirely within the dermis remain benign, but a small percentage of the junctional naevi, so called because they are seen in the basal layer of the epidermis at its junction with the dermis, may undergo malignant change (Fig. 7.1).

Intradermal melanoma or naevus

This is the commonest variety of mole.

The naevus may be light or dark in colour and may be flat or raised, hairy or hairless. A hairy mole is nearly always intradermal. They may be found in every situation except the palm of the hand, the sole of the foot or the scrotal skin.

Histologically, there is a nest of melanocytes situated entirely within the dermis where the cells form non-encapsulated masses. They never undergo malignant change, and need no treatment unless the diagnosis is uncertain.

Junctional melanoma or naevus

The junctional naevus is pigmented to a vari-

Fig. 7.1 (a) The normal skin contains melanocytes (shown as cells) and melanin pigment shown as dots. The pigment increases in sunburn and freckles. (b) A benign intradermal naevus; the melanocytes are clumped together in the dermis to form a localized benign tumour. (c) A junctional naevus with melanocytes clumping together in the basal layer of the epidermis. These are usually benign but may occasionally give rise to an invasive malignant melanoma (d).

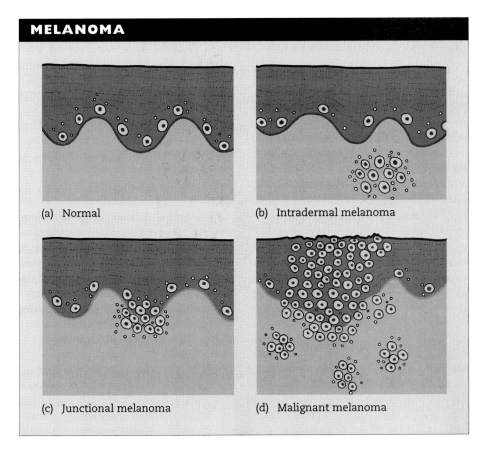

MELANOMA

(a) Normal

(b) Intradermal melanoma

(c) Junctional melanoma

(d) Malignant melanoma

able shade from light brown to almost black. It is nearly always flat, smooth and hairless. It may occur anywhere on the body and, unlike the intradermal naevus, may be found on the palm of the hand, sole of the foot and the genitalia.

Histologically, naevus cells are seen in the basal layers of the epidermis from which the cells may spread to the surface.

Only a small percentage of junctional naevi undergo malignant change, but it is from this group that the vast majority of malignant melanomas arise.

Compound melanoma or naevus

Clinically, this is indistinguishable from the intradermal naevus, but histologically it has junctional elements that make it potentially malignant.

Juvenile melanoma

Melanomas before puberty are relatively unusual, and may present as a dark nodule. Microscopically, they may be indistinguishable from malignant melanoma; yet fortunately and surprisingly these usually pursue a completely benign course. Melanomas in children should therefore always be dealt with by conservative surgery in spite of their frightening histological appearance.

Malignant melanoma

Malignant melanomas arise in pre-existing naevi, either junctional naevi or compound naevi where there is a junctional component. They occur in white people on light-exposed areas, hence the higher incidence on the legs of females. It is rarely found in the pigmented skin of dark-skinned races, tending to be found in the non-pigmented skin on the sole of the foot. A premalignant form, the *lentigo maligna*, also exists.

Presentations

The two main presentations of malignant melanoma are the superficial spreading type, and the nodular type. Several other presentations also occur.

Superficial spreading melanoma. The commonest presentation of malignant melanoma is of a previously dormant naevus starting to spread superficially. The surface has patches of deep pigmentation.

Nodular melanoma. The naevus is nodular and deeply pigmented and may bleed or ulcerate. Such a nodule may occur on a pigmented background such as the lentigo maligna. It tends to invade deeply rather than spread superficially, and carries a poorer prognosis with earlier lymphatic involvement.

Acral melanoma. These are so called because they occur at the extremities, commonly on the palms and soles of feet. It is this type that occurs in dark-skinned races. The subungual melanoma is a variant of acral melanoma (see p. 40).

Lentigo maligna. This is a brown pigmented patch with an irregular outline and is usually found on the cheeks of elderly women, often called a *Hutchinson's freckle.** The pale patch appears over several years; malignant change is indicated by deeper pigmentation or nodule formation.

Mucosal melanoma. Malignant melanoma may be found on the mucous membranes of the nose, mouth, anus and intestine.

Choroid melanoma. Melanomas may arise from melanocytes in the pigment layer of the retina. These are renowned for presenting many years after enucleation with hepatic metastases, hence the aphorism 'beware the patient with the large liver and the glass eye'.

Amelanotic melanoma. Paradoxically, melanomas are not always pigmented, but they remain DOPA positive.

---

*Sir Jonathan Hutchinson (1828–73), Surgeon, The London Hospital, London. Described numerous conditions and was first to perform a successful operation for reduction of an intussusception in a child.

Signs of malignant change in a naevus

- Increase or irregularity in size.
- Increase or irregularity in pigmentation.
- Bleeding or ulceration.
- Spread of pigment from the edge of the tumour.
- Itching or pain.
- Formation of daughter nodules.
- Lymph-node or distant spread.

Pathology

Microscopically, pleomorphic cells are seen, which spread through the layers of the epidermis and which are usually pigmented (occasionally the cells are amelanotic).

Spread. As well as local growth and ulceration, malignant melanomas seed by lymphatic permeation, which produces cutaneous nodules by progressive proximal spread, and by lymphatic emboli to the regional lymph nodes. There is also widespread dissemination by the blood stream to any and every organ in the body. Free melanin in the blood may produce generalized skin pigmentation and melanuria in late cases.

Staging

The prognosis of malignant melanoma depends upon its degree of invasion, which is measured by the depth of invasion. The depth may be measured either by reference to the normal skin layers (Clark's levels), or more simply according to its measured depth (Breslow). Because of its simplicity Breslow's method is now routinely adopted.

Treatment of pigmented lesions

The following is a general guide to the management of pigmented lesions of the skin.

Prophylactic removal. Any pigmented tumour on the hand, sole or genitalia, or any that, in other situations, are subjected to trauma should be excised; these are the commonest among the small percentage of naevi to undergo malignant change. In addition, pigmented lesions should be removed for cosmetic reasons or if the patient is acutely anxious about their presence — this is a particularly common phenomenon among doctors, nurses and medical students. Such lesions are sent for careful histological examination and should always be removed in their entirety.

Suspicious naevi. If the pigmented lesion shows any of the features already listed that suggest that malignant change has taken place, the naevus is first removed for urgent histological examination (frozen section). If malignant melanoma is confirmed, a wide local excision of the area is performed, with a margin of clearance proportional to the depth of invasion (Breslow thickness). This is commonly translated into a centimetre margin for every millimetre of invasion; primary skin grafting may be required.

Regional lymph nodes. If the regional nodes are involved, these are treated by block dissection. If impalpable, they are kept under careful surveillance and block dissection performed if subsequent enlargement takes place.

Adjuvant therapy. Malignant melanoma deposits often show regression when the primary lesion is excised, implying an immunological component. Direct immunotherapy, such as interferon-γ and interleukin-2 administration, has had some success.

Melanomas are generally radio resistant, but chemotherapy, particularly high-dose isolated perfusion of a limb with cytotoxic chemotherapeutic agents, has a place.

Prognosis

Prognosis depends on large number of factors.
- *The thickness* of the primary lesion. Prognosis is good when this is less than 1.5 mm in depth. The deeper the lesion, the greater the risk of lymph-node metastasis.
- *Type of lesion.* A superficial spreading melanoma has a better prognosis than a penetrating and ulcerating lesion.
- *The anatomical site.* Tumours on the trunk and scalp have a poor prognosis.

• *Lymph-node metastases* indicate poor prognosis, more so if there are cutaneous deposits.

The most important factor is the depth of invasion by Breslow thickness, usually divided into band widths. In the absence of satellite or lymph-node involvement, the 5-year survival is:

Depth	5-year survival
<0.75 mm	>95%
0.75–1.5 mm	90%
1.5–4.0 mm	70%
>4.0 mm	<50%

In the presence of nodal involvement, or satellite lesions, survival at 5 years is under 30%.

Tumours of sweat glands and sebaceous glands

Benign and malignant tumours of these glandular adnexae of the skin are rare.

Sebaceous adenomas

These are more in the nature of a hyperplasia of the glands than true tumours. They occur as pink or yellow nodes on the nose, cheek and forehead. Microscopically, they are merely overgrowths of sebaceous glands.

Sebaceous carcinoma

Found rarely on the face and scalp in elderly subjects. Carcinomatous change may rarely occur in sebaceous cysts.

Sweat-gland adenomas or carcinomas

May occur on the face and scalp and in the apocrine sweat glands of the axilla, vulva and scrotum. They are composed of columns or cylinders of clear cells and the descriptive term 'cylindroma' is applied to these tumours for this reason. On the scalp they may form masses of large nodules ('turban tumour'), but tumours of similar appearance may also be of basal cell origin.

Dermal tumours

Tumours of blood vessels usually lie in the dermis, although the underlying muscles and soft tissues may be involved. The abdominal viscera, central nervous system and bone may also be the sites of these lesions. The terminology of blood-vessel tumours is confusing and is bedevilled with picturesque descriptive terms. Most benign blood-vessel 'tumours' are indeed congenital malformations or hamartomas.

Classification
• Capillary haemangioma.
• Cavernous haemangioma.
• Sclerosing angioma (fibrous histiocytoma).
• Glomus tumour.
• Haemangiosarcoma.
• Kaposi's sarcoma.

Capillary haemangioma

A variety of types of congenital capillary malformation may be found in the skin, usually at birth.

Salmon pink patch is a common blemish on the head or neck of a new-born child and rapidly disappears spontaneously.

Strawberry naevus is bright red, raised, and usually disappears during the first few years of life, although there may at first be a rapid alarming enlargement, even with ulceration, before involution occurs.

Port-wine stain, flush with the skin, usually on the face, lips and buccal mucosa, produces an extensive area of dark-red, blue or purple discoloration. It is present from birth and shows no tendency to regress with age.

Note that port-wine stain of the face may have a segmental distribution corresponding to the cutaneous branches of the trigeminal nerve and may be associated with angiomas of the cerebral pia-arachnoid, which may manifest themselves by focal epileptic attacks (the Sturge–Weber syndrome*).

---

*William Allen Sturge (1850–1919), Physician, Royal Free Hospital, London. Frederick Parkes Weber (1863–1962), London Physician with a life-long interest in rare diseases.

Campbell de Morgan spots[*] are found on the trunk of middle-aged and elderly subjects. They are bright-red aggregates of dilated capillaries, which can be emptied by pressing on them with the tip of a pencil. They are of no significance.

Spider naevus is another example of a capillary haemangioma. Isolated 'spiders' are present in normal people, but they are more common during pregnancy and in chronic liver disease. They comprise a central arteriole from which radiate capillaries. Pressure on the central arteriole with a pinhead causes the lesion to disappear while pressure is maintained.

Treatment
Most strawberry naevi disappear spontaneously, but diathermy coagulation, application of CO_2 snow or excision and grafting may be required. The port-wine stain may respond to cutaneous laser therapy, but the simplest treatment remains camouflage with cosmetics.

Cavernous haemangioma
These are made up of large blood spaces lined with endothelium. They occur on the skin, lip and, quite commonly, as multiple nodules in the liver. They are usually present at birth, and grow to keep pace with normal body growth.

The lesions are blue, may be raised and may partly empty on pressure. They may infiltrate the underlying tissues and may be associated with unsightly overlying cutaneous thickening.

Treatment
This is often difficult. The condition may be disguised by the use of cosmetics, or thrombosis can be encouraged by injection of sclerosing agents. Very unsightly small lesions may be excised and skin grafted.

Sclerosing angioma (fibrous histiocytoma)
This is a pigmented tumour of the skin that may easily be confused with a malignant melanoma with which it has a close macroscopic resemblance. Palpation, however, reveals a typically hard consistency due to the dense fibrous stroma. It is probably produced as a result of fibrosis of a capillary haemangioma. The pigment is due to iron and not to melanin: this is easily shown with specific histological staining.

Glomus tumour
Glomus bodies are found in the subcutaneous tissues of the limbs, particularly the fingers, the toes and their nail beds. They are convoluted arterio-venous anastomoses with a cellular wall comprising a thick layer of cuboidal 'glomus' cells, which are modified plain muscle; between these cells are abundant nerve fibres. These structures are perhaps concerned with cutaneous heat regulation. Glomus tumours are blue or reddish, small, raised lesions, which occur in young adults at the common sites of glomus bodies. Their characteristic is exquisite tenderness, which makes their slightest touch agonizing.

Treatment
Treatment is excision of the lesion, which is rewarded by the heartfelt gratitude of the patient.

Haemangiosarcoma
Malignant tumours of the vascular endothelium are extremely rare, although they do occur at any site where haemangiomas are found. In the past, the term has been applied to many highly vascular sarcomas simply because they contained large vascular spaces. Haemangiosarcoma of the liver has been reported in workers in the plastics industry exposed to vinyl chloride.

---

*[*] Campbell de Morgan (1811–76), Surgeon, Middlesex Hospital, London.

Kaposi's sarcoma*

This tumour has a multi-centric origin. It used to be most common in the elderly in central Europe, particularly Ashkenazi Jews†; now it is a common tumour in patients with acquired immune deficiency syndrome (AIDS), in whom it is very aggressive. Recent work has demonstrated that DNA extracted from Kaposi's sarcoma tissue is homologous with some herpes viruses, indicating a viral origin for the disease. It presents as a number of bluish red or dark-blue nodules scattered over the extremities of one or more of the limbs. The nodules spread centrally along the limb, may ulcerate and can metastasize to the liver and lungs. In the aggressive form, which occurs in the immunosuppressed, visceral involvement occurs with bowel perforation, haemorrhage or intussusception.

Histologically, there are two components: blood vessels and fibroblasts. The latter show the malignant features, thus distinguishing this tumour from a haemangiosarcoma. The tumour can be kept under control for long periods by local radiotherapy or cytotoxic drugs.

Telangiectasia

Telangiectases, although not truly tumours, are conveniently mentioned in this section. They are dilatations of normal capillaries and are seen in a number of circumstances, e.g. on the weather-beaten faces of country people and on the legs of young women, who may complain of their cosmetic appearance.

Hereditary haemorrhagic telangiectasia (Osler–Weber–Rendu syndrome‡) is an inher-ited autosomal dominant disease characterized by tiny capillary angiomas of the skin, lips and mucous membranes; they may give rise to repeated nose-bleeds and gastrointestinal haemorrhage. Typically, the telangiectases are visible around the mouth and in the fauces.

Lymph-vessel tumours

Lymphangiomas are congenital in origin and similar to haemangiomas; they are lined by endothelium but contain lymph. They are relatively uncommon, but occur mainly on the lips, tongue and cheek, resulting in macrocheilia or macroglossia.

Cystic hygroma

This arises from the jugular lymph sac in the neck, the embryonic precursor of the jugular part of the thoracic duct. It consists of a multilocular cystic mass, which is often present at birth or noticed in early infancy. Character-istically, it is supremely transilluminable. It may respond to injection of hypertonic saline as a sclerosant. Surgical treatment consists of ex-cision, but this is a difficult procedure, as the cysts ramify throughout the structures of the neck.

Nerve tumours

Tumours of the peripheral nerves arise from the neurilemmal sheath of Schwann,§ hence the terms neurilemmoma, neurofibroma or Schwannoma. They push the fibres of the nerve to one side or actually grow within the sub-stance of the nerve. The tumours may be soli-tary or multiple and may involve any peripheral nerve in the body. Of the cranial nerves, the eighth is most commonly involved, often as a solitary tumour (the acoustic tumour, see p. 99). Tumours may arise within the spinal canal, particularly from the dorsal nerve roots,

*Moritz Kaposi (1837–1902), Professor of Derma-tology, Vienna, Austria.

†Ashkenazi Jews: Contrast Sephardic and Oriental Jews. Migrated to Germany, Poland and Russia.

‡Sir William Osler (1849–1919), Canadian, Profes-sor of Medicine successively at McGill, Montreal, Johns Hopkins, Baltimore and the University of Oxford. Frederick Parkes Weber (1863–1962), London Physician. H. J. L. Rendu (1844–1902), Physi-cian, Hôpital Neckar, Paris, France.

§Theodor Schwann (1810–82), Professor of Anatomy, Louvain and then Liège, Belgium.

resulting in an extramedullary, intrathecal, slow-growing spinal tumour (see p. 127). Part of this tumour may protrude through the intervertebral foramen, producing a dumb-bell tumour, which projects either into the thoracic cavity or the abdominal cavity.

In the skin and subcutaneous tissues there is a wide range of presentations from a solitary tumour arising from a peripheral nerve to uncountable numbers involving the whole of the body (*von Recklinghausen's disease**; his name is also applied to the osteitis fibrosa cystica of hyperparathyroidism, p. 308).

Clinical features

The tumours may appear in childhood and there is often a family history, von Recklinghausen's disease being an autosomal dominant condition. The cutaneous lesions are soft and often pedunculated. They are usually painless, although pressure may produce pain along the line of the nerve, particularly when larger nerve trunks are involved. The tumour is mobile from side to side but not longitudinally, in the line of the nerve to which is it attached. There may be associated café-au-lait patches of pigmentation. In some cases there are disfiguring masses of neurofibromatous tissue over which the thickened skin hangs in ugly folds. The 'Elephant Man' of the London Hospital was a gross example of the disease.

Treatment

Where the neurofibromas are solitary or few in number, removal can be performed, either by enucleation, if the nerve fibres are pushed to one side, or resection with suture of the divided nerve. Incomplete removal must not be performed, as sarcomatous change may follow. Where the whole body is covered by these lesions, some cosmetic improvement can be effected by excising the more noticeable lesions from the face and hands.

*Friederich Daniel von Recklinghausen (1833–1910), Professor of Pathology successively at Königsberg, Würzburg and Strasbourg.

Neurofibrosarcoma is uncommon. It may arise *de novo* or as malignant change in a neurofibroma. Clinical features are pain, rapid growth and peripheral anaesthesia or paralysis. Treatment is wide excision.

Fatty tumours

Lipoma

Lipomas are the commonest of benign tumours. They usually occur in adults, and the sex distribution is equal, although females are more likely to present to the surgeon for cosmetic removal of these lesions. Lipomas may arise in any connective tissue but especially in the subcutaneous fat, particularly around the shoulder and over the trunk. They do not occur in the palm, sole of the foot or in the scalp, because in these areas the fat is contained within dense fibrous septa. Occasionally, lipomas appear in large numbers subcutaneously and are tender (Dercum's disease†) and it is sometimes quite difficult to differentiate them from neurofibromas. Elsewhere it is useful to remember 'lipomas occur beneath everything'; thus, in addition to being subcutaneous, they may be subfascial, subperiosteal, subperitoneal, submucosal and subpleural.

The diagnosis is rarely in doubt with this soft, lobulated, fluctuant tumour. The fluctuation is interesting; it is often said to be due to the fat being liquid at body temperature, but anyone observing an operation will notice that fat within the body certainly does not flow out in liquid form over the surgeon's boots when the skin is incised. The fluctuation can be explained by the histological structure of the lipoma, which consists of aggregates of typical fat cells; each cell itself forms a microscopic cyst. This is very much like the fluctuation that can be elicited in a colloid goitre made up of thyroid vesicles distended with colloid material.

†Francis Xavier Dercum (1856–1931), Neurologist, Jefferson Medical College, Philadelphia, USA.

Treatment

Treatment consists of excision if the lipoma is cosmetically troublesome.

Liposarcoma

A rare tumour, which probably arises as an unusual event in a pre-existing benign lipoma. The retroperitoneal site is commonest, but it may also occur around the thigh region and should be suspected if the tumour is very large, firmer than usual, vascular or rapidly growing.

Treatment

Treatment comprises wide excision if this is possible.

CHAPTER 8

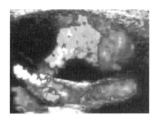

The Chest and Lungs

Injury to the chest

Ventilation of the lungs depends on a patent main airway and pulmonary alveoli, a rigid bony skeleton of the thorax, and on the integrity of the nerves and muscles that control the movements of the ribs and diaphragm. Traumatic disruption of the chest wall is likely to be lethal unless treatment is instituted rapidly.

Dangerous complications of chest injury are:
• paradoxical respiration;
• pneumothorax;
• penetration of the lung;
• haemothorax;
• cardiac tamponade due to laceration of the heart;
• large-vessel damage.
Serious harm can also result from crush injuries that do not penetrate the chest; thus, a main bronchus or the aorta may be ruptured, the lung contused and papillary muscles of the heart or the coronary arteries may be damaged.

Fractures of the ribs
Clinical features
The commonest injury to the chest is fracture of the ribs by a direct blow. The most commonly affected ribs are the seventh, eighth and ninth in which the fracture usually occurs in the region of the mid-axillary line. The patient complains of pain in the chest overlying the fracture and this pain is intensified by springing the ribs with gentle but sharp pressure on the sternum.

Special investigations
• *Chest X-ray* may confirm rib fractures, and will identify underlying lung damage or haemorrhage that would not have been suspected from the trivial nature of the patient's symptoms. However, an X-ray may not always demonstrate a fracture, and if the patient has clinical signs of fractured ribs, he or she should be treated for this condition in spite of a negative X-ray. A repeat X-ray at 2 weeks may show fracture callus and confirm the diagnosis.
• *Bone scan* is more sensitive at detecting fractures, especially pathological fractures, when it may reveal metastatic tumour deposits elsewhere in the skeleton, or be suggestive of metabolic bone disease.

Complications
Flail chest (Fig. 8.1)
Crush injuries of the chest, in which multiple ribs are fractured at both ends or the whole sternum loosened by fractured ribs on either side, result in the condition of flail chest. On inspiration, the flail part of the chest wall becomes indrawn by the negative intrathoracic pressure, as it is no longer in structural continuity with the bony thoracic cage. Similarly, in expiration the flail part of the chest is pushed out whilst the rest of the bony cage becomes contracted. This is termed *paradoxical move-*

FLAIL CHEST

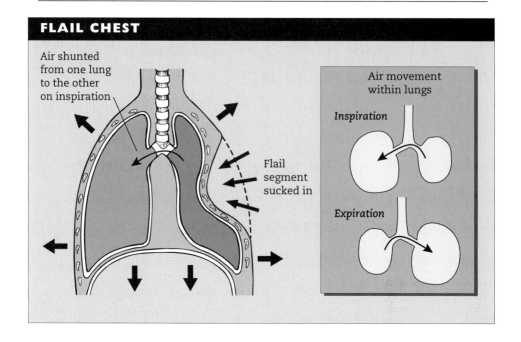

Air shunted from one lung to the other on inspiration

Flail segment sucked in

Air movement within lungs

Inspiration

Expiration

Fig. 8.1 Flail chest. On inspiration, the detached segment of the chest wall is sucked inwards, producing paradoxical movement, and inhaled air shunts back and forth between lungs.

ment. The patient becomes grossly anoxic due to failure of adequate expansion of the affected side and also because of shunting of deoxygenated air from the lung on the side of the fracture into the opposite side. The pendulum movements of the mediastinum also produce cardiovascular embarrassment so that the patient becomes rapidly and progressively shocked.

Pneumothorax (Fig. 8.2)

If a bony spicule penetrates the lung, air escapes into the pleural cavity and will result in a pneumothorax. If the pleural tear is valvular, a *tension* pneumothorax result, where air is sucked into the pleural cavity at each inspiration but cannot return into the bronchi on expiration. A tension pneumothorax produces rapidly increasing dyspnoea; the trachea and the apex beat are displaced away from the side of the pneumothorax and, on the left

side, cardiac dullness may be absent. The chest on the affected side gives a tympanitic percussion note with bulging of the intercostal spaces.

Subcutaneous emphysema (surgical emphysema)

When a fractured rib tears the overlying soft tissue and allows air to enter the subcutaneous tissues, subcutaneous emphysema will result. The skin over the trunk, neck and sometimes face gives a peculiar crackling feel to the examining fingers (*crepitation*) and, in severe cases, the face and neck may become grossly swollen. The alternative name, surgical emphysema, is misleading as it is rarely caused by surgeons.

Sucking wound of the chest

A pneumothorax will also result from a penetrating wound of the chest wall produced, for example, by a knife stab or gunshot wound. The lips of the wound may also have a valvular effect so that air is sucked into the cavity at each inspiration, but cannot escape on expiration, thus resulting in another variety of tension

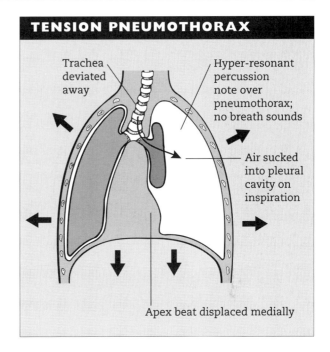

TENSION PNEUMOTHORAX

Trachea deviated away

Hyper-resonant percussion note over pneumothorax; no breath sounds

Air sucked into pleural cavity on inspiration

Apex beat displaced medially

Fig. 8.2 Tension pneumothorax produced by a valvular tear in the lung. Air is sucked into the pleural cavity on inspiration and cannot escape on expiration.

pneumothorax, which has been vividly named a sucking wound of the chest.

Haemothorax

A haemothorax often accompanies a chest injury and may indeed be associated with a pneumothorax (haemo-pneumothorax). The bleeding is usually from an intercostal artery in the lacerated chest wall or from underlying contused lung, but on occasions may result from injury to the heart or great vessels. Retropleural bleeding may compress the thoracic viscera without breaching the pleural cavity.

Traumatic asphyxia

With severe crush injuries of the chest, the sudden sharp rise in venous pressure produces extensive bruising and petechial haemorrhages over the head, neck and trunk. There are often subconjunctival haemorrhages and nasal bleeding. Any area of the skin that has been subjected to compression at the time of injury (e.g. from a tight collar, braces or spectacles) is

protected and these areas remain mapped out on the body as strips of normal skin, giving a completely characteristic appearance to the patient.

Other visceral injury

It is important to remember that penetrating wounds of the chest may also injure the underlying diaphragm and thence the abdominal viscera. Thus, it is not uncommon for a knife or bullet wound of the left chest to penetrate the spleen or, on the right side, to damage the liver.

Treatment

The priorities in the management of chest injuries are as follows.
• *Airway control.* This may involve the passage of an endotracheal tube particularly where a head injury coexists with chest trauma. Aspiration of vomit is prevented by passing a naso-gastric tube to empty the stomach.
• *Breathing.* Ensure the patient is breathing and maintaining adequate oxygenation. A saturation monitor should be employed and

intubation and ventilation considered. Oxygen saturation below 80% or a $P\text{co}_2$ above 7.3 kPa (50 mmHg) are indications for this.

• *Sucking wounds* should be closed. In an emergency, a dressing pad should be applied over the hole.

• *Lung expansion* should be achieved by insertion of an intercostal drain with underwater drainage.

• *Stop bleeding*. A haemothorax should be drained, and large haemothoraces may require multiple drains, all placed on underwater seals as for a pneumothorax (Fig. 8.3). Continued bleeding is an indication for an exploratory thoracotomy.

Simple rib fracture

• *Pain relief* may be achieved by analgesics, particularly non-steroidal anti-inflammatory drugs (NSAIDs), by the injection of local anaesthetic in the para-vertebral region to block the intercostal nerves or by a thoracic epidural block, which can be repeated by means of an indwelling plastic catheter.

• *Vigorous physiotherapy* is administered to encourage deep breathing.

• Strapping of the chest wall inhibits thoracic movement and encourages pulmonary collapse so that most surgeons have abandoned this practice.

Flail chest

• *Support the flail segment* in an emergency by means of a firm pad held by strapping. This stops the paradoxical movement and air shunting.

• *Endotracheal intubation* and *positive-pressure ventilation* on admission to hospital will stop the paradoxical movement, as the chest wall now moves as a single functional unit. The treatment is continued for about 10 days until fixation of the chest wall occurs. In cases of gross instability, wire fixation of the chest wall may be necessary.

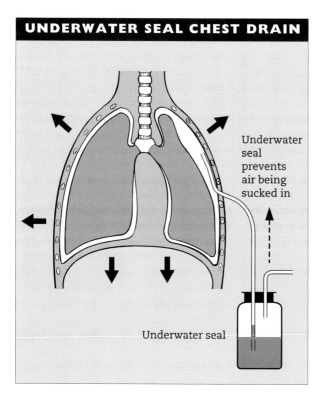

UNDERWATER SEAL CHEST DRAIN

Underwater seal prevents air being sucked in

Underwater seal

Fig. 8.3 Underwater seal chest drain in the treatment of a pneumothorax. Air escapes from the pleural cavity on expiration but cannot be sucked back through the water seal on inspiration (as shown here).

- Tracheostomy may be indicated for prolonged periods of intubation.

Tension pneumothorax

Urgent emergency treatment is required. An *intercostal tube drain* is inserted by means of a trocar and cannula. The tube is then led to an underwater seal. When the pressure in the pleural space is increased on expiration, the air escapes through the water but air cannot enter the chest at inspiration as this is prevented by the water seal. This essential safety valve has been a most important step in the development of safe thoracic surgery (Fig. 8.3). If a pneumothorax persists, a broncho-pleural fistula due to rupture of a bronchus should be suspected and bronchoscopy carried out, followed, if confirmed, by thoracotomy and repair.

Penetrating wounds of the chest

Immediate application of a dressing is required in order to prevent suction of air into the pleural space. Minor cases require only wound toilet with an underwater intercostal drain to allow escape of any accumulated blood or air in the pleural space. Large wounds demand formal exploration with excision or repair of damaged lung tissue, repair of any diaphragmatic tear and exclusion of injury to underlying abdominal viscera.

Cardiac tamponade

This may follow open or closed injuries to the chest or upper abdomen. It is characterized by a rise in venous pressure and a fall in arterial pressure. The heart sounds are distant and the cardiac shadow enlarged on chest X-ray. Treatment is emergency surgical exploration; the pericardium is opened, the blood is evacuated and the cardiac laceration sutured.

Lung abscess

Aetiology

- Bronchial obstruction secondary to carcinoma of the lung.
- Inhalation pneumonitis, e.g. inhaled vomit or pus.
- Inhaled foreign body, e.g. at dental extraction.
- Infected cyst.
- Infected pulmonary infarct.
- Blood-borne, secondary to staphylococcal septicaemia.
- Secondary to pulmonary infection, e.g. pneumonia, bronchiectasis or tuberculosis, especially in immunocompromised patients.

Clinical features

The history may suggest the primary cause. There is usually acute fever and toxaemia, although the disease may sometimes run a more chronic course. If the abscess ruptures into the bronchus there is a foul productive cough.

Complications

- Empyema.
- Metastatic cerebral abscess (a feared complication of all pulmonary sepsis).

Special investigations

- *Chest X-ray* shows a solid opacity or a fluid level if the abscess communicates with the bronchus.
- *Bronchoscopy* may demonstrate the primary cause if this is a foreign body or carcinoma.
- *Computed tomography (CT)* will accurately locate the abscess and confirm the diagnosis. Percutaneous CT-guided drainage may be possible and effective.

Treatment

The underlying cause may itself require treatment. The mainstay of therapy for lung abscess is postural drainage combined with antibiotics. Surgical excision is only required for the small percentage that fail to respond to this therapy, where some underlying cause needs to be treated, or where, in a late case, there is a complicating empyema that requires drainage.

Empyema

An empyema (pyothorax) is a collection of pus in the pleural cavity.

Aetiology
- Underlying lung disease: pneumonia, bronchiectasis or carcinoma of the lung; tuberculous empyema is now uncommon.
- Penetrating wounds of the chest wall or infection following a trans-thoracic operation.
- Perforation of the oesophagus.
- Trans-diaphragmatic infection from a subphrenic abscess.
- Haematogenous.

Complications
- Rupture into a bronchus (broncho-pleural fistula).
- Discharge through the chest wall (empyema necessitans).
- Cerebral abscess.

Clinical features
There is usually a history of the underlying cause. The patient is febrile, toxic and may be anaemic. There are signs of fluid in the chest on the affected side. In chronic cases, finger clubbing may be present.

Special investigations
- *Full blood count* will reveal a leucocytosis.
- *Chest X-ray* demonstrates an effusion and there may be evidence of the underlying lung disease.
- *Bronchoscopy* is useful in determining the primary pathology.
- *Aspiration* of the chest confirms the diagnosis and identifies the responsible bacteria. The infecting organisms are usually *Pneumococcus*, *Streptococcus* or *Staphylococcus*.

Treatment
An acute empyema may respond to repeated aspirations together with antibiotic therapy, based on the sensitivity of the responsible organism and given both systemically and into the pleural cavity. If the condition fails to respond to this treatment, drainage by means of excision of a rib overlying the empyema becomes necessary. An intercostal tube is inserted and progress followed by repeated sinograms to ensure adequate drainage and ultimate obliteration of the empyema cavity. In more chronic cases, the fibrous wall of the empyema cavity may require excision (decortication).

Lung tumours

Classification
Benign
- Adenoma.
- Carcinoid (occasionally malignant).
- Hamartoma.
- Haemangioma (rare).

Malignant
1 Primary:
    (a) squamous cell carcinoma;
    (b) adenocarcinoma;
    (c) small-cell carcinoma;
    (d) large-cell carcinoma;
    (e) carcinoid.
2 Secondary:
    (a) carcinoma (especially breast, kidney);
    (b) sarcoma (especially bone);
    (c) melanoma.

Adenoma
Pathology
Adenomas account for about 4% of lung primary tumours. Two-thirds of the patients are female and the average age is 40 years.

The tumour arises from the mucosa usually of the main bronchus as a cherry-red swelling, which ulcerates and bleeds (hence the common presenting symptom of haemoptysis). The growth may eventually block the bronchus with resulting pulmonary collapse and infection. Although slow growing, it cannot be considered benign, as infiltration and metastases may eventually take place.

Occasionally, serotonin is secreted, producing attacks of flushing and dyspnoea (carcinoid syndrome, see p. 192).

Treatment
Removal by local resection, lobectomy or pneumonectomy.

Carcinoma

This is the commonest cancer affecting male adults and accounts for some 40 000 deaths a year in England and Wales, with an age-standardized incidence for males of over 70 per 100 000 per year.

Aetiology

In the UK the main aetiological factor is the smoking of cigarettes. Passive smoking, air pollution with diesel, petrol and other volatile hydrocarbon fumes, asbestos exposure and exposure to radioactive gases such as radon in uranium mines are also predisposing factors. The incidence is higher in urban than in rural populations.

Carcinoma of the lung has an extremely poor prognosis, and the gravity of this condition should be impressed on all patients who are inveterate smokers. The decision whether or not to continue smoking depends on the patient, but there is no doubt that the doctor's advice should be against it. There is an increased incidence of carcinoma of the lung even in patients who smoke only a few cigarettes a day and this danger is greatly increased in patients smoking more than 20 cigarettes a day for a number of years.

Pathology

There is considerable predominance of males over females in this disease (six to one), but the ratio is decreasing as women tend to smoke more. It is uncommon before the fifth decade and peaks in the 60s.

Macroscopic appearance

About half the tumours arise in the main bronchi (particularly squamous carcinoma), and 75% are visible at bronchoscopy. The growth may arise peripherally (particularly adenocarcinoma) and some appear to be multifocal.

The bronchial wall is narrowed and ulcerated. Surrounding lung tissue is invaded by a pale mass of tumour, which may undergo necrosis, haemorrhage or abscess formation. The lung segments distal to the occlusion may show collapse, bronchiectasis or abscess formation.

Microscopic appearance

Squamous cell carcinoma (40%). Mostly poorly differentiated and arising in an area of squamous metaplasia of bronchial epithelium. Following successful resection, new primaries are common (10%), reflecting the 'field change'.

Adenocarcinoma (30%). Very rapidly growing tumour often found in the periphery of the lung, associated with a large fibrotic (desmoplastic) reaction. This type of lung primary is common in non-smokers.

Large-cell carcinoma (10%). Large cells containing abundant cytoplasm and without evidence of squamous or glandular differentiation.

Small-cell carcinoma (20%) (also known as oat-cell carcinoma) has neuro-endocrine properties and produces peptides giving rise to paraneoplastic syndromes (see p. 26). The tumour comprises small cells with little cytoplasm. It has a poor prognosis, has generally spread by the time of diagnosis, and is best treated by chemotherapy.

Spread

• *Local*, to pleura, left recurrent laryngeal nerve, pericardium, oesophagus (broncho-oesophageal fistula) and brachial plexus (Pancoast's tumour*).
• *Lymphatic*, to mediastinal and cervical nodes. Compression of the superior vena cava by massive mediastinal node involvement produces gross oedema and cyanosis of the face and upper limbs (superior vena cava syndrome).
• *Blood*, to bone, brain, liver and suprarenals.
• *Trans-coelomic*, pleural seedlings and effusion.

---

*Henry Pancoast (1875–1939), Professor of Radiology, University of Pennsylvania, Philadelphia, USA.

Clinical features

Carcinoma of the lung may present with the following.

• *Local features*, namely cough, dyspnoea, haemoptysis or lung infection.

• *Secondaries*, which are especially likely to occur in the brain, suprarenal, liver and bones; thus, the patient may present with evidence of a space-occupying lesion within the skull, pathological fracture, jaundice and hepatomegaly, or adreno-cortical failure.

• *Paraneoplastic syndromes* due to the remote effects of a hormone or cell product produced by the tumour. Small-cell carcinomas often produce adrenocorticotrophic hormone (ACTH), while squamous carcinomas may produce parathormone (PTH) and present with hypercalcaemia.

• *The general effects of neoplasm*: loss of weight, anaemia, cachexia and also peripheral neuropathies, myopathies and endocrine disturbances.

Unfortunately, by the time carcinoma of the lung is diagnosed, most cases are quite incurable. About half the patients will be found to have inoperable growths when they have had no symptoms at all, with a lesion discovered on routine chest X-ray. Certainly any middle-aged or elderly person presenting with a respiratory infection that has continued for more than 2 weeks should have a chest X-ray, and, if the symptoms persist and nothing shows on the chest X-ray, he or she should be bronchoscoped.

Patients may present with bizarre neuropathies and myopathies that can occur with cancer anywhere, but these are especially common in growths of the lung. Cancer of the lung is likely to lead to pulmonary infection and the patients often develop clubbing of the fingers, which are usually nicotine-stained.

On examination, special attention should be paid to evidence of stridor or hoarseness of the voice due to recurrent laryngeal nerve involvement with growth. The heart may be invaded, resulting in atrial fibrillation or cardiac failure. There may be enlarged lymph nodes, especially at the root of the neck, and signs in the chest of consolidation, fluid or collapse.

Special investigations

• *Chest X-ray* and *thoracic CT scan* may show an opacity in the lung and enlargement of the hilar lymph nodes. There may be paralysis of one side of the diaphragm due to involvement of the phrenic nerve. In addition to imaging the chest, a CT scan should also image the liver and suprarenal glands for evidence of secondary spread.

• *Cytology* of the sputum may identify malignant cells, particularly sensitive in proximal exuberant bronchial growths.

ABNORMAL SHADOW IN THE MEDIASTINUM

• Retro-sternal thyroid.
• Aneurysm of the thoracic aorta.
• Thymic tumour and cysts.
• Carcinoma of the lung with a mediastinal mass.
• Heart enlargement:
    cardiac failure;
    valve incompetence;
    pericardial effusion;
    left–right shunts;
    cardiomyopathies.
• Enlarged lymph nodes:
    sarcoid;
    Hodgkin's disease;
    non-Hodgkin's lymphoma;
    leukaemia;
    secondary deposits.
• Oesophageal enlargement:
    tumour;
    hiatus hernia;
    mega-oesophagus in achalasia of the cardia.
• Paravertebral abscess, particularly due to tuberculosis.
• Scoliosis.
• Dumb-bell tumour of neurofibroma.
• Dermoid cyst or teratoma.

• *Fine-needle aspiration cytology* of a peripherally placed lesion under X-ray guidance.

• *Bronchoscopy and biopsy.* Bronchoscopy may reveal an ulcerating or exuberant growth, and involved lymph nodes may widen the carina.

• *Mediastinoscopy*, performed through a small suprasternal incision, may be indicated to remove lymph nodes from the region of the carina for histological examination to aid in staging.

Treatment
Surgery
The possibility of curative surgery is assessed by biopsy of all suspicious nodes to exclude spread, as well as radiological imaging and bronchoscopy. Removal of a lobe, or of the whole lung, is performed where there is a possibility of cure, and, in these highly selected cases, the 5-year survival rate of this disease is in the order of 20–30%.

Sometimes, with a technically resectable early tumour, the patient's general respiratory reserve is so limited by years of tobacco abuse as to make resection impossible on these grounds, and pulmonary function tests should be performed on all patients.

Radiotherapy
Radiotherapy may give useful palliation in the inoperable cases. Although it may not prolong life, it may stop distressing haemoptysis, cure the pain from bone secondaries and produce dramatic improvement in a patient with acute superior vena caval obstruction. It may also give some relief from the irritating cough and dyspnoea resulting from early bronchial obstruction.

Cytotoxic chemotherapy
Cyclical cytotoxic therapy combined with radiotherapy gives improved survival in small-cell tumours but the other types of primary carcinoma of the lung are not responsive to chemotherapy.

Secondary tumours
The lung is second only to the liver as the site of metastases, which may be from carcinoma (especially breast, kidney), sarcoma (especially bone) or melanoma. Spread may be either as a result of vascular deposits or retrograde lymphatic permeation from involved mediastinal nodes—lymphangitis carcinomatosa.

Pulmonary metastases are so common that it should be routine practice to X-ray the chest in every case of malignant disease.

CHAPTER 9

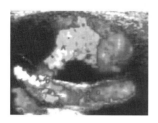

The Heart and Thoracic Aorta

Cardio-pulmonary bypass

Background

Prior to the development of cardio-pulmonary bypass, surgery on the heart was limited to procedures that could be performed rapidly on a beating heart, such as mitral valvotomy to relieve mitral stenosis, where a finger is passed blindly through the left atrial appendage and through the stenotic mitral valve. If the circulation is temporarily stopped at normal body temperature, organs suffer ischaemic damage due to lack of oxygen, the extent varying according to the metabolic demand of the organ. The brain is the most sensitive tissue in this respect and is liable to irreversible changes after 3 minutes of ischaemia. The spinal cord is next, followed by heart muscle, which will tolerate between 3 and 6 minutes of ischaemia at normal temperature. The tolerance to ischaemia can be increased slightly by lowering the metabolic rate by hypothermia; at 28°C up to 10 minutes of circulatory arrest can be tolerated.

With the development of cardio-pulmonary bypass, the heart may be stopped for prolonged periods while a machine is used to take over the pumping and oxygenation of the blood. Generally, a combination of hypothermia and cardio-pulmonary bypass is used.

Technique (Fig. 9.1)

After full heparinization, cannulae are inserted into the venae cavae via the right atrium to syphon off the venous return from the systemic circulation. The blood is then pumped through an oxgenator and a heat exchanger before returning to the systemic circulation via a catheter in the ascending aorta or femoral artery. This form of bypass will perfuse the whole body with oxygenated blood at an adequate pressure while diverting it from the heart and lungs. The heart may now be stopped and cooled by infusion via the coronary arteries of cold 'cardioplegic' solution containing potassium, to produce rapid cardiac arrest in diastole. If the aorta is cross-clamped, the heart may be opened in a bloodless field with access to all chambers.

Complications

• *Emboli.* Air entrapped during formation of the bypass circuit or entering during bypass, or thrombus forming in the bypass circuit, may embolize into the cerebral and peripheral circulation with catastrophic results.

• *Haemorrhage* post-operatively may result in cardiac tamponade. Passage through the bypass circuit activates the clotting cascade and consumes platelets, thus increasing the risk of haemorrhage.

CARDIO-PULMONARY BYPASS

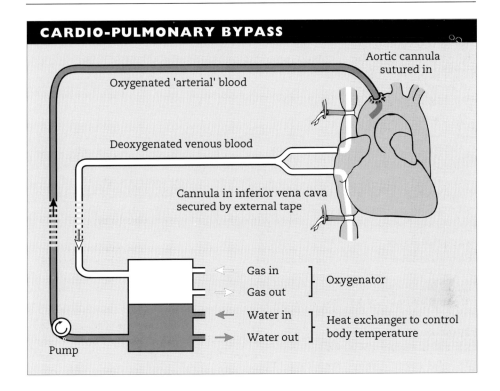

Fig. 9.1 Cardio-pulmonary bypass.

• *Hypothermic and ischaemic injury* may result in pancreatitis and contribute to the occurence of peptic ulceration and mesenteric ischaemia.

Valvular disease

Valve repair and replacement
With the advent of cardio-pulmonary bypass, it has become possible to remove diseased valves and replace them with artificial ones, either prosthetic, human or xenograft. In mitral valve regurgitation, if the valve is not heavily distorted or calcified, repair may be undertaken in preference to replacement.

Prosthetic valves
Many examples exist, such as the St Jude bileaflet valve, where the valve comprises two semicircular tilting leaflets. Prosthetic valves may become obstructed by thrombus due to turbulent flow across the valve, therefore recipients should be indefinitely anticoagulated.

Xenograft valve
Commonly of pig origin, this comprises a porcine valve suspended on a prosthetic ring to allow it to be sewn in place; once implanted, the recipient does not require anticoagulation. The lifetime of such valves is generally shorter than prosthetic valves, but the avoidance of anticoagulation makes them the preferred choice in the elderly.

Complications of valve replacement
• *Valve thrombosis and embolus formation*, especially if not on anticoagulation.

• *Mechanical failure* with embolus of valve fragments, out-flow obstruction or massive valve incompetance.
• *Anticoagulation* with the risks of haemorrhage due to over-anticoagulation.
• *Paraprosthetic leaks*, where blood leaks between the artificial valve ring and the outflow tract.
• *Infection of valve*, a situation akin to infective endocarditis of a native valve.

Mitral stenosis

Mitral stenosis is a consequence of rheumatic valve disease and is much less common since the widespread use of penicillin. The original infection is due to a group A β-haemolytic *Streptococcus* and may have been so mild that only half the patients give a previous history of rheumatic fever or chorea.

Pathology

Pathological changes consist of fusion of the valve commissures with shortening of the chordae tendinae. As the mitral valve opening narrows, blood flow across the valve is impaired and the left atrium, particularly the atrial appendage, dilates, and with the dilatation atrial fibrillation follows. Thrombus may form in the atrial appendage. In time, the valve narrows critically and prevents adequate ventricular filling, resulting in exertional dyspnoea.

Clinical features

Patients usually present between the 20th and 40th year, females more commonly than males. The usual presenting feature is increasing dyspnoea due to progressive cardiac failure. There may be nocturnal dyspnoea and episodes of pulmonary oedema with recurrent lung infections.

On examination, the patient may have the typical malar flush. There is a mid-diastolic murmur in the mitral area and the opening snap of the mitral valve may be audible and palpable as a tapping apex beat. Atrial fibrillation is common and this is accompanied by the disappearance of the pre-systolic murmur as effective atrial contraction ceases.

Complications

• Right-heart failure.
• Peripheral arterial embolism (particularly in atrial fibrillation).
• Infective endocarditis—likely wherever there is a valve abnormality.

Treatment

In the absence of mitral regurgitation, evidence of valve calcification or history of emboli, an open valvotomy is perfomed to split the fused commissures. If unsuccessful, or in the presence of calcified and distorted valves or regurgitation, valve replacement is performed.

Aortic stenosis

Stenosis of the aortic valve may be congenital or acquired. The acquired variety may be due to rheumatic heart disease, but in older patients it is more commonly due to calcification of bicuspid valves. Unfortunately, no matter what the cause, the aortic valve when stenosed is usually grossly distorted and calcified and unsuitable for valve repair; replacement is the treatment of choice.

Clinical features

The three presenting symptoms of aortic stenosis are angina, dyspnoea due to cardiac failure, and syncope (occasionally sudden death). Examination reveals a slow rising pulse, a low blood pressure and left-ventricular hypertrophy, as shown on electrocardiogram (ECG) and echocardiogram. Chest X-ray may show valve calcification and post-stenotic dilatation of the aorta. Once the gradient across the valve exceeds 50 mmHg, or the patient is symptomatic, surgery is advised.

Treatment

Valve replacement on cardio-pulmonary bypass.

Ischaemic heart disease

Severe angina due to myocardial ischaemia may

be alleviated by increasing the arterial supply to the muscle. Two treatment options exist: endoluminal intervention with balloon angioplasty and stenting, and direct reconstructive surgery using the internal mammary (thoracic) artery and aorto-coronary bypass grafts.

Aetiology

The risk factors for coronary artery disease are those for atheroma in general (see box, p. 75). In particular, raised serum cholesterol, hypertension and cigarette smoking each double the risk of coronary artery disease. The presence of all three increases the risk eightfold.

Special investigations

• *Exercise ECG* shows whether there is myocardial ischaemia on exercise.
• *Coronary arteriography* is performed on patients with ischaemic responses to exercise.

It is important for accurate anatomical diagnosis, and may be combined with endoluminal therapy.

Treatment

• *Angioplasty.* Isolated stenoses in proximal vessels are most appropriate for percutaneous transluminal coronary angioplasty (PTCA). Where the stenosis recurs after initial dilatation, endoluminal stenting may prolong patency.
• *Surgical revascularization.* For total occlusions or stenoses in multiple vessels, the procedure of choice is surgery. This involves joining one (sometimes both) internal mammary (internal thoracic) arteries to the diseased coronary artery distal to the blockage. For multiple grafts, autogenous reversed saphenous vein is also used as an aorto-coronary bypass conduit (Fig. 9.2).

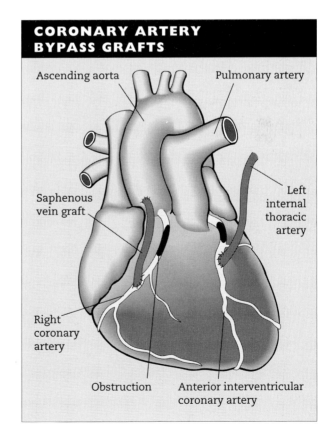

CORONARY ARTERY BYPASS GRAFTS

Ascending aorta

Pulmonary artery

Saphenous vein graft

Left internal thoracic artery

Right coronary artery

Obstruction

Anterior interventricular coronary artery

Fig. 9.2 A saphenous vein graft from the aorta to the right coronary artery and a direct left internal mammary (thoracic) artery graft to the anterior interventricular coronary artery.

As with all arterial surgery for atherosclerosis, there is a tendency for recurrent disease with the passage of time. This may require repeat surgery, or may be amenable to endoluminal procedures. In young patients crippled by angina in whom direct bypass surgery is impossible or in those with gross myocardial disease, cardiac transplantation may be the only treatment that can give relief of symptoms and a return to normal life.

Surgery for the complications of myocardial infarction

Acute ventriculo-septal defect. Where the infarcted ventricular muscle was part of the septum and undergoes necrosis, septal rupture may occur. This occurs 1–2 weeks after myocardial infarction in 1% of patients and requires urgent repair.

Ventricular aneurysm. If the infarcted wall is apical, it may necrose and rupture, leading to rapid death by tamponade. Alternatively, a ventricular aneurysm may form, which may require excision if paradoxical movement or thrombus become symptomatic.

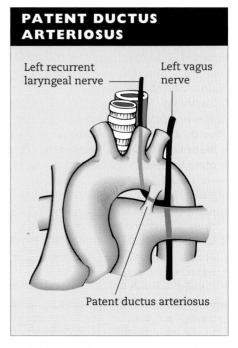

PATENT DUCTUS ARTERIOSUS

Left recurrent laryngeal nerve

Left vagus nerve

Patent ductus arteriosus

Fig. 9.3 A patent ductus arteriosus—note its close relationship to the left recurrent laryngeal nerve.

Thoracic aortic disease

Persistent ductus arteriosus (Fig. 9.3)
Pathology
If the channel between the aorta and pulmonary artery fails to close at the time of birth, blood will be shunted from the systemic circulation with its higher pressure into the pulmonary circulation, resulting in pulmonary hypertension. In time, pulmonary vascular resistance increases and exceeds peripheral resistance, at which time the shunt reverses, deoxygenated blood from the pulmonary artery passes into the systemic circulation, and the patient becomes cyanosed.

Clinical features
In neonates with a large duct, shunting may progress rapidly and cardiac failure may occur in infancy. A duct with moderate flow tends to present later with exertional dyspnoea. Most commonly, the patient is asymptomatic and the condition is diagnosed because of finding the characteristic machinery-like continuous murmur with systolic accentuation best heard over the second left space anteriorly. In infants, the bruit may be purely systolic.

Special investigations
• *Chest X-ray* will usually show left ventricular hypertrophy and increased pulmonary arterial markings.
• *Echocardiography and angiocardiography* will demonstrate the patent ductus and indeed the cardiac catheter can often be manipulated through the ductus into the aorta.

Treatment
Operative ligation and division of a persistent ductus should be undertaken on diagnosis, and before irreversible pulmonary hypertension or

cardiac failure have occurred. Percutaneous endovascular insertion of an occlusive device into the ductus may achieve a cure without surgery.

Coarctation of the aorta
Pathology
This is a congenital narrowing of the aorta, which, in the majority of cases, occurs in the descending aorta just distal to the origin of the left subclavian artery close to the obliterated ductus arteriosus. Indeed, the pathogenesis of coarctation formation may be related to the presence of abnormal ductus tissue. Coarctation can rarely occur in other sites up and down the aorta. The stenosis is usually extreme, only a pinpoint lumen remaining.

Blood reaches the distal aorta via collateral connections between branches of the subclavian, scapular and intercostal arteries, and by the anastomosis between the internal thoracic and inferior epigastric arteries. Although the blood supply to the lower part of the body is diminished, patients with coarctation seldom suffer from peripheral gangrene, although occasionally they complain of intermittent claudication. The danger of coarctation is due to the effects of hypertension, which is often severe and is likely to result in cerebral haemorrhage or left-ventricular failure. The mechanism of the hypertension is probably due to the relatively poor blood supply to the kidneys, which results in release of renin and renal hypertension (see p. 69).

Patients also run the risk of developing infective endarteritis.

Clinical features
The diagnosis is usually made on account of hypertension in a young adult or a child. In addition to the hypertension, the most characteristic physical sign is absent, diminished or delayed femoral pulsations in relation to the radial pulse, and confirmed by a large difference in the blood pressure between arm and leg. A systolic murmur is sometimes present in the left chest, and large collateral blood vessels may be seen or felt in the subcutaneous tissues of the chest wall.

Special investigations
• *Chest X-ray* will show left-ventricular hypertrophy, and often the ribs are notched by the large intercostal collateral blood vessels bypassing the stenotic area.
• *Echocardiography* in an infant to exclude coexisting cardiac anomalies.
• *Angiography* will confirm the diagnosis.

Treatment
This is desirable before complications arise and consists of excision of the stenotic segment and either end-to-end anastomosis of the proximal and distal aorta or, if the gap to bridge is too great, an arterial graft is interposed between the two aortic ends.

Thoracic aortic aneurysms
Aneurysms can occur in any situation in the body (see p. 84) but the aorta is particularly liable to be affected. Aneurysms of the arch of the aorta were once commonly syphilitic but now are mainly due to Marfan's syndrome,* medial degeneration or atherosclerosis. Aneurysms of the descending thoracic aorta may be traumatic, syphilitic or atherosclerotic. With the exception of aneurysms with a very narrow neck, those involving the thoracic aorta require some form of vascular bypass in order to treat them surgically.

A thoraco-abdominal aneurysm is an aneurysm extending across the diaphragm and involving the coeliac, superior mesenteric and renal artery origins.

Clinical features
Aneurysms of the ascending aorta may present with chest pain, aortic regurgitation, obstruction of the superior vena cava, obstruction of the right main bronchus and eventually a pulsating mass in the front of the

*Antonin Marfan (1858–1942), Professor of Paediatrics, Hospital for Sick Children, Paris, France.

chest, which may even ulcerate through the chest wall, resulting in exsanguination.

Aneurysms of the arch of the aorta may compress the trachea or ulcerate into it; they are liable to stretch the left recurrent laryngeal nerve leading to hoarseness and may obstruct the left lower lobe bronchus, producing an area of collapse.

Aneurysms of the descending thoracic aorta may produce pain in the back, erosion of vertebrae, or may press on the oesophagus producing dysphagia and even rupture into it. Not surprisingly, this is the most lethal cause of haematemesis.

Special investigations
• *Chest X-ray* may show the extent of the aneurysm due to calcification in its walls.
• *Computed tomography (CT) and magnetic resonance imaging (MRI)* are useful in demonstrating the size and extent of the aneurysm and its relation to the major vessels of the neck.
• *Aortography* may be dangerous and often does not help in establishing the diagnosis, as the lumen of the aneurysm is narrowed by thrombus.
• *Echocardiography* is important to diagnose aortic incompetance caused by aneurysmal dilatation of the valve ring.

Treatment
Aneurysms of the ascending aorta and arch require total cardio-pulmonary bypass for adequate surgical treatment, which consists of partial excision of the aneurysm and insertion of a prosthetic graft with appropriate junction limbs to the main aortic branches. Aneurysms of the descending thoracic aorta require a left-heart bypass for their surgical treatment, which is similar in principle to those of the arch.

Complications
• *Spinal ischaemia* due to loss of flow in the great radicular artery (of Adamkiewicz), which arises from the aorta near T10 and supplies the lower part of the spinal cord. This results in paraplegia.

Aortic dissection (Fig. 9.4)
Pathology
An aortic dissection (dissecting aneurysm) consists of a tear in the wall of the aorta, usually in the region of its arch, which allows blood to dissect along a plane of cleavage in the media. The false passage thus formed may rupture internally into the true lumen, thus decompressing itself and resulting in an aorta with a double lumen. Such a case may survive. However, more commonly, the aneurysm ruptures externally into the pericardium producing cardiac tamponade, or into the mediastinum or abdominal cavity with fatal haemorrhage.

Aetiology
Cystic medial degeneration weakens the wall of the aorta and enables the splitting to occur. It is usually found in arteriosclerotic, hypertensive subjects.

Classification
Aortic dissection has been classified into type A and type B.
• *Type A dissection* affects the ascending aorta and arch and occurs in two-thirds of cases.
• *Type B dissection* has an initial tear distal to the left subclavian origin and only the decending aorta is affected. It occurs in one-third of cases.

Clinical features
The patient usually presents with a sudden severe pain in the chest, which may radiate to the arms, neck or abdomen, or with a tearing interscapular pain. In addition, there may be signs of surgical shock, either from cardiac tamponade or from external rupture of the aneurysm. Patients with dissecting aneurysm are therefore usually initially diagnosed as suffering from coronary thrombosis, and an ECG may not help differentiate between the two conditions. Indeed, if the coronary sinus is involved, coronary occlusion may

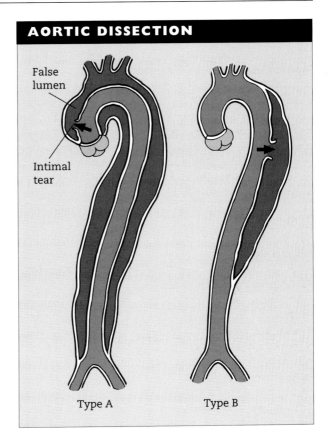

AORTIC DISSECTION

False
lumen

Intimal
tear

Type A

Type B

Fig. 9.4 Classification of aortic
dissection.

have occured. In type A dissections, the aortic
valve may become incompetent as the root
dilates.

As the dissection in the wall of the aorta
progresses, the origins of main arterial
branches may become blocked, producing
progression of symptoms and the disappearance and reappearance of peripheral
pulses. If the renal vessels are involved, there
may be haematuria or anuria. One or both
femoral pulses may disappear with leg
ischaemia. Mesenteric ischaemia is usually
diagnosed late.

Special investigations

• *Chest X-ray* shows widening of the mediastinum in two-thirds of patients and a small
left pleural effusion.

• *Contrast-enhanced CT* shows a flap across the
lumen with distal aneurysmal change, and this
may be confirmed by aortography.

• *Echocardiography* may also demonstrate a
flap and aortic regurgitation. *Trans-oesophageal
echocardiography* is probably the investigation
of choice.

Treatment

Once the diagnosis is made, treatment
depends largely upon the type of dissection.

Type A dissections should be managed surgically because of the risk that the dissection may
extend back across the aortic root resulting
in tamponade, and to correct aortic incompetence where present. The surgery aims to
interpose a tube of Dacron at the aortic root

to prevent further dissection (and tamponade), and carries a high mortality.

Type B dissections are usually treated conservatively, and hypotensive drugs are used, reducing systolic pressure to 100–120 mmHg to prevent further extension of the dissection. The dissected portion may then thrombose. Any organ, limb or mesenteric ischaemia resulting from the dissection is treated by revascularization. An aneurysm resulting from a chronic dissection may require treatment if it enlarges or produces pressure symptoms.

Hypertension

This section summarizes raised blood pressure in its surgical aspects.

Classification
- Primary (cause unknown).
- Secondary (causes at least partially understood).

Primary hypertension
Primary hypertension is a disease of middle-aged and elderly patients, which tends to run in families. It is a very common condition and may be compatible with few symptoms and a long life. There is an increase in the peripheral resistance due to arteriolar thickening or spasm, but as arteriolar thickening is a consequence of hypertension the argument of which is the primary factor has not been resolved in this disease.

The kidney may be an important contributor to the hypertension when its blood supply is impaired due to arteriolar narrowing. There is a vicious circle of arteriolar spasm, arteriolar thickening, renal ischaemia and further hypertension, which leads to a progressive increase in the severity of this condition.

Secondary hypertension
This may be due to the following.
1 Renal disease.
2 Coarctation of the aorta (p. 65).

3 Endocrine causes:
  (a) phaeochromocytoma (p. 314);
  (b) Cushing's syndrome (p. 312);
  (c) Conn's syndrome (p. 313).
4 Raised intracranial pressure (p. 109).
5 Toxaemia of pregnancy.

Renovascular hypertension
Mechanism of renal hypertension
(Fig. 9.5)
Ever since the experiments of Goldblatt,* it has been known that impairment of blood perfusion to the kidneys can result in hypertension, which, if the renal perfusion remains impaired, may become permanent, due to the vicious circle that has already been mentioned. The mechanism of renal hypertension appears to be the release of the hormone renin from the juxta-glomerular cells in the renal cortex. Renin acts on the serum protein angiotensinogen to give rise to a physiologically inactive decapeptide, angiotensin I. Angiotensin I is then converted to the octapeptide angiotensin II by the action of angiotensin-converting enzyme (ACE). Angiotensin II is a potent vasoconstrictor and causes an increase in peripheral resistance (and thus hypertension) and acts on the suprarenal cortex to release aldosterone (which causes sodium retention). The features of hypertension are thus set in motion, and renal perfusion is further impaired. This renin mechanism is protective as far as the kidney is concerned and is one method by which the kidney maintains its circulation. How important renin is in the maintenance of normal blood pressure has not been established. All forms of renal parenchymal disease are likely to produce hypertension. Especially common are chronic glomerulonephritis and chronic pyelonephritis.

ACE inhibitors, such as captopril, are effective at reducing blood pressure in patients with renal disease. However, where renal insufficiency is due to renal artery stenosis their use will exacerbate the impaired per-

*H. Goldblatt (1891–?), Professor of Experimental Pathology, University of Southern California, USA.

RENAL HYPERTENSION

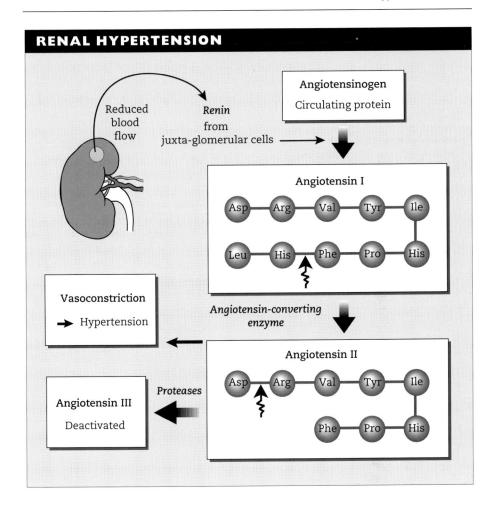

Fig. 9.5 Mechanism of renal hypertension.

fusion and result in deterioration in renal function.

Unilateral renal diseases producing hypertension

These are of particular surgical importance, as they may sometimes be amenable to curative treatment either by nephrectomy or by reconstructive procedures on the kidney or on its blood supply.

Unilateral pyelonephritis

Rarely, pyelonephritis may affect one kidney only, especially if this kidney has been the site of previous trauma or of congenital malformation, if the ureter on that side has been blocked or if there is unilateral hydronephrosis. If the condition is diagnosed early, before the hypertension has reached the chronic established stage and before hypertensive changes have taken place in the opposite kidney, removal of the affected kidney may result in a return to normal blood pressure. Presence of a functioning contralateral kidney should be confirmed first.

Renal artery stenosis

This is a fairly common cause of secondary hypertension. It occurs in two age groups: the elderly (70%), where the cause of the narrowing is atherosclerosis, and young people, especially women, in whom the cause appears to be the thickening of the intima and media by hyperplasia of collagen and muscle — fibromuscular dysplasia.

Special investigations
• *Arteriography* should be performed in young patients where fibro-muscular dysplasia characteristically shows up as a string of beads in the distal part of the renal artery, and is bilateral.
• *Duplex scanning* may permit diagnosis of a significant stenosis.
• *Renin estimation* should be performed by selective renal vein catheterization. Renin concentration is at least 1.5 times higher on an affected side.
• *DTPA radionuclide scan* will show renal blood flow difference, especially if the patient has been given an ACE inhibitor like captopril to exaggerate the condition.

Treatment
• *Angioplasty.* In suitable cases, a localized stenosis can be dilated by a balloon angioplasty. This is particularly successful in fibromuscular dysplasia.

• *Renal artery bypass.* If the stenosis is fairly proximal and the distal vessels relatively healthy, it may be possible to remove the stenotic portion of the artery or bypass it, e.g. on the left side by joining the splenic artery to the renal artery distal to the blockage.
• *Autotransplantation* of the kidney may be performed after excising the stenosed portion of the artery.
• *Unilateral nephrectomy* is appropriate where the small intrarenal branches of the renal artery are also diseased.

Other lesions of the renal arteries, for instance aneurysm and congenital bands, may also result in hypertension, which can be cured by unilateral nephrectomy or direct arterial surgery.

It should be noted that since the introduction of effective anti-hypertensive drugs (in particular ACE inhibitors), enthusiasm for surgery in unilateral renal disease has waned apart from cases where the kidney's function is grossly impaired.

Other unilateral renal diseases can cause hypertension, including hydronephrosis, tuberculosis of the kidneys or tumours of the kidney; nephrectomy is indicated in these conditions.

CHAPTER 10

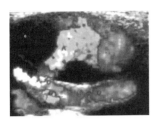

Arterial Disease

Assessing the patient with arterial disease

Arterial disease may result in impaired blood supply to the limbs or other end organs, aneurysm formation, or haemorrhage due to trauma or disease. The commonest causes of arterial disease are:
- atherosclerosis;
- embolus;
- thrombosis;
- spasm—Raynaud's phenomenon;
- diabetes;
- Buerger's disease;
- ergot poisoning — usually iatrogenic from migraine therapies;
- vessel injury due to trauma, cold or chemicals.

In addition, there is a genetic component predisposing to both occlusive disease and aneurysm formation. Although there are a large number of diseases that can cause impaired arterial blood flow to the limbs, three conditions are relatively common in the UK. First, and most important, atherosclerotic disease including the premature atherosclerosis seen in diabetics; second, embolism; and third, arteriolar spasm in Raynaud's phenomenon.

Clinical features

Accurate pathological and anatomical diagnosis can be made by careful history taking and clinical examination.

History

The time course of the symptoms is important, ranging from the insidious progression of intermittent claudication of the calves over a period of months or years to the acute onset of ischaemia following an embolus. Sudden onset of pain in the leg suggestive of an embolus should prompt the student to seek a likely source such as atrial fibrillation, recent myocardial infarction or aortic aneurysm. Acute deterioration in a patient with claudication is suggestive of thrombosis on the background atherosclerotic occlusive disease. A history of cold, painful hands since childhood, especially in the female, will be suggestive of Raynaud's disease, and coexistence of connective tissue disorders, such as systemic lupus erythematosus (SLE) or systemic sclerosis (scleroderma) favours Raynaud's phenomenon. The change in colour (pale and deathly white, then blue and finally a dusky red) precipitated by cold immersion is typical.

The symptoms of atherosclerosis occurring

SIGNS IN VASCULAR DISEASE

General signs
- Xanthelasma and evidence of hyperlipidaemia.
- Pulse rhythm—fibrillation or other arrhythmia.
- Blood pressure—low or high.

Appearance of limb
- Colour.
- Hair loss.
- Nutrition of skin.
- Evidence of ulceration or gangrene.
- Temperature.
- Presence of pulses.
- Auscultation of bruits.
- Venous guttering.
- Capillary return.
- Buerger's test.
- Ankle brachial pressure index measurement.

in a young person, especially a heavy smoking male, is typical of Buerger's disease.

Ergot poisoning is occasionally seen in patients with migraine who are consuming large doses of ergotamine.

It is important to determine the degree of handicap produced by the symptoms, for on this will depend the selection of patients for reconstructive surgery. Similarly, if a patient suffers from angina pectoris as well as intermittent claudication, there may be more handicap from the angina than the claudication, and more benefit from coronary revascularization (see p. 63).

Atherosclerosis is a generalized disease, and the cerebral circulation is often affected in addition to the circulation in the legs. Thus, a history of intermittent loss of consciousness, blindness and hemiparesis is of importance and may indicate coexisting carotid artery disease.

Examination

Careful clinical examination will usually provide a very clear indication of the severity and nature of the ischaemic disease. It is important that attention should be directed to other systems of the body, especially the heart and blood pressure (is the poor circulation due to a poor cardiac output?).

Heart rhythm. The presence of atrial fibrillation or other cardiac arrhythmias should be

noted, particularly if there is a history of acute limb ischaemia or stroke. The heart should be examined with particular attention to the apex beat (ventricular aneurysm) and auscultated for evidence of valvular disease (e.g. mitral stenosis).

Peripheral pulses. The peripheral pulses throughout the body should be examined. Whereas normal pulsation can be appreciated easily, palpation of weak pulsation requires practice, care and, above all, time. The presence of a weak pulse that is definitely palpated is of considerable significance diagnostically and can be important prognostically, as even a weak pulse means the vessel is patent.

Careful recording of the peripheral pulses will often clearly delineate a blockage in the arterial system. For instance, the presence of a good femoral pulse and absence of pulses distal to the femoral suggests a superficial femoral arterial block. Presence of all pulses including the radial and ulnar pulses, yet obvious ischaemia of the digits is a typical finding in Raynaud's phenomenon.

Aortic pulsation. The abdomen should be examined for any evidence of abnormal aortic pulsation, and the popliteal and femoral arteries are also often aneurysmal and should be examined with this in mind. If distal pulses are absent then it is possible that no aortic pulsation will be felt due to thrombosis of the terminal aorta.

Auscultation of vessels. In all areas where pulses are felt, auscultation should be performed. Partial blockage of arteries very often causes bruits, which are usually systolic in timing. They may even be felt as thrills. Arterio-venous communications will produce continuous bruits with systolic accentuation (machinery murmur), and pulsating dilated veins.

Inspection of limbs. Attention is then directed to the legs. Inspection may reveal marked skin pallor, an absence of hairs, ulcers (usually lateral malleolus and often in the interdigital clefts) and gangrene, all being evidence of impaired circulation. *Fixed staining* (purpuric areas not blanching on pressure) in the context of an acutely ischaemic limb is a sign of irreversible tissue injury. A tense, tender calf with impaired dorsiflexion in acute ischaemia signifies compartment compression and requires urgent fasciotomy in addition to revascularization.

Capillary return. The speed of return of capillary circulation after the blanching produced by pressure is a very useful gauge of the peripheral circulation.

Skin temperature. In addition to the pulses, skin temperature can be readily assessed by palpation, which is especially sensitive when the dorsum of the hand is used. A difference between the temperatures of one part of the leg and another or between the two legs can be ascertained when it is as small as 1°C. A clearly marked change of temperature may reveal the site of blockage of a main artery.

Venous guttering. The veins of the foot and leg in a patient with diminished arterial supply are often very inconspicuous compared with normal veins. Indeed, the veins may be so empty that they appear as shallow grooves or gutters, especially in the elevated limb.

Buerger's test.* Buerger's test should be performed, which involves raising the legs to 45° above the horizontal and keeping them there for a couple of minutes. A poor arterial supply is shown by rapid pallor. The legs are then allowed to hang dependent over the examination couch. The feet reperfuse with a dusky crimson colour in contrast to a normally perfused foot, which has no colour change. In severe cases, the foot may remain pale and some time may pass before the reactive hyperaemia appears.

Ankle brachial pressure index (ABPI). The ABPI should be measured in each leg as part of the routine examination. A Doppler probe† is held over the brachial artery and a blood-pressure cuff inflated to occlude the blood flow. As the blood-pressure cuff is deflated, a Doppler signal reappears and a systolic pressure can be recorded. Similar pressure readings are taken from the dorsalis pedis and posterior tibial arteries with a cuff just above the ankle. The ABPI is the ratio of pressure at the foot pulse to that at brachial artery. Values less than 0.5 indicate significant ischaemia. Heavily calcified vessels may be incompressible and give false high readings.

Exercise test. If it is difficult to obtain a clear history of the exact severity of intermittent claudication, the patient should be taken for a walk with the doctor who observes the time and nature of the onset of symptoms. Measurement of the ABPI pre- and post-exercise may show a significant fall from normal after exercise indicating a critical stenosis in the proximal vessels.

Cervical rib. Raynaud's phenomenon may be secondary to a cervical rib or band. In this circumstance the rib may be palpable, or a sensation of fullness experienced in the affected supraclavicular fossa as the vessels are displaced. Palpate the radial pulse while asking the

*Leo Buerger (1879–1943), Born in Vienna; Urologist, Mount Sinai Hospital, New York, USA.

patient to hyperabduct the arms, or brace the shoulders and the pulse on the affected side may disappear. A supraclavicular fossa bruit may also be audible.

Special investigations
• *Urine for sugar and blood glucose* to exclude diabetes, a common accompaniment of peripheral artery disease. If necessary, a fasting blood glucose estimation or glycosylated haemoglobin (HbA1c) may be necessary.
• *Haemoglobin estimation* to exclude anaemia or polycythaemia. Anaemia may sometimes precipitate angina or claudication.
• *Serum cholesterol* is often raised in atherosclerosis, and is treatable.
• *Electrocardiogram (ECG)* to exclude associated coronary disease.
• *Echocardiogram* to confirm valvular lesions, mural thrombus on an akinetic ventricular wall, ventricular aneurysm and atrial myxoma.
• *Chest X-ray.* Bronchial carcinoma is a common finding in end-stage vascular disease, both caused by smoking. Chest X-ray also allows assessment of the cardiac silhouette.
• *Doppler ultrasound.*[*] The Doppler ultrasonic probe can be used to generate a waveform of the arterial pulse in the peripheral vessels in addition to allowing the measurement of pressure and derivation of the ABPI. The waveform is biphasic in normal elastic arteries, but becomes monophasic in hardened arteries.
• *Duplex sonography.* Combining Doppler ultrasound with real time produces duplex scanning, which is a sensitive method of imaging blood vessels. By measuring flow patterns it can quantify the degree of stenosis of a vessel because the blood velocity increases as it crosses a stenosis in order to maintain the same flow rate. Summation of scans produces a result similar to angiography, but noninvasively. It is particularly useful in assessing carotid artery disease.

[*]C. J. Doppler (1803–53), Professor of Physics, University of Vienna, Austria.

• *Arteriography* is used to determine the site and extent of a blockage, and is performed if reconstructive surgery or angioplasty is contemplated to identify the severity and distribution of disease, whether atheromatous plaques, stenoses, or complete blocks as well as demonstrating run-off (Fig. 10.1).
• *Angioplasty.* At the time of arteriography, a stenosed segment of artery may be dilated using a specially designed balloon catheter. This percutaneous transluminal angioplasty (PTA) is now commonly undertaken for coronary as well as peripheral arteries. It may be combined with endoluminal stenting to maintain the patency of the dilated segment.
• *Computed tomography (CT) and ultrasound scanning.* These are useful in determining the presence and extent of aneurysmal disease, and their relation to other structures.

Principles of treatment
There are two treatment principles underlying the management of patients with vascular disease, both come under the adage of *primum non nocere* (first do no harm).
1 *Treat handicap not disability.* Treatment must be tailored to the patient. If a patient claudicates at 500 metres (the disability), but seldom needs to walk that distance, there is no handicap with this disability and therefore the patient needs no treatment. However, if the patient is young and work requires him or her to walk 500 metres (e.g. on a milk round) then the patient is handicapped by the disability and merits treatment.

There are usually two treatment options: conservative management and surgery. Reconstructive surgery can produce dramatic results but at a risk.
2 *Prophylactic surgery is only appropriate when the risk of the event outweighs the risk of the procedure.* For example, surgical repair of an aortic aneurysm is advised when the risk of rupture (which is usually fatal) outweighs the operative mortality. If the patient is a poor operative risk then the threshold for surgery increases.

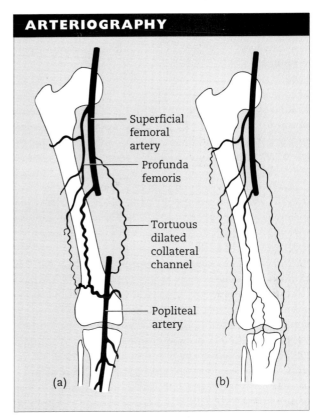

ARTERIOGRAPHY

Superficial femoral artery

Profunda femoris

Tortuous dilated collateral channel

Popliteal artery

(a) (b)

Fig. 10.1 Tracings of arteriograms. (a) An example of a good 'run-off' with a patent popliteal artery; this is suitable for reconstructive surgery. (b) The main arterial tree is obliterated and reconstruction cannot be carried out.

Atherosclerotic arterial disease

Arterial disease may be divided into occlusive disease and aneurysmal disease, the commonest cause of both being atherosclerosis. This common aetiology results in both manifestations coexisting, hence the patient with an abdominal aortic aneurysm frequently also has coronary artery disease.

Aetiology

Many factors have been shown to contribute to the genesis of atherosclerosis. While there is a familial tendency to the disease, the most common aetiological factors are smoking, hyperlipidaemia and hypercholesterolaemia, hypertension and diabetes. It is a disease that affects predominantly males, although with increasing age females become more susceptible.

Smoking

There are three components of the serious effects of smoking in atherosclerotic disease.

1 Nicotine, which induces vasospasm.

2 Carbon monoxide, present in inhaled smoke, is taken up by haemoglobin to form carboxyhaemoglobin, which dissociates slowly and is, therefore, unavailable for oxygen carrying, resulting in relative tissue hypoxia.

RISK FACTORS FOR ATHEROSCLEROTIC DISEASE

- Smoking.
- Hyperlipidaemia.
- Hypertension.
- Diabetes mellitus.
- Male sex.
- Increasing age.
- Family history.

3 Increased platelet stickiness, with increased risk of thrombosis formation.

Hyperlipidaemia

Raised cholesterol and raised triglycerides are both implicated in vascular disease and cholesterol-lowering agents have been shown to reduce the risk of death from coronary artery disease in patients with hypercholesterolaemia.

Diabetes

Diabetic patients are prone to higher incidence of atherosclerosis, and also are at risk of diabetic micro-angiopathy resulting in poor tissue perfusion, ulceration and gangrene, due to both tissue perfusion and the neuropathy that accompanies diabetes.

Atherosclerotic occlusive arterial disease

Occlusive disease results in ischaemia of the end organ or tissue that is supplied. In the peripheral arteries the three cardinal features are exercise-induced pain (intermittent claudication), which may progress as the disease progresses to pain at rest and gangrene. The progression is not necessarily a smooth one in the early stage, with deterioration in claudication distance followed by some improvement as collateral circulation develops, before further deterioration due to thrombosis.

Parallels to peripheral artery occlusive disease are present in the other circulatory systems.

Coronary occlusive disease

Angina pectoris is the coronary circulation's equivalent of intermittent claudication, with pain on exertion as oxygen demand exceeds supply, and rest pain being analogous to unstable angina with resultant infarction if the coronary circulation is not revascularized either by thrombolysis or bypass surgery.

Mesenteric occlusive disease

Mesenteric angina occurs when the blood supply to the gut is impaired and follows the ingestion of food. Patients present with pain after meals, a history of marked weight loss and fear eating because of pain. Acute occlusion results in infarction.

Cerebral occlusive disease

In the cerebral circulation, progressive occlusive disease manifests as dementia, while small emboli causing occlusion of small vessels may appear as transient ischaemic attacks, complete occlusion resulting in cerebral infarction in the absence of a collateral circulation.

Intermittent claudication

Intermittent claudication manifests as a gripping, tight, cramp-like pain in the calf on exercise, and usually affects one leg in advance of the other. The pain disappears on resting. Pain that is present on standing and that requires the patient to sit down before it is relieved is more typical of cauda equina compression (spinal claudication) (p. 126).

The pathology lies in one of the main arteries supplying the leg. Calf claudication is usually due to a lesion in the thigh, while buttock claudication is due to a reduced blood flow down the internal iliac arteries, either due to a lesion there or higher up in the common iliac artery or the aorta. Bilateral buttock claudication is associated with impotence, as both internal iliac arteries are compromised (Leriche's syndrome*: absent femoral pulses, intermittent claudication of the buttock muscles, pale cold legs and impotence).

Management
Conservative treatment

If patients stop smoking and continue exercise, or better still are enrolled into a programme of supervised exercise, over one-third of patients will extend their claudication distance due to the development of collateral vessels that bypass the blockage. Only one-third will deteriorate. In addition to cessation of smoking, the other risk factors for the development of arterial disease should be treated, so diabetes should be sought and treated

*Rene Leriche (1870–1955), Professor of Surgery successively at Lyon, Strasbourg and Paris, France.

TREATMENT OF CLAUDICATION

Conservative
- Stop smoking.
- Exercise to increase the collateral circulation.
- Learn to live within a claudication distance, involving a change in lifestyle and perhaps employment.
- Weight loss—less effort for the muscles.
- Raising the heel of shoe—less effort for the calf muscles.
- Foot care to prevent minor trauma that may lead to gangrene.
- Treat coexisting conditions such as diabetes, hypertension and hyperlipidaemia.

Interventional
- Angioplasty.
- Endoluminal stenting.
- Bypass surgery, but only if severely handicapped.

---

aggressively and hyperlipidaemia if present should be treated.

The work performed by the legs is greater if the patient is overweight so strict dieting may well improve exercise tolerance. If the claudication is limited to the calf, raising the heels of the shoes 2 cm will relieve the work performed by the calf muscles, and therefore allow the patient to walk greater distance. Careful chiropody is important. Gangrene can commence from a minor trauma such as faulty nail or corn cutting and may result in limb loss.

Interventional treatment

If claudication is a significant handicap to the patient, the possibility of reconstructive surgery or angiographic intervention should be considered.

Special investigations

Special investigations detailed above should be arranged. The following in particular:
- *Arteriography*. This should include the aorta, iliac, femoral, popliteal and distal arteries on the affected side. In particular, this should look for short (less than 10 cm) occlusions or significant (greater than 70%) stenoses, which would be amenable to angioplasty.
- *Duplex sonography*. Duplex scanning is now replacing angiography in many centres. It takes longer to perform and is more subjective but can give better information as to the

significance of stenoses and has the benefit of being non-invasive.

Treatment choices

- *Angioplasty*. Angioplasty involves blowing a balloon up within the vessel to stretch and fracture the stenosis or blockage, and allow more blood to pass through. This is most successful with concentric stenoses or blocks in the iliac system and is less successful with long blocks over 10 cm, particularly in the distal femoral and popliteal arteries. An endovascular stent may be used to maintain patency. Angioplasty carries the risk of distal embolization and vessel perforation.
- *Thrombolysis*. Where there has been an acute deterioration in claudication distance due to thrombosis occuring on a background of pre-existing disease, thrombolysis may be appropriate. A fibrinolytic enzyme such as streptokinase or tissue plasminogen activator (TPA) is infused into the clot, which it dissolves. Complete dissolution of thrombus takes time, so the technique is not appropriate where limb viability is acutely threatened.
- *Bypass surgery*. Bypass surgery should not be undertaken for minimal symptoms and is now generally reserved for limiting claudiction or rest pain. Complications include intimal dissection, distal embolization and graft thrombosis, which worsen the initial situation.

Critical ischaemia

Critical ischaemia may be defined as rest pain, ulceration or gangrene associated with absent pedal pulses.

Rest pain
Rest pain occurs when the blood supply to the leg is insufficient. Initially the pain occurs at night after the foot has been horizontal for a few hours in bed. The patient gains relief by sleeping with the leg hanging out of bed. As the disease progresses the pain becomes continuous.

Gangrene
The presence of gangrene indicates a severe degree of vascular impairment. Typically, it occurs in the toes or at pressure areas on the foot, particularly the heel, over the malleoli or on the plantar aspect of the ball of the hallux. Gangrene results from infection of ischaemic tissues. Minimal trauma, such as a nick of the skin while cutting the toenails or an abrasion from a tight shoe, enables ingress of bacteria into the infarcted tissues; the combination of these two factors results in clinical gangrene.

Investigation
Critical ischaemia needs investigating with great urgency to relieve the patient's pain and to prevent irreversible damage leading to limb loss. The investigations are the same as those used to evaluate claudication.

Treatment
Non-operative treatment
Arteriography and angioplasty. Arteriography should be performed with a view to angioplasty or stenting where possible, and to identify surgically reconstructable disease.

Lumbar sympathectomy. Sometimes, palliation may be achieved by lumbar sympathectomy, which increases the blood supply to the skin, and which may be performed percutaneously. The small increase in blood supply may be sufficient to allow an ulcer to heal but will not generally improve rest pain.

Operative treatment
Amputation. Pain that is not controlled by sympathectomy or reconstructive surgery, and gangrene that is associated with life-threatening infection are indications for amputation of the limb or part of the limb. The general principle is to achieve a viable stump that heals primarily, and a secondary goal is to make the stump as distal as possible.

Reconstructive surgery. Successful surgical reconstruction demands four things.
1 *In-flow.* A good arterial supply up to the area of blockage is necessary to ensure that enough blood can be carried distally via the conduit to the ischaemic area.
2 *Out-flow (run-off).* There should be good vessels below the area of disease on to which a conduit can be anastomosed. If there is nowhere for the blood to go the conduit will occlude.
3 *The conduit.* A graft of saphenous vein, reversed or used *in situ* with valve destruction, or an inert prosthetic material such as polytetrafluoroethylene (PTFE), may be used for the conduit to take blood from the proximal artery to distal around the blockage. In grafts that start and finish above the knee there is little to choose between PTFE and vein in terms of long-term patency; but a graft that crosses the knee is much more likely to remain patent if it is saphenous vein rather than PTFE. Infection is less likely with autologous vein.
4 *The patient.* Critical ischaemia is often the first sign of the end-stage vascular disease which inevitably results in death. Surgery for critical ischaemia has a high mortality reflecting this general deterioration.

Carotid artery disease
(Fig. 10.2)

Like atheroma elsewhere, the disease affects the bifurcation of arteries, in this case of the

INTERNAL CAROTID ARTERY STENOSIS

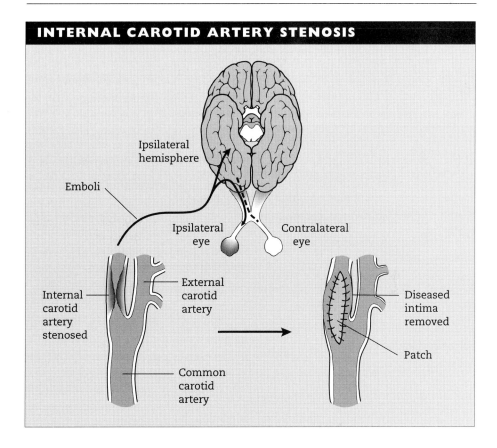

Ipsilateral hemisphere

Emboli

Ipsilateral eye

Contralateral eye

Internal carotid artery stenosed

External carotid artery

Diseased intima removed

Patch

Common carotid artery

Fig. 10.2 Symptoms and treatment of carotid artery stenosis.

carotid artery into the internal and external carotid arteries. Atheromatous plaques may ulcerate and thrombus form on their surface. If this thrombus breaks off, it forms an embolus comprising platelet clumps or atheromatous debris. This may impact in the ipsilateral retinal artery producing ipsilateral blindness, or the cerebral arteries of the ipsilateral hemisphere producing contralateral paralysis. Alternatively, the atheroma may so narrow the artery that blood flow is critically limited or totally occluded, producing similar symptoms.

Clinical features
• *Amaurosis fugax*. The patient commonly complains of a loss of vision like a curtain coming down across his or her visual field. The blindness is unilateral and usually lasts a few minutes.
• *Cerebro-vascular accidents (stroke)*. Emboli in the carotid territory of the cerebral circulation of the ipsilateral hemisphere will result in symptoms affecting the contralateral side of the body, commonly loss of use of the arm. If the dominant hemisphere is involved, speech may be affected.
• *Transient ischaemic attack (TIA)*. By definition, these mimic strokes but last less than 24 hours.
• *Cerebral hypoperfusion*. Bilateral severe stenoses may result in critical ischaemia in the brain such that cerebral or physical exertion may result in relative hypoperfusion and confusion or TIA.

Examination may reveal a bruit over the

affected side (although very tight stenoses are often silent) and evidence of vascular disease elsewhere. During an attack, unilateral weakness affecting arm or leg, dysphasia, and retinal emboli and infarction may be noted.

Differential diagnosis

Other causes of focal neurological deficits include hypoglycaemia, focal epilepsy, migraine, intracerebral neoplasm and emboli secondary to cardiac arrhythmias and valve disease.

Special investigations

• *Duplex sonography*. This gives a non-invasive assessment of degree of stenosis and is useful to screen for the disease.
• *Angiography* allows accurate assessment of the degree of stenosis, but carries the risk of dislodging thrombus and precipitating an embolic stroke.
• *Magnetic resonance imaging (MRI) angiography* can also give good images of the carotid vessels and also allows good visualization of the vertebral system to assess the complete cerebral perfusion. It is less accurate in the measurement of the degree of stenosis.
• *MRI/CT of the brain* is indicated if any doubt over symptoms exists, as intracranial tumours may mimic carotid artery disease, and may coexist.
• *Cerebral reactivity*. If cerebral perfusion is marginal, with bilateral stenoses or an occlusion on one side and stenosis on the other, the haemodynamic response to stress can be gauged by measuring the change in cerebral blood flow using intracranial duplex scanning while the patient breathes CO_2, which causes vasodilatation so intracranial blood flow should increase. However, if there is a critical stenosis affecting the carotid artery, and the collateral cerebral circulation provided by the circle of Willis* is not intact or sufficient, there will be no reactive increase in perfusion.

*Thomas Willis (1612–75), Physician and Anatomist, first in Oxford then London.

• *ECG/echocardiography*. This may be necessary to exclude a cardiac cause of cerebral symptoms.

Treatment

Patients who have had recent TIA, amaurosis fugax, or stroke with full recovery in the presence of an internal carotid stenosis of 70% or more are at high risk of a subsequent stroke in the months following. These patients benefit from endarterectomy to remove the diseased intima and re-establish normal carotid flow. All patients should be started on aspirin upon diagnosis, and this should be continued indefinitely as prophylaxis against further events. Patients with asymptomatic stenoses may also benefit from surgery, but here the risk/benefit ratio is not as favourable.

Carotid endarterectomy is performed as prophylaxis against future stroke. The diseased intima is removed, and peroperatively a shunt is used to keep blood flowing to the brain.

Complications of carotid endarterectomy

• *Death and disabling stroke*. Up to 5% of patients will suffer a stroke, some of whom will die as a consequence.
• *Haemorrhage*. Bleeding is common, as the patients are on aspirin therapy. Occasionally, post-operative haemorrhage requires re-exploration.
• *Hypoglossal neuropraxia*. The hypoglossal nerve crosses the upper part of the incision and may be damaged during surgery resulting in a hypoglossal palsy, manifested by protrusion of the tongue to the ipsilateral side.
• *Reperfusion syndrome*. The sudden increase in blood flow to the brain may result in cerebral oedema and fitting or haemorrhage. Good post-operative blood-pressure control is therefore vital.
• *Re-stenosis*. The vessel may re-stenose at the site of the arteriotomy. To overcome this, a patch is usually used, made from saphenous vein or prosthetic material such as PTFE or Dacron.

Raynaud's phenomenon*

Chnical features
The syndrome occurs due to intermittent spasm of the small arteries and arterioles of the hands (and feet). Spasm is usually precipitated by cold exposure. During the spasm the hands go white. As the vasospasm resolves, the pallor changes to cyanosis and then crimson red as reperfusion and hyperaemia occurs, the process commonly taking 30–45 minutes.

Aetiology
This may be *primary Raynaud's disease*, almost invariably in females, or *Raynaud's phenomenon*, secondary to some other lesion, particular connective tissue disorders such as scleroderma and polyarteritis nodosa, the other symptoms of which it may precede by several years. It may occur in patients with cryoglobulinaemia or it can result from work with vibrating tools. It is important to exclude other causes of cold, cyanosed hands, for instance pressure on the subclavian artery from a cervical rib (sometimes complicated by multiple emboli arising from the damaged artery wall at the site of rib pressure), or blockage of a main artery in the upper limb due to atherosclerosis or Buerger's disease.

Treatment
Conservative
The management should initially be conservative. Patients should be exhorted to keep their hands and feet warm, to wear gloves and fur-lined boots in the winter, and make sure that the house, especially the bed, is warm at night. They should also avoid immersion of the limbs in cold water. Treatment with vasodilator drugs is usually tried but the results are often disappointing. Smoking must be stopped.

Surgery
Sympathectomy almost invariably produces a dramatic improvement in the symptoms, but unfortunately may not be long-lasting in the upper limbs. Rarely, Raynaud's phenomenon or disease leads to actual necrosis of tissues and gangrene of the digits. If this occurs, local amputation may be necessary, but as the circulation of the proximal part of the hand is usually satisfactory, major amputations are seldom required.

Buerger's disease†

Buerger's disease (thromboangiitis obliterans) is a rather poorly defined entity, usually affecting males (90%), the salient features of which are similar to atherosclerosis but the age incidence is much younger and the association with heavy smoking is almost invariable. Peripheral vessels tend to be affected earlier in Buerger's disease and the veins may be inflamed together with the arteries. It is more an inflammatory condition than atherosclerotic, although the symptoms of distal claudication and ischaemic ulceration of the toes are similar. It tends to affect the hands and fingers more commonly than atheroma.

Embolism (Fig. 10.3)

An embolus is abnormal undissolved material carried in the blood stream from one part of the vascular system to impact in a distant part. While the embolus may comprise air, fat or tumour (including atrial myxoma), it is most commonly thrombus that becomes dislodged from its source, usually the heart or the major vessels.

Emboli tend to lodge at the bifurcation of vessels; their danger will depend upon the

*Maurice Raynaud (1834–81), Physician, Paris, France.

†Leo Buerger (1879–1943), Born in Vienna; Urologist, Mount Sinai Hospital, New York, USA.

SOURCES OF EMBOLI

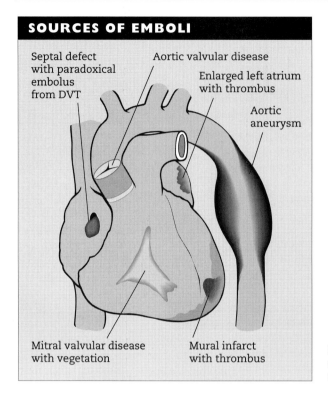

Septal defect with paradoxical embolus from DVT

Aortic valvular disease

Enlarged left atrium with thrombus

Aortic aneurysm

Mitral valvular disease with vegetation

Mural infarct with thrombus

Fig. 10.3 Sources of peripheral emboli. DVT, deep vein thrombosis.

POTENTIAL SOURCES OF EMBOLI

- *Left atrium*: atrial fibrillation and mitral stenosis, atrial myxoma.
- *Heart valves*: infective endocarditis.
- *Left ventricular wall*: mural thrombus after myocardial infarction or from ventricular aneurysm.
- *Aorta*: from aneurysm or atheroma.
- *Interventricular septum*: rare paradoxical embolus via a septal defect, originating in the systemic veins.

anatomical situation. Blockage of arteries of the central nervous system, retina and small intestine will produce dramatic effects. Emboli in the renal arteries will produce haematuria and pain in the loin. Emboli in the splenic artery will produce pain under the left costal margin. Large emboli straddling the aortic bifurcation (a saddle embolus) may cause bilateral signs.

The late results of embolism in limb vessels are similar to those of atherosclerosis and may, in fact, be associated or caused by this condition. However, acute embolism is a surgical emergency and prompt adequate treatment may produce a complete recovery.

Clinical features

The history and physical signs may reveal a cause for the embolus. The commonest causes of arterial emboli are atrial fibrillation due to rheumatic heart disease or myocardial ischaemia and dislodgement of a mural clot from a myocardial infarct, often occurring around 10 days previously. The history in acute blockage of a limb is usually one of sudden pain in the limb, which soon becomes white and cold. Sensation may disappear and the muscles may become rapidly paralysed. As time progresses, the limb becomes anaesthetic, fixed muscular contractures develop and skin staining appears, which does not blanch on pressure (fixed staining). Aortic dissection is an uncommon differential diagnosis, when ischaemia may progress down the body, often with spontaneous recovery corresponding to the intimal flap dissecting away from the true lumen (see p. 66). Paradoxical emboli are also uncommon. In patients with a patent foramen ovale, or other septal defect, a clot originating in the veins may pass up towards the chest. In addition to impacting in the pulmonary arterial tree, it may pass across the septal defect and lodge in the arterial system. This is particularly likely after a pulmonary embolus, as the raised pulmonary artery pressure results in increased shunting across a septal defect if present.

On examination, the site of the block will usually be considerably proximal to the site at which pain is experienced. It is fairly common for the block to travel distally in the course of the first few hours, due to the embolus being dislodged or fragmented.

Treatment
Urgency
The likelihood of surgical removal of an embolus being successful is inversely proportional to the time interval from the onset of the block to the operation, and after 24 hours have elapsed successful disobliteration of the artery becomes less likely. Fixed staining of the skin is a sign that it is too late for revascularization.

Heparinization
As soon as the diagnosis is made, the patient should be systemically heparinized, so as to prevent propagation of clot from the site of blockage.

Assessment
The limb is exposed to room temperature and observed for signs of impairment to the circulation. If the block seems to be resolving, with the appearance of pulses that had previously been absent, the collateral circulation may produce adequate distal arterial blood supply and surgery may not be required; thrombolysis may be an appropriate alternative. If the distal limb has apparently no blood supply and there are neurological changes, urgent surgery is indicated. Absent femoral, popliteal or aortic pulsations are indications that operation will probably prove necessary.

Surgical procedure
The approach to the involved vessel will depend on physical findings indicating the level of the block. The operative treatment is relatively simple: the vessel is exposed, opened and the clot removed. A special balloon catheter (designed by Thomas Fogarty* when he was a medical student) is passed into the vessel with the balloon collapsed. The balloon is then inflated and pulled back, the clot being expelled by the balloon via the arteriotomy. Poor results will be due to propagation of clot beyond the embolus, particularly down the branches of the popliteal artery, and local thrombolysis may be required. Emboli in the upper limb vessels usually produce less disability than those in the lower limb, as a collateral circulation in the upper limb is better. Surgery is therefore indicated less often.

Where there is no obvious cause for an embolus, a spontaneous thrombosis in situ must be considered. This is more likely if the patient has a previous history of occlusive symptoms such as claudication. In this case, collaterals have already developed and the limb remains viable. Thrombolysis may restore patency followed by angioplasty to treat the

ACUTE LIMB ISCHAEMIA

- Pain.
- Pallor.
- Pulselessness.
- Paraesthesiae.
- Paralysis.
- Perishingly cold.

*Thomas Fogarty (Contemporary), Surgeon, Portland, Oregon, USA.

underlying disease. Occasionally, *in situ* thrombosis may be a manifestation of malignancy.

It is most important that after the successful outcome of an embolectomy the cause of the embolism be treated if this is possible.

Aneurysm

An aneurysm is an abnormal permanent dilatation of a vessel or part of a vessel. Morphologically it may be fusiform or saccular. The term aneurysm is also used to describe any condition in which there is a sac communicating with an arterial lumen, in which case the aneurysms are false or pseudo-aneurysms. These false aneurysms may also involve arterio-venous fistulae (arterio-venous aneurysms) and dissecting aneurysms, although the latter is now more usually termed aortic dissection rather than a dissecting aneurysm.

Aneurysm types (Fig. 10.4)
Saccular aneurysms
A dilated portion of the artery joins the main lumen by a narrow neck. Mycotic aneurysms are often of this sort, where infection causes a local weakness of the wall which gives way to aneurysmal dilatation.

Fusiform aneurysm
A generalized dilatation of the artery exists, and this is the commonest type of aneurysm to affect the abdominal aorta.

False (pseudo-) aneurysm
Blood leaks out of an artery and is contained by the surrounding connective tissue lined with thrombus. The resultant blood collection communicates with the artery so it is pulsatile and expansile. It will either thrombose spontaneously or enlarge and rupture.

Arterio-venous aneurysm
A communication between adjacent artery and vein, this is essentially a false aneurysm intervening between artery and vein.

Dissecting aneurysm
Blood forces a passage through a break in the intima of a vessel, creating a separate 'false'

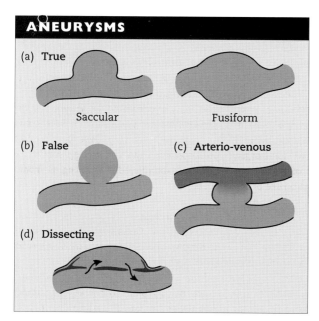

Fig. 10.4 The types of aneurysm.

channel between the external layers of the arterial wall. This false channel may then either rupture back into the lumen, or rupture out of the adventitia externally. Over the arterial segment where flow is extraluminal, vessels taking their origin from the true lumen will be deprived of blood (see aortic dissection, p. 66).

Aetiology
Congenital
The small berry aneurysms that occur intracranially on the circle of Willis and also the less common arterio-venous aneurysms and fistulae in the limbs are congenital.

Degenerative
Atheromatous degeneration of the vessel wall is the commonest cause of a true aneurysm.

Traumatic
Penetration or weakening of the arterial wall by a penetrating wound such as a bullet or knife, or iatrogenic injury during catheterization for angiography and angioplasty, may result in a true aneurysm or false aneurysm, possibly with an associated arterio-venous fistula.

Infection
Mycotic aneurysms, previously seen in the thoracic aorta of patients with tertiary syphilis, are now more commonly seen in the abdominal aorta or femoral artery as a consequence of salmonellosis, or resulting from mycotic emboli in patients with infective endocarditis. Patients with immunodeficiency, whether as a result of immunosuppression for organ transplantation or as a result of human immunodeficieny virus (HIV) infection are prone to mycotic aneurysms from unusual bacteria or fungi.

Inflammatory
This is a subtype of atherosclerotic and mycotic aneurysms in which there is an immune response to components in the aneurysm wall resulting in a dense inflammatory response with a rind of inflammatory tissue surrounding the lumen. In non-infective cases this may subside with corticosteroid treatment. It is also associated with retroperitoneal fibrosis and ureteric obstruction.

Clinical features of true aneurysms
The clinical features of an aneurysm depend on its location, and it may present with symptoms far distant from the aneurysm itself. Abdominal aortic aneurysms may present with back pain but they are frequently asymptomatic and picked up on routine examination for other reasons, such as during the investigation of prostatic symptoms. The patient may feel a sensation of abdominal bloating or may have noticed the pulsatile swelling, or may present with distal emboli from the sac contents. When the peripheral arteries are involved it is more common to find a complaint of a pulsatile mass or distal ischaemia. On examination there is a dilatation along the course of the artery. The aneurysm itself is both pulsatile and expansile. In smaller peripheral aneurysms, direct compression may empty the sac or diminish its size, and pressure on the artery proximal to the aneurysm may reduce its pulsation. If the feeding vessel has a narrow orifice there may be a thrill and bruit, and if there is an arterio-venous communication a machinery murmur is audible.

Differential diagnosis
• A dilated, tortuous, atheromatous artery common in elderly subjects.
• A mass overlying or displacing the artery superficially. In the abdomen a carcinoma of the pancreas may have a transmitted pulsation from the underlying aorta but will not be expansile, distinguishing it from an aneurysm.

Complications
• *Rupture.* The likelihood of rupture increases as the diameter of the artery increases relative to its normal size.
• *Thrombosis.* Thrombus lines the wall of the aneurysm, and may dislodge or extend to completely occlude the artery. This results in acute impairment of the distal circulation.

• *Embolism.* Lining thrombus may detach and embolize to distal circulation, either as small emboli resulting in digital ischaemia or as a large mass of thrombus threatening the entire limb.

• *Pressure.* Adjacent structures may be eroded or displaced. Hence backache and sciatica are common in patients with large abdominal aortic aneurysms, and occlusion of the femoral vein is common with large femoral aneurysms.

• *Infection.* An aneurysm may become infected or arise secondary to infection and consequent weakening of the arterial wall.

Special investigations

• *Abdominal X-ray.* This may show calcification in the wall of the aneurysm. A lateral film is particularly helpful in demonstrating aortic aneurysm calcification.

• *CT, MRI and ultrasound scanning* may delineate the size and extent of an aneurysm, its relationship to other structures and evidence of leakage.

• *Angiography* underestimates the size and extent of a true aneurysm, as it images the lumen, which is usually narrowed by thrombus. In addition, it may be dangerous, as the guide wire or cannula may perforate the aneurysm wall. It is useful in false aneurysms to identify the connection.

Treatment

The treatment of an arterial aneurysm depends on its nature (true or false), location, size and symptoms. Abdominal aortic aneurysms should be resected when they become symptomatic or reach a size at which the risk of rupture outweighs the likely operative mortality for the individual. Aneurysms of other large vessels, such as the femoral and popliteal arteries, may be replaced with a prosthetic graft or saphenous vein, while a small peripheral aneurysm can usually be excised without endangering the distal circulation assuming an adequate collateral circulation. False aneurysms and mycotic aneurysms are more prone to rupture and require urgent attention.

Abdominal aortic aneurysm

Dilatation of the abdominal aorta is a common finding in older males, and in those with a positive family history. Around 10% will have a coincidental popliteal aneurysm. Small aneurysms (less than 4 cm), are generally benign and grow slowly (1–2 mm per annum). As they enlarge, the growth rate increases, and the risk of symptoms increases. The most feared complication is rupture. This has an incidence of around 5% per annum once the aneurysm reaches 6 cm in antero-posterior diameter. With operative mortality at or below 5%, resection of the aneurysm is advised at 5.5–6 cm as prophylaxis against rupture.

Management

Patients with asymptomatic aortic aneurysms are followed up by regular screening scans to monitor the rate of growth. Once the threshold diameter is reached, or the aneurysm becomes symptomatic, elective surgical resection is advised. Pre-operative assessment includes evaluating the patient's operative risk by screening for coincident cardiac disease (by ECG, echocardiography or MUGA scan to assess the ventricular ejection fraction) and for carotid arterial disease. This information may affect the decision to operate.

Operative management

Surgery involves replacement of the aneurysmal aorta with an artificial graft, usually made of Dacron. Endoluminal repair of some aneurysms may be possible in some patients by passing a graft via the femoral artery up to the aorta, anchoring it proximally and distally with self-expanding stents. This avoids a major abdominal procedure.

Complications of surgery

• *Renal failure.* The renal arterial ostia are often compressed when the aorta is clamped and are thus rendered ischaemic for the duration of cross-clamping. The left renal vein may be ligated and divided as part of the operative procedure. Hypotension pre- or post-operatively may exacerbate the renal injury.

• *Distal embolization.* Thrombus from the sac may disperse distally and block the small vessels in the foot and lower leg causing acute ischaemia, in this context called 'trash foot'.

• *Myocardial infarction.* Coronary artery disease is common in the population who develop aortic aneurysms. Cross-clamping the aorta during surgery dramatically increases the peripheral resistance against which the heart must work, and this extra stress, coupled with the metabolic stress that occurs when the legs are reperfused, may precipitate a myocardial infarct.

• *Graft infection.* This occurs in about 1% of cases and may lead to an aorto-enteric fistula.

Ruptured abdominal aortic aneurysm

A patient with a ruptured aneurysm usually presents with severe back pain, frequently with radiation to the groin, and the diagnosis is often confused with renal colic, although renal colic is less likely in the elderly population (60 years and over) than a ruptured aneurysm. Occasionally, only groin or iliac fossa pain may be the presenting symptom. Sometimes, the pain is confined to the epigastrium leading to the mistaken diagnosis of myocardial infarction.

Fifty per cent of patients die from the initial rupture and never reach hospital. Those which do reach hospital are usually profoundly shocked (cold, clammy, tachycardic, hypotensive) with generalized abdominal tenderness. A pulsatile mass is an indication for immediate laparotomy. In most patients reaching hospital, the rupture is contained by the retroperitoneum, helped by the hypotension following rupture. Injudicious fluid replacement to restore normal blood pressure prior to surgery may lead to further bleeding and breaching of the retroperitoneum resulting in haemoperitoneum and exsanguination. Occasionally, the aortic aneurysm may rupture into the inferior vena cava (aorto-caval fistula, diagnosed by a machinery murmur and pulsatile veins) or into the duodenum (aorto-duodenal fistula, diagnosed by coexistence of an aneurysm and brisk haematemesis).

Acute aortic expansion

The aneurysm may expand acutely and result in the typical pain of rupture but without the haemodynamic consequences of a bleed. Indeed, some patients are paradoxically hypertensive during this phase. At laparotomy the aneurysm sac is found to be oedematous or a local rupture is found.

Special investigations

Investigation of a patient with a suspected rupture should only be performed if there is reasonable doubt about the diagnosis, as delay may be fatal. Investigation should answer two questions.

1 *Does the patient have an aneurysm?* Often an aneurysm is difficult to feel because of hypotension and a large retroperitoneal haematoma masking the sac. A plain X-ray will frequently show calcification in the wall of an aneurysm, particularly in an aortic aneurysm. A dorsal decubitus film is particularly valuable, showing the calcified sac displacing the bowel anteriorly.

2 *Is the aneurysm bleeding?* A patient known to have an aneurysm presents with abdominal pain and is normotensive. In this context a CT is useful to identify a leak, but no modality will distinguish an uncomplicated aneurysm from one that has acutely expanded and that may imminently rupture.

Popliteal aneurysm

Popliteal aneurysms are the most common peripheral aneurysms, and historically were the first to be diagnosed and treated surgically. They are usually associated with other aneurysms, and are frequently bilateral.

Clinical features

Generally asymptomatic, when they do present it is either in association with distal embolization of sac contents leading to claudication or digital infarction, acute occlusion or rupture (uncommon). Examination confirms a prominent pulsation in the popliteal fossa, often extending proximally. Distal pulses should be sought for evidence of embolization.

Special investigations
- *Duplex*. Delineates the extent and size of the aneurysm.
- *Angiography*. To examine the arterial tree distal to the aneurysm.

Treatment
Symptomatic aneurysms should be treated by femoral to distal popliteal bypass, with ligation of the feeding vessels. Aneurysms containing clot should be repaired electively. Distal emboli may be treated by thrombolysis at the time of surgery.

Arterial trauma

Traumatic arterial injuries are due to either closed (blunt) trauma or open (penetrating) trauma.

Closed injuries
The artery is injured by extraneous compression such as a crush injury, fractures of adjacent bones with displacement of the artery (e.g. supracondylar fracture of the humerus in children) or joint dislocation. Iatrogenic causes include a tight plaster of Paris cast where no consideration has been made for post-traumatic oedema.

Penetrating injuries
Penetrating arterial injuries may result from gunshot wounds, stabbing, penetration by bone spicules in fractures, or iatrogenic injury.

Types of arterial injury
- *Mural contusion with secondary spasm.*
- *Intimal tear*. This injury is usually a result of distraction, where the artery is stretched and the intimal layer tears, while the surrounding adventitia remains intact. The intima then buckles and causes a localized stenosis, which may or may not result in thrombosis or dissection.
- *Full-thickness tear*. All layers of the artery are divided, and this may be partial or complete. Partial tears bleed copiously, while complete division of the artery often results in contraction and spasm of the divided vessel with surprisingly little blood loss.

Consequences of injury
- *Haemorrhage*. This may be concealed or overt.
- *Thrombosis*. Immediate or delayed.
- *Arterio-venous fistula formation.*
- *False (pseudo-) aneurysm formation.*
- *Arterial dissection.*
- *Compartment syndrome*. Ischaemic muscle swells and if the muscle is contained by a fibrous fascial compartment, such as in the forearm or in the lower leg, the swelling further exacerbates the ischaemia by an increased compartment pressure. Volkmann's ischaemic contracture* is a result of compartment syndrome.

Clinical features
The features of arterial injury may be those of acute ischaemia, haemorrhage or often both. Acute ischaemia is characterized by pain (in the limb supplied, starting distally and progressing proximally), pallor, pulselessness, paraesthesiae, paralysis and coldness. Haemorrhage may be overt (bright-red blood), or concealed (e.g. closed limb fractures). Symptoms are those of rapidly developing hypovolaemic shock (cold, clammy, tachycardia, hypotension, loss of consciousness, oliguria progressing to anuria).

Treatment
Closed injuries
- *Treat causative factors*. If the cause of ischaemia is a tight plaster cast, remove or split the cast. If due to a supracondylar humeral fracture, the peripheral pulses return within an hour of fracture reduction, the delay being attributable to spasm.
- *Angiography*. An angiogram will reveal whether ischaemia is due to spasm, intimal tear or arterial disruption. It may be performed in

*Richard von Volkmann (1830–89), Professor of Surgery, Halle, Germany.

a radiology suite, or intra-operatively. Partial tears in large vessels may be amenable to intravascular stenting.

• *Operative exploration*. If a limb fails to reperfuse after a fracture or dislocation is reduced, and angiography is unhelpful or shows a tear or block, exploration is mandatory. The affected vessel is either repaired directly or a segment of saphenous vein interposed to replace the injured area.

• *Fasciotomy*. Muscle ischaemia leads to swelling and compartment syndrome. The fascial compartments should be opened to relieve compartment pressure.

Open injuries

• *Direct compression*. Primary measures to staunch haemorrhage should include direct pressure. The use of a proximal tourniquet usually exacerbates blood loss, as it seldom generates sufficient pressure to occlude arterial flow, but does block venous return, which results in increase blood loss.

• *Resuscitation*. Replace blood loss.

• *Exploration*. Small vessels that are part of a large collateral supply may be sacrificed and ligated above the site of injury. Partial tears may be directly sutured or closed with a vein patch; complete division often requires interposition of reversed saphenous vein. The use of prosthetic material after trauma is avoided if possible due to the risk of contamination and graft infection.

CHAPTER 11

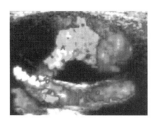

Venous Disorders of the Lower Limb

Anatomy of the venous drainage of the lower limb

In order to understand the various manifestations of venous disease in the lower leg it is essential to understand the functional anatomy of the venous system. There are two venous systems taking blood from the skin and muscles of the lower limb back to the trunk: the deep system and the superficial system (Fig. 11.1).

The deep venous system

This comprises a network of veins lying deep to the deep fascia that envelops the muscular compartments of the leg. Smaller tributaries drain into the popliteal vein behind the knee, which then ascends as the femoral vein to the inguinal ligament, where it becomes the external iliac vein. From there, blood passes up the common iliac vein, via the inferior vena cava, to the right atrium.

The superficial venous system

This comprises the medially placed great (long) saphenous vein, draining from the dorsum of the foot to the sapheno-femoral junction in the groin, and the small (short) saphenous vein, which drains the lateral aspect of the lower limb into the popliteal vein behind the knee. The superficial system lies outside the deep fascia, and drains the skin and superficial tissues.

Perforating veins

Beside the sapheno-femoral and sapheno-

popliteal junctions, there are additional communications between superficial and deep veins with valves allowing blood in the superficial system to pass into the deep system, and preventing blood flowing out from deep to superficial. These are called perforating veins, or perforators. Typically, there is one mid-thigh (called the Hunterian perforator on account of its relationship to Hunter's canal*), and several running up the medial and lateral aspect of the tibia just above the ankle.

The calf pump

All the major leg veins have valves that prevent blood flowing away from the heart. As the calf muscles contract, the deep veins within them are squeezed and emptied, the blood passing upwards, directed towards the heart by the non-return valves. As the muscles relax, blood flows in from the superficial system via perforators as well as from more distal segments of the vein, only to be pumped upwards again by the next contraction of the calf muscles, which are thus acting as a pump.

Pathology of venous disease

Venous disorders, whether in the superficial veins (e.g. varicose veins) or deep veins (venous insufficiency), share the same underlying pathology: valvular incompetence resulting

*John Hunter (1728–93), Surgeon, St George's Hospital, London.

in a disturbance of the normal flow of blood (Fig. 11.2). This haemodynamic disturbance is due either to a physical obstruction such as a thrombosis, or a functional obstruction leading to high pressure as occurs when valves are incompetent or, rarely, when an arterio-venous fistula exists. When valves are incompetent there is a greater resistance to return flow (the functional obstruction). One incom-petent valve will put extra pressure on the next and will tend to make this incompetent and so once defects have arisen there is a tendency for the condition to get worse as further valves are involved.

There are no valves in the vena cava, and none in the common iliac vein. The first valve usually occurs in the external iliac vein. Congenital absence of this, or destruction following disease, imposes increased pressure on the next in line, commonly the one guarding the sapheno-femoral junction. The pressure on this valve is then equivalent to a column of blood from the sapheno-femoral junction to the right atrium. This absence of valves and the tendency to develop varicose veins is the unfortunate legacy from the days before humans adopted the upright posture.

VEINS OF THE LEG

Valve at sapheno-femoral junction

Great saphenous vein

Mid-thigh perforator

Femoral vein

Deep fascia

Small saphenous vein

Ankle perforators

Lateral malleous

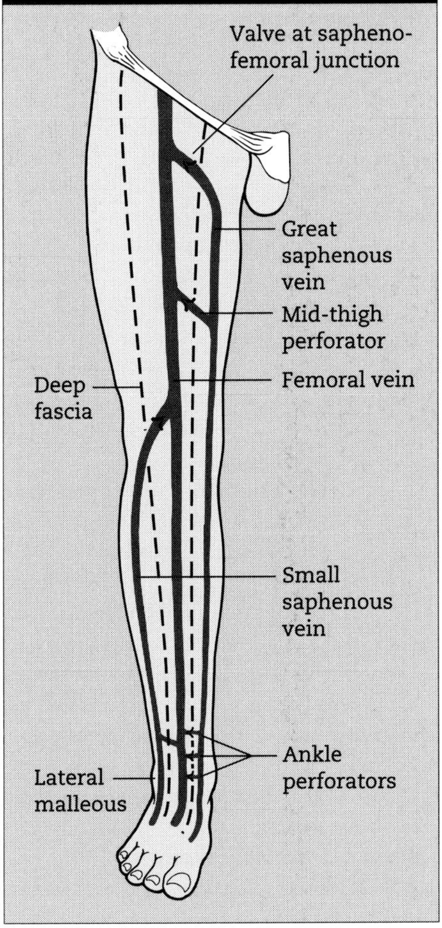

Fig. 11.1 A diagram of the superficial and deep veins of the leg. Note the two superficial systems—the great saphenous and small saphenous—each of which communicates with the deep veins by piercing the deep fascia.

Varicose veins

Definition
Varicose veins are abnormally dilated and lengthened superficial veins. They should be distinguished from the clusters of small dilated venules that occur subcutaneously as a result of hormonal change, pregnancy or trauma, and prominent normal veins which are most obvious over the muscular calves of an athlete.

Classification
Primary or idiopathic
The great majority of cases are idiopathic. This probably represents a primary valve defect and may be familial. Females are affected twice as commonly as males. Symptoms are often accentuated by pregnancy, partly as a result of pressure of the enlarged uterus on the iliac veins and partly due to relaxation of smooth muscle under the influence of hormones such as progesterone.

Secondary
• *Previous deep vein thrombosis.* Occluded veins may subsequently recanalize but their valves are rendered incompetent.

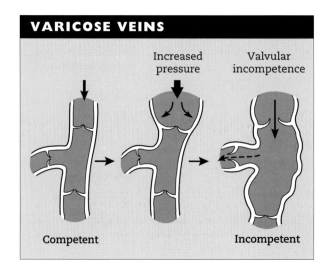

VARICOSE VEINS

Increased pressure   Valvular incompetence

Competent   Incompetent

Fig. 11.2 Normal veins and incompetent varicose veins. Note the vein dilates under pressure and the valve becomes incompetent.

• *Raised venous pressure* due to compression (e.g. by a pelvic tumour including a pregnant uterus), congenital venous malformation (e.g. Klippel–Trenaunay syndrome), arterio-venous fistula (congenital or acquired following trauma) or severe tricuspid incompetence. The last two cause pulsating varicosities.

Clinical features
History
Varicose veins are prominent and unsightly, and patients may seek treatment on account of the unpleasant appearance. Other symptoms are of tiredness, aching or throbbing in the legs and swelling of the ankles, particularly after long periods of standing. Other points to note are a history of deep vein thrombosis, or a history suggestive of thrombosis such as swelling and pain post-operatively, or after a long period of immobilization. If the deep veins are still blocked, the varicose veins that are visible may represent the sole venous drainage of the leg. A history of any complications arising from the veins (e.g. thrombophlebitis) should be sought.

Examination
A patient with varicose veins must be examined whilst standing. Examination of the legs should include inspection of the medial gaiter area for evidence of deep venous insufficiency (haemosiderosis, eczema, lipodermatosclerosis — see later). Overlying port-wine stains or similar pigmentation may suggest underlying arterio-venous malformation, especially in young patients. Auscultation over such areas may be diagnostic.

A *saphena varix*, a prominent dilatation of the vein (varicosity) at the sapheno-femoral junction, may be present. It gives a characteristic thrill to the examining fingers when the patient coughs, quite different from a femoral hernia. It disappears when the patient lies flat.

The tap test involves placing the fingers of one hand over the sapheno-femoral (or sapheno-popliteal) junction and tapping over distally placed varicosities. In the absence of valves there will be a continuous column of blood and a transmitted thrill will be palpated proximally.

*Trendelenburg's test** detects reflux from deep into superficial veins, and when carefully performed can identify the site of the incompetent connections. The patient lies flat and the leg is elevated to empty the superficial veins. A tourniquet is placed around the upper thigh

*Friedrich Trendelenburg (1844–1924), successively Professor of Surgery in Rostock, Bonn and Leipzig, Germany.

and the patient stands up. If sapheno-femoral junction incompetence is the cause of the superficial venous reflux, this high thigh tourniquet will control it and the varicose veins will remain empty. If this high tourniquet does not control the varices, the tourniquet test can be repeated with progressively lower placement of the tourniquet until the varicosities are controlled, and the level of the incompetent connection between deep and superficial veins identified.

Perthe's test* evaluates the deep veins, and is appropriate for patients with a history of deep-vein thrombosis. A rubber tourniquet is placed around the leg at the level found to *control* the veins in the Trendelenburg test. The patient is asked to stand up and down on tiptoes repeatedly, thus exercising the muscles of the calf pump. This results in venous blood being pumped up normal deep veins, emptying of superficial veins via perforators, and the disappearance of superficial varicosities. In the presence of blocked deep veins, venous return via the deep system is occluded so blood fills superficial veins via perforators, and varicosities become more prominent. This is accompanied by a burning sensation in the exercising calf. A similar test involves walking with a tourniquet around the leg. If the tests suggest an occluded deep system this should be confirmed by venography or duplex scanning.

Special investigations
• *Hand-held Doppler probes* are useful to diagnose reflux at sapheno-femoral and saphenopopliteal junctions. Identifying perforating veins is more difficult, and the device is not as sensitive as duplex scanning or venography.
• *Venography* involves placing a tourniquet around the ankle to occlude superficial veins and injecting contrast medium into the dorsum of the foot such that it will pass through the deep system up the leg. Its progress is followed on sequential X-rays. Reflux through perforating veins and deep vein occlusion are readily detected.
• *Duplex scanning* can accurately map the veins in the leg and diagnose both valvular and perforator incompetence, as well as occlusion of large veins. Like hand-held Doppler it allows accurate pre-operative localization of perforating veins.

Treatment
Graded compression stockings
Indicated for minor varicosities, and for the elderly, the pregnant and the unfit. The stocking is elasticated and specially fitted to ensure that it delivers graduated compression along its length, such that at the ankle the elastic compression of the leg is much higher than that at the thigh.

Sclerotherapy
Superficial varicosities that are cosmetically undesirable may be obliterated by injection of a small volume of sclerosant with the vein emptied. The vein is kept compressed with firm pressure bandaging for a period of 2 weeks to enable fibrosis to take place. This out-patient treatment is used for small- or moderate-sized varices below the knee. Recurrences can be treated by further injections. Complications include bruising, phlebitis with unsightly skin staining, ulceration and deep-vein thrombosis.

Surgical treatment
Varicose vein surgery is one of the most commonly performed elective surgical procedures in the UK. More recently, the indications for the procedure have come under fresh scrutiny on account of their cosmetic nature, the need for the great saphenous vein as a conduit for future arterial surgery such as coronary artery bypass, and cost.

Indications for varicose vein surgery include:
• haemorrhage occurring from a varicosity;
• varicosities being grossly dilated or otherwise symptomatic;
• incompetent perforator veins. These should be identified pre-operatively and ligated by

*Georg Clemens Perthes (1869–1927), Professor of Surgery at Tübingen. Also described osteochondritis of the femoral capital epiphysis.

a conventional open technique or subfascial ligation performed via an endoscope, assuming the deep system is patent.

Surgery involves disconnecting the great saphenous vein from the femoral vein; the terminal branches of the great saphenous vein are individually ligated and divided. This may be combined with stripping of the veins. If there are other incompetent communications (perforators), these need to be individually ligated or avulsed. Small varicose venules can be avulsed via a small skin incision.

Recurrence of varicose veins after operation is due either to a failure in the original diagnosis (underlying deep vein incompetence or arterio-venous fistula), or a defect in operative technique, particularly a failure to divide and excise all the groin tributaries of the saphenous vein. If this error is made, these tributaries will dilate and form new varices. However, recurrence may also be due to the development of further varices *de novo*, despite an adequate operation.

Complications of varicose veins
Haemorrhage
This is usually due to minor trauma to a dilated vein. The bleeding is profuse due to the high pressure within the incompetent vein. The treatment is very simple; the patient is laid recumbent with the leg elevated, and a pressure bandage is applied. Subsequent to the emergency, the varicose veins should be treated by operation.

Phlebitis
This may occur spontaneously or may be secondary to trauma to the leg. A mild phlebitis is produced by the sclerosing fluid used in the injection treatment of varicose veins. Occasionally, the reaction to this is quite violent and alarming; the varicose vein becomes extremely tender and hard and the overlying skin may be inflamed. The patient may have a constitutional disturbance with pyrexia and malaise. Secondary bacterial infection may occasionally complicate the thrombosis.

Treatment
Bed rest with the foot of the bed elevated and a pressure bandage on the leg, which compresses the superficial veins and increases the speed of flow of blood in the deep veins. If infection is present, antibiotics may be necessary, but this is unusual. In severe cases, systemic anticoagulation may alleviate pain and prevent spread of the condition. Non-steroidal anti-inflammatory drugs may give relief of symptoms but they can cause peptic ulceration.

Deep venous insufficiency

Varicose veins appear when superficial veins are dilated by blood entering via incompetent perforating veins or incompetent superficial valves. Deep venous insufficiency (also known as chronic venous insufficiency, post-thrombotic limb and post-phlebitic limb) is the term given to the situation where the valves of the deep venous system are incompetent. In the normal patient, there is a pressure in the veins at the ankle of around $100\,cmH_2O$, equivalent to the height of the column of blood from the right atrium to the ankle. Upon walking, this pressure drops to around $20\,cmH_2O$ as the calf pump drives the blood upwards. In the presence of incompetent valves, blood is no longer pumped back efficiently, and the venous pressure remains at the high resting state. This raised hydrostatic pressure causes an increase in fluid transudation across the capillaries following Starling's forces (p. 7).

Aetiology
Primary
• Congenital valveless syndromes where valves are absent.

Secondary
• Venous hypertension. Deep-vein thrombosis is the major cause of deep venous insufficiency, where the previous thrombosis has recanalized but left the valves incompetent.
• Arterio-venous fistula.

Features of venous hypertension in the leg

- *Swelling*, particularly of the lower leg, is due to transudation of fluid across capillaries causing oedema, which takes on a brawny character with time.
- *Superficial varicose veins*, caused by perforator incompetence secondary to the raised venous pressure.
- *Pigmentation of skin*, particularly the medial gaiter area (just above the medial malleolus). The pigment is haemosiderin and appears brown.
- *Eczema*, particularly over the pigmented area, causing pruritus. When the patient succumbs to the temptation to scratch this skin it is further damaged and predisposed to ulcer formation.
- *Lipodermatosclerosis*. The soft subcutaneous tissue is replaced by thick fibrous tissue, a consequence of inflammation and fibrin exudation. In time this forms a hard enveloping layer around the lower leg through which the veins pass, forming prominent gutters when the leg is elevated. The appearance of the lower leg has been likened to an inverted champagne bottle, with the narrow ankle below and soft oedematous limb above.
- *Ulceration* occurs as a consequence of the poor skin nutrition. Repeated excoriations due to the irritation of the eczema, and the impaired nutrition of the fibrotic subcutaneous tissue lead to epithelial damage and ulceration.

Special investigations

- *Venography* to detect perforators that may be treated, and identify occlusions that may explain the aetiology of the condition.
- *Duplex sonography*, in the hands of an experienced operator, will demonstrate deep venous reflux as well as detecting occlusions.

Treatment

There is no successful way to repair or replace the valves of the deep veins. If there is incompetence in the superficial veins they may be removed, and incompetent perforators ligated.

Venous ulceration

As described above, ulceration due to venous hypertension is generally due to incompetence of the deep veins, although superficial vein incompetence may be present. All patients with such an ulcer (also called varicose or gravitational ulcers), should be asked if there has been any previous history of venous thrombosis, suggested by painful swelling of the leg after an operation, childbirth or immobilization in bed for any reason.

Why the ulcer occurs around the malleoli and not in the foot itself is not fully explained. It is probable that in this area the subcutaneous tissue is less well supported than in the foot. The pressure of the column of blood and the consequent oedema and pericapillary fibrin cuffs result in ischaemia and very poor nutrition to this area so that the skin may break down either spontaneously or more commonly after minor trauma.

Venous ulcers have an edge which is either ragged or, where the ulcer is healing, the margins will be shelving with a faint-blue rim of advancing epithelium. Previous scarring

DIFFERENTIAL DIAGNOSIS OF LEG ULCERS

- *Ischaemic ulcer*, due to impaired arterial blood supply; the peripheral pulses must always be examined.
- *Neuropathic ulcer*: particularly common in diabetics where they are often compounded by ischaemia due to diabetic micro-angiopathy.
- *Venous ulcer* complicating venous insufficiency.
- *Malignant ulcer*: a squamous carcinoma, often arising in a pre-existing chronic ulcer, or an ulcerated melanoma.
- *Ulcer complicating systemic disease*, e.g. acholuric jaundice, ulcerative colitis and rheumatoid arthritis.
- *Arterio-venous fistula*-associated ulcer.
- *Repetitive self-inflicted injury*.
- *Gummatous ulcer* of syphilis: usually affects the upper one-third of the leg.

appears as a white rim around the ulcer, known as *atrophie blanche*. Rarely, a squamous carcinoma can develop in the edge of a long-standing ulcer (*Marjolin's ulcer**).

Treatment

If the patient is confined to bed with the foot of the bed elevated, so that the high venous pressure is abolished, venous ulcers will heal fairly quickly, provided they are kept clean by careful toilet. Antibiotics should be administered only in the unusual circumstances of the ulcer being grossly infected with a surrounding cellulitis. The antibiotics used will depend on the sensitivity of the bacteria cultured from the ulcer. Topical antibiotic chemotherapy should be avoided; the incidence of sensitivity reaction is high.

Unfortunately, this simple treatment is often not a practical one. The patients are mostly elderly, and prolonged recumbency is obviously of some danger in these cases. Younger patients, from the economic point of view, do not wish to spend several weeks in hospital in bed.

In such cases, healing can be obtained by

either tight elastic bandaging of the leg or by using proprietary paste bandages over which elastoplast is applied. This firm pressure empties the dilated superficial veins and enables the calf muscle pump to act more efficiently. Oxygenated blood is therefore able to reach the previously ischaemic tissues. A split-skin graft may be useful in indolent cases, but grafting must only supplement the other treatment modalities.

Once the ulcer has healed, the patient is fitted with a firm elastic graduated compression stocking or advised to continue with the elastic bandage. Incompetent perforating veins are ligated. Unless the incompetent veins are treated thus, either by support, or operation, recurrence is inevitable.

Venous ulcers account for approximately 90% of all ulcers of the legs, but other, rarer, causes should always be considered (see box, p. 95).

Deep vein thrombosis

Spontaneous deep vein thrombosis generally presents to, and is managed by, general physicians. To surgeons it is usually a post-operative complication, which is where it is discussed in full (p. 15).

---

*Jean Nicholas Marjolin (1780–1850), Surgeon, Hôpital Sainte-Eugénie, Paris, France.

CHAPTER 12

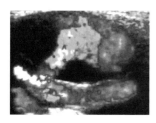

The Brain and Meninges

Space-occupying intracranial lesions

Space-occupying lesions within the skull may be caused by the following.

1 Haemorrhage:
  (a) extradural;
  (b) subdural—acute or chronic (see p. 115);
  (c) intracerebral.
2 Tumour.
3 Hydrocephalus.
4 Brain swelling (oedema), e.g. head injury, encephalitis.
5 Cerebral abscess.

Other causes are rare and include hydatid cyst, tuberculoma and gumma.

Clinical features

A space-occupying lesion manifests itself by the general features of raised intracranial pressure and by localizing signs.

Raised intracranial pressure

A space-occupying lesion within the skull produces raised intracranial pressure not only by its actual volume within the closed box of the cranium, but by provoking oedema, and sometimes by impeding the circulation or absorption of cerebrospinal fluid (CSF) causing hydrocephalus (see p. 103). For example, a tumour in the posterior fossa

may rapidly present with severe symptoms of raised intracranial pressure secondary to hydrocephalus.

A slowly progressive rise in intracranial pressure may lead to the following presenting features.

• *Headache*: may be severe, often present when the patient wakes and is aggravated by straining or coughing.
• *Vomiting*: often without preceding nausea.
• *Papilloedema*: which may be accompanied by blurring of vision and may progress to permanent blindness.
• *Depressed conscious level.*
• *Neck stiffness*: particularly if the lesion is in the posterior fossa.
• *Diplopia, ataxia.*
• *Enlargement of the head*: in children before the sutures have fused.

A rapid rise in intracranial pressure results in a clinical picture of intense headache with rapid progression into coma.

Localizing signs

Having diagnosed the presence of raised intracranial pressure, an attempt must be made on clinical findings to localize the lesion, although in some cases this is not possible. There may be upper motor neurone weakness indicating a lesion of the pyramidal pathway; there may be cranial nerve signs, e.g. a bitemporal hemianopia indicating pressure on the optic chiasma. A lesion of the post-central cortex may produce loss of fine discrimination and of stereognosis. Cerebellar lesions may produce coarse ataxia, muscular hypotonia, incoordination and often nystagmus. A focal fit may provide valuable localizing data. Motor aphasia (the patient knows what he or she wishes to say but cannot do so) suggests a lesion in Broca's area on the dominant side of the lower frontal cortex of the cerebrum. Pupillary dilatation is a late sign, and is caused by the uncus of the temporal lobe being displaced through the tentorial hiatus where it compresses the oculomotor nerve.

Special investigations
The following investigations are required in the study of a suspected space-occupying lesion.
• *Computed tomography (CT)*, with intravenous contrast enhancement, is a non-invasive and extremely accurate investigation for all cerebral tumours and other space-occupying lesions.
• *Magnetic resonance imaging (MRI)* gives superb 'anatomical' localization of intracerebral space-occupying lesions.
• *Chest X-ray* should always be performed if tumour is suspected to exclude a symptomless primary bronchogenic carcinoma.
• *Burr-hole biopsy* may be appropriate to establish a tissue diagnosis.
• *Skull X-ray* has been largely superseded in the diagnosis of space-occupying lesions by the newer cross-sectional imaging techniques (CT and MRI). Ten per cent of tumours show calcification, most commonly craniopharyngiomas and oligodendrogliomas. It is occasionally found in astrocytomas, meningiomas and vascular malformations.

The pineal gland may be calcified (30% of 30-year-olds, 70% of 70-year-olds). Inspection of the films of the skull may show a shift of the pineal to one side, indicating a space-occupying lesion on the other.

The sella turcica should be examined; decalcification is evidence of raised intracranial pressure, and expansion of the sella with erosion of the clinoid processes suggests the presence of a pituitary tumour. In children, widening of the coronal sutures and increased convolutional markings may be seen (the 'beaten brass' appearance).

Intracranial tumours

Intracranial tumours can be divided into intrinsic tumours of the brain arising usually from the supporting (glial) cells, and extracerebral tumours, which originate from the numerous structures surrounding the brain. In addition, 15% of cerebral tumours presenting to neurosurgical units are metastatic from distant sites, but many patients dying of widespread metastases have cerebral deposits and do not come under specialist care. The overall incidence of central nervous system (CNS) tumours is around 5 per 100 000 population.

The symptoms of intracranial tumours are those of a progressive increase in intracranial pressure, those attributable to their location within the brain, and seizures. Cerebellar tumours therefore lead to ataxia, occipital lobe tumours result in visual field disturbance and tumours in the posterior aspect of the frontal lobe affecting the motor cortex will result in weakness. Investigation is outlined above.

Classification
Common tumours include the following:

Intracerebral tumours
• Gliomas (45%) include astrocytoma, oligodendroglioma, ependymoma, medulloblastoma.
• Lymphoma.
• Pineal gland tumour.
• Metastases (15%).

Extracerebral
• Meningioma (15%).
• Neuroma, e.g. acoustic neuroma (5%).
• Pituitary tumour (5%) includes pituitary adenomas and craniopharyngioma.

Gliomas

Gliomas arise from the glial supporting cells and are usually supratentorial. They are classified according to the principal cell component. The four important subgroups are as follows.

Astrocytomas (80%)

These vary considerably in their histological differentiation and invasiveness, and about half are the highly anaplastic *glioblastoma multiforme*, the name referring to the primitive cell structure of this tumour. The more benign forms are often cystic and are slow growing, although they may change over the years into less differentiated and more invasive tumours. Often a glioma may have cells of different grades of differentiation in different areas of the tumour. It is interesting that the glioblastoma tends to occur in the adult and in the cerebrum, whereas the well-differentiated cystic glioma (juvenile pilocystic astrocytoma) occurs frequently in children and usually arises in the cerebellum.

Medulloblastomas (10%)

These are rapidly growing small-cell tumours generally affecting the cerebellum in children, usually boys. They may block the fourth ventricle producing an obstructive hydrocephalus and may spread via the CSF to seed over the surface of the spinal cord. The cells appear to be embryonal in origin and form characteristic rosettes under the microscope. They are often referred to as primitive neuroectodermal tumours (PNET).

Ependymomas (5%)

These arise from the lining cells of the ventricles, the central canal of the spinal cord or the choroid plexus. They usually occur in children and young adults.

Oligodendrogliomas (5%)

These are relatively slow growing and are usually found in the cerebrum and in adults.

Treatment

Only the well-differentiated lesions are amenable to surgical removal. The more anaplastic growths have an extremely poor prognosis and are treated by palliative radiotherapy, which may be combined with surgical decompression and/or chemotherapy.

Meningioma

Meningiomas arise from arachnoid cells in the dura mater to which they are almost invariably attached and typically are found in middle-aged patients. Special sites are one or both sides of the superior sagittal sinus, the lesser wing of the sphenoid, the olfactory groove, the suprasellar region and within the spinal canal. The majority are slow growing and do not invade the brain tissue but involve it only by expansion and pressure, so they may become buried in the brain. The tumour may, however, invade the skull, producing a hyperostosis, which may occasionally be enormous.

Treatment

Most meningiomas are surgically removable.

Acoustic neuroma

Neuromas are benign tumours that arise from the Schwann cells of a cranial nerve. The great majority arise from the eighth cranial nerve at the internal auditory meatus (acoustic neuroma). They are usually found in adult patients between the ages of 30 and 60 years and are occasionally associated with neurofibromatosis type II when they may be bilateral.

Neurofibromatosis has two forms. Type II is characterized by neurofibromas on cranial nerves, mental retardation and a tendency to form gliomas and meningiomas, in contrast to type I neurofibromatosis where there is a peripheral distribution with tumours on spinal roots and peripheral nerves, and skin signs such as café-au-lait spots. Both forms have an autosomally dominant inheritance.

As the acoustic tumour slowly enlarges, it

stretches the adjacent cranial nerves, VII and V anteriorly, and IX, X and XII over its lower surface. It also presses on the cerebellum and the brain stem, producing the 'cerebello-pontine angle syndrome' with the following features:
• unilateral nerve deafness often associated with tinnitus and giddiness (VIII) is the first symptom;
• facial numbness and weakness of the masticatory muscles (V);
• dysphagia, hoarseness and dysarthria (IX, X and XII);
• cerebellar hemisphere signs and, later, pyramidal tract involvement;
• eventually features of raised intracranial pressure;
• facial weakness with unilateral taste loss (VII) is very uncommon (<5%).

Treatment

Acoustic neuromas can be removed completely but with some risk to facial nerves. Alternatively, stereotactic radiosurgery (gamma knife) is now being used to treat some smaller tumours.

Pituitary tumours

Pituitary tumours have two special features.
1 Endocrine disturbances: the tumour may produce excessive and unregulated amounts of a hormone, or as it grows it may suppress production of other hormones both in the anterior pituitary (hypopituitarism) and the posterior pituitary and hypothalamus (e.g. diabetes insipidus)
2 Visual field disturbance (bitemporal hemianopia) due to optic chiasma compression.
They are named according to their staining on light microscopy.

Chromophobe adenoma (80%)

This is the commonest pituitary tumour which, as it enlarges, compresses the optic chiasma, producing a bitemporal hemianopia. Half are non-secretory tumours, which gradually destroy the normally functioning pituitary, producing hypopituitarism with loss of sex charac-teristics, hypothyroidism and hypo-adrenalism. In childhood there is arrest of growth together with infantilism. Half produce prolactin, which causes infertility, amenorrhoea and galactor-rhoea. These tumours may extend to involve the hypothalamus, producing diabetes insipidus and obesity.

Eosinophil (acidophil) adenoma (15%)

These are slow-growing tumours, which secrete growth hormone. If they occur before puberty, which is unusual, they induce gigan-tism. After puberty, acromegaly results.

Basophil adenoma (5%)

Small, produces no pressure effects and may be associated with Cushing's syndrome (adrenocorticotrophic hormone production, see p. 312).

Treatment

Pituitary tumours which are producing pressure symptoms on the optic chiasma are treated by intracapsular removal through a trans-sphenoidal (or occasionally trans-cranial) route. Prolactin-secreting tumours (prolactinomas) may respond to treatment with a dopamine agonist (e.g. bromocriptine) to suppress prolactin secretion and reduce tumour size.

Craniopharyngioma

Craniopharyngioma (suprasellar cyst, or cyst of Rathke's pouch) is a benign tumour, usually cystic, which arises in the remnant of the craniopharyngeal duct (the precursor of the anterior pituitary). It may present in childhood or early adult life and lies above and/or within the sella turcica.

The tumour produces hypopituitarism, raised intracranial pressure and optic chiasmal involvement. Treatment involves removal and/or radiotherapy. Craniopharyngiomas may be very difficult to remove completely because of their close relationship to the hypothalamus.

Secondary tumours

These account for about 15% of intracranial

tumours seen on a neurosurgical unit but are more common on the general wards. Common primary tumours are lung, breast, kidney and melanoma, the last occasionally presenting with intracranial haemorrhage.

Cerebral abscess

Aetiology
There are three common causes of brain abscess.

1 *Penetrating wound* of the skull, usually with a staphylococcal secondary infection.

2 *Direct spread*—the cause in 75% of cases:
   (a) an infected middle ear or mastoid, spreading to either the temporal lobe or the cerebellum;
   (b) an infected frontal or ethmoid sinus to the frontal lobe.

3 *Blood-borne spread*. A septic embolus, especially from a lung focus of infection such as bronchiectasis or lung abscess, or occasionally from the systemic circulation in the presence of congenital cyanotic heart disease where there is a right-to-left shunt. Such abscesses commonly occur in the middle cerebral artery territory.

An abscess localized to the extradural or subdural space may result from the same aetiological factors, particularly direct spread of infection.

Clinical features
The clinical features are those of the following.
• The underlying cause (e.g. chronic mastoiditis).
• Evidence of the development of an intracerebral space-occupying lesion (raised intracranial pressure).
• Localizing features (e.g. epilepsy or a focal neurological defect).
• Toxaemia, fever, meningism and a leucocytosis particularly if there is rapidly spreading cerebral infection. Often the abscess is walled off by a relatively thick capsule so that the general manifestations of infection (fever, and toxaemia) are not evident.

Special investigations
• *Skull X-ray* may show evidence of frontal sinus or mastoid infection.
• *CT scan and MRI* provide accurate diagnosis and localization of the abscess, typically appearing as a ring-enhancing lesion with extensive oedema.

Treatment
In the first instance, the abscess is aspirated through a burr-hole by means of a brain needle. Antibiotics are instilled into the abscess cavity and resolution is followed by serial CT scans. The aspirations may require to be repeated and systemic antibiotics are given, depending on the bacteriology report on the pus. Occasionally, the abscess fails to respond to aspiration and its capsule must be excised.

Epilepsy develops in one-third of patients and anticonvulsant therapy is therefore given prophylactically.

Intracranial vascular lesions

Intracranial vascular lesions may present either as subarachnoid or intracerebral haemorrhage, or a combination of the two. There are two primary lesions: an aneurysm of a cerebral artery or an arterio-venous malformation.

Intracranial aneurysms
Pathology
Intracranial (berry) aneurysms are primary aneurysms of the cerebral arteries. They are saccular, generally arise near the bifurcation of an artery, and are probably due to aplasia or hypoplasia of the tunica media. Eighty-five per cent occur in the anterior half of the circle of Willis, with equal distribution between anterior communicating artery, internal carotid artery and middle cerebral artery. The internal carotid artery aneurysms occur at its terminal bifurcation, origin of the posterior communicating artery, and occasionally in the cavernous sinus or at the origin of the ophthalmic

artery. Fifteen per cent occur on the basilar or vertebral arteries. About 20% are multiple. Males and females are equally affected, and they may be familial. They are occasionally associated with polycystic kidneys, coarctation of the aorta and collagen disorders such as the Ehlers–Danlos syndrome. They are rarely due to arteriosclerosis, trauma or infection (mycotic aneurysms).

Clinical features

These can be divided into two groups.

1 *Subarachnoid haemorrhage*: bleeding into the CSF from a ruptured intracranial aneurysm is the commonest cause of spontaneous subarachnoid haemorrhage. It presents with:
- sudden onset of a severe headache ('as if I was hit across the back of my head');
- vomiting;
- photophobia;
- irritability;
- neck stiffness and a positive Kernig's sign (flexion of the hip with extension of the leg causes pain when meningeal irritation present);
- Impairment of consciousness — drowsy, unconscious;
- focal neurological signs.

Rupture may also cause intracerebral or subdural bleeding with neurological signs depending on the site of the haematoma. Most cases occur after the age of 40 years, where increasing atheromatous degenerative changes in the arteries and hypertension are probably precipitating factors. The clinical diagnosis is confirmed by CT, or, if CT is negative, lumbar puncture will reveal blood-stained CSF.

2 *Pressure symptoms due to the aneurysm*: especially third-nerve palsy from an aneurysm of the posterior communicating artery.

Haemorrhage from a ruptured aneurysm is serious and one-quarter of the patients die without recovering consciousness. Further deterioration results from the intense spasm that follows several days after the haemorrhage, and from further bleeding. About 50% will bleed again within 6 weeks of the initial haemorrhage and the mortality of such bleeds is high.

Treatment

If the patient is in coma or has significant neurological deficit, but does not have hydrocephalus or a significant intracerebral bleed, conservative management is adopted initially. This involves flat bed rest, adequate fluid replacement and analgesia, and nimodipine to reduce the risk of development of delayed cerebral ischaemia from vasospasm.

If the patient recovers from the initial bleed, cerebral angiography is performed to locate the site of the aneurysm. If the aneurysm is demonstrated, treatment comprises craniotomy with the direct application of a clip across the base of the aneurysm. Endovascular approaches using platinum coils are currently under evaluation. The results of clipping are good in 80% of patients, with a 2–8% mortality.

About 15% of the angiograms are negative and probably indicate that thrombosis has taken place in a micro-aneurysm. Such cases are treated conservatively and the prognosis is good.

Arterio-venous malformations

Developmental vascular malformations may occur in any part of the CNS, particularly over the surface of the cerebral hemispheres in the distribution of the middle cerebral artery. They comprise a tangle of abnormal vessels, ranging from telangiectasia to cavernous and venous malformations often with arterio-venous fistulae.

They may produce focal epilepsy, headaches or slowly progressive paralysis, and 50% present with subarachnoid or intracerebral bleeding. The subarachnoid haemorrhage is less catastrophic than in rupture of an aneurysm, but accounts for about 10% of all cases of spontaneous subarachnoid bleeding. Half of the cases have a bruit, which may be heard over the eye, the skull vault or over the carotid arteries in the neck. Exact diagnosis and localization is made by cerebral angiography.

The haemorrhage rate is around 4% per year. Accessible malformations in non-eloquent parts of the brain are often treated by surgery, while stereotactic radiosurgery (involving multiple columnated beams of gamma rays, the gamma knife) is now employed for the majority of patients, inducing endarteritis obliterans in the nidus of the lesion. Both surgery and stereotactic radiosurgery may be facilitated by prior embolization.

*Sturge–Weber syndrome** is an association between a port-wine stain localized to one or more segments of the cutaneous distribution of the trigeminal nerve with a corresponding extensive venous angioma (which may cause contralateral focal fits).

Hydrocephalus

The circulation of CSF

CSF is produced by the choroid plexuses of the lateral, third and fourth ventricles. It escapes from the fourth ventricle through the median foramen of Magendie and the lateral foramina of Luschka into the cerebral subarachnoid space. About 80% of the fluid is reabsorbed via the cranial arachnoid villi. The remaining 20% of the CSF is absorbed by the spinal arachnoid villi or escapes along the nerve sheaths into the lymphatics.

Obstruction along the CSF pathway produces a rise in pressure and dilatation within the system proximal to the block. Hydrocephalus may be classified according to whether the block occurs within the ventricular system or outside it.

Non-communicating or obstructive hydrocephalus

CSF cannot escape from within the brain to the basal cisterns. This may be due to congenital

*William Allen Sturge (1850–1919), Physician, Royal Free Hospital, London. Frederick Parkes Weber (1863–1962), Physician, London.

narrowing of the aqueduct of Sylvius or the Arnold–Chiari malformation, which is a congenital downward protrusion of the cerebellum into the foramen magnum (with consequent occlusion of the foramina of the fourth ventricle) frequently associated with spina bifida. It may also be acquired as a result of cerebral abscess or tumour either within or adjacent to a ventricle.

Communicating hydrocephalus

CSF can escape from within the brain but absorption via the villi is prevented as a result of the obliteration of subarachnoid channels. It may be congenital as a result of failure of development of the arachnoid villi, or it may be secondary to meningitis or bleeding into the subarachnoid space (head injury, aneurysm rupture, arterio-venous malformation).

Clinical features

Clinically, hydrocephalus may be divided into two important groups. The first is the acquired variety, which presents with features of raised intracranial pressure described on page 97. The second comprises the congenital hydrocephalics who show the characteristic picture of enlargement of the skull (comparison should be made with the size of an infant's skull of the same age obtained from standard charts), over which the scalp is stretched with dilated cutaneous veins. The fontanelles are enlarged, tense and fail to close at the normal times. Typical of this condition is the downward displacement of the eyes ('sun setting') and there may be an associated squint and nystagmus. Papilloedema is not present in these cases. There may be late epilepsy, and mental impairment may be considerable where there is extensive thinning of the cerebral cortex. There may be associated congenital deformities, especially spina bifida.

In some infants with congenital hydrocephalus, natural arrest occurs, presumably as a result of recanalization of the subarachnoid spaces. In the remainder there is steady progression with inevitable mental deterioration and high mortality unless adequate treatment is instituted.

Special investigations
- *CT scan* confirms ventricular enlargement
- *Cranial ultrasound* through the fontanelle is useful in the child.

Treatment
The goal of treatment is to divert the CSF around the blockage by means of a shunt. For non-communicating (obstructive) hydrocephalus, direct removal of the occluding mass lesion is desirable.

Decompression of the hydrocephalus can be achieved by diverting CSF into the peritoneum (ventriculo-peritoneal shunt) or right atrium via the internal jugular vein (ventriculo-atrial shunt). The shunts comprise silicone catheters with a regulator valve mechanism in the middle to permit CSF flow at a certain ventricular pressure without over-drainage of the CSF.

In non-communicating (obstructive) hydrocephalus, an artificial outlet may be created through the floor of the third ventricle into the basal cisterns (endoscopic third ventriculostomy).

CHAPTER 13

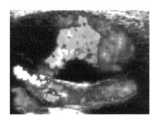

Head Injury

Head injury is a major cause of death in children and young adults. Many survivors of head injury are catastrophically disabled. Recognizing a severe head injury and administering prompt and appropriate care is important for all medical practitioners who, if not receiving patients with such injuries under their care, may nevertheless be bystanders witnessing such an injury. If presented with a patient in 'coma' other causes of unresponsiveness should be considered.

Head injuries are generally classified as closed (concussional) or open (penetrating).

Types of injury

Injuries are usefully classified according to the structures involved (scalp, skull and underlying brain) together with the mechanism of the injury, be it penetrating or blunt, and whether an acceleration/deceleration and/or a rotational brain injury occurred. In reality, isolated injuries are uncommon, and patients more typically experience blunt injury fracturing the skull in which acceleration/deceleration of the brain also occurs.

Scalp injuries

Most scalp injuries are simple penetrating injuries, which are readily managed by debridement and suture. When the skull is also penetrated, the brain may be lacerated. However, if the injury occurred when the head was stationary, in the absence of acceleration and deceleration, consciousness may not be lost and neither the patient nor the doctor may appreciate the true extent of the injury.

Skull injuries

Injuries to the skull are a result of crushing or other severe force. The skull fractures along its weakest plane, which varies according to the position of the injuring force. Typically this is a linear fracture of the skull vault, but may extend into the skull base. A simple crush injury to a stationary head may leave the scalp intact and not disturb consciousness in the absence of acceleration and deceleration forces, although the subsequent skull X-ray may show extensive fractures.

A skull fracture is most important as an indicator of the force of the injury, and the risk of intracranial haemorrhage. There are several other facets of a skull fracture that are important to note.

CAUSES OF COMA

The casualty officer is often called upon to make a diagnosis of a patient in coma. The following are the common causes to be considered, the first three groups accounting for the great majority of cases.
- Central nervous system:
  (a) trauma;
  (b) disease (e.g. cerebro-vascular accident (the commonest), epilepsy, subarachnoid haemorrhage, cerebral tumour, abscess, meningitis, etc.)
- Drugs etc.:
  (a) alcohol;
  (b) carbon monoxide;
  (c) barbiturates, aspirin, opiates, etc.

- Diabetes:
  (a) hyperglycaemia;
  (b) hypoglycaemia.
- Uraemia.
- Hepatic failure.
- Hypertensive encephalopathy.
- Profound toxaemia.
- Hysteria.

It is usually easy enough to determine that unconsciousness is due to trauma, but it is important to remember that a drunk or epileptic person, for example, may have struck his or her head in falling so that the condition is complicated by a head injury.

Fractures involving paranasal air sinuses: cerebrospinal fluid rhinorrhoea

Fractures extending through any of the paranasal air sinuses (frontal, ethmoid or sphenoid) communicate with the outside and are therefore compound (open) fractures, as the overlying dura is usually breached. This external communication may manifest as a runny nose, the clear cerebrospinal fluid (CSF) being rich in glucose and low in mucin content (and positive for Tau protein), compared with the normal nasal secretion, which contains no sugar and is rich in mucin. Such a connection may also be indicated by intracranial air (aerocele), or fluid in one of the sinuses on a computed tomography (CT) scan or skull X-ray. Anosmia may occur if the fracture crosses the cribriform plate. Such patients are at risk of meningitis. Some CSF leaks heal spontaneously, particularly those involving the temporal bone, but a persistent leak will require dural repair.

Fractures of the petrous temporal bone: CSF otorrhoea or rhinorrhoea

Fractures through the petrous temporal bone may result in CSF otorrhoea, as CSF passes through into the external auditory meatus either directly or via the mastoid air cells or middle ear in the presence of a ruptured tympanic membrane. If the tympanic membrane is intact, CSF rhinorrhoea occurs. Involvement of the inner ear will result in deafness. Spontaneous resolution of the leak is usual.

Depressed fractures

A localized blow drives a fragment of bone below the level of the surrounding skull vault. Such fractures are often compound, as the overlying scalp is torn. The depressed bone may be left if it is not deeply depressed (less than the skull thickness) and not otherwise troublesome. Indications for elevation include the debridement of a contaminated wound, depression greater than the bone thickness, associated intracranial haematoma or epileptic focus.

Fractures through the temporal bone: middle meningeal vessels

A fracture through the temporal bone may disrupt the middle meningeal artery and/or vein as they traverse the bone, and result in an extradural haemorrhage, which may not manifest immediately (see p. 113).

Orbital haematoma

Fractures of the anterior and middle cranial fossae are very frequently associated with orbital haematoma; blood tracks forward into the orbital tissues, into the eyelids and behind the conjunctiva. It may be difficult to differentiate this from a 'black eye', which is a superficial haematoma of the eyelid and surrounding soft tissues produced by direct injury.

An orbital haematoma is suggested by the following features:
• there is an associated subconjunctival haemorrhage, the posterior limit of which cannot be seen;
• absence of grazing of the surrounding skin;
• the haematoma is confined to the margin of the orbit (due to its fascial attachments), whereas a black eye frequently extends onto the surrounding cheek;
• there is usually an associated mild exophthalmos and a degree of ophthalmoplegia;
• the orbital haematoma is usually bilateral.

There may also be some confusion in making a diagnosis between a subconjunctival and conjunctival haemorrhage. The *subconjunctival haemorrhage* extends from the orbit forwards deep to the conjunctiva; there is therefore no posterior limit to the haemorrhage. A *conjunctival haemorrhage* results from a direct blow on the eye and produces a small haematoma clearly delimited on the conjunctiva itself.

Brain injuries

Brain injury can be divided into *primary brain injury*, occurring directly as a result of trauma, and *secondary brain injury*, which occurs later as a result of hypoxia, hypercapnia, ischaemia, intracranial haemorrhage or meningitis.

Primary brain injury may have several components, which, apart from direct penetrating injuries, are the result of the brain being relatively mobile within the skull and it being violently forced into sudden acceleration and deceleration. These result in both diffuse and local effects.

Diffuse brain injury

Diffuse neuronal injury occurs as a result of

PHYSICAL SIGNS OF SKULL FRACTURES

Anterior fossa
• Nasal bleeding.
• Orbital haematoma (see text).
• Cerebrospinal fluid rhinorrhoea.
• Cranial nerve injuries, nerves I to VI.

Middle fossa
• Orbital haematoma.
• Bleeding from the ear.
• Cerebrospinal fluid otorrhoea (rare).
• Cranial nerve injuries, nerves VII and VIII.

Posterior fossa
• Bruising over the suboccipital region, which develops after a day or two (Battle's sign).
• Cranial nerve injuries—nerves IX, X and XI (rare).

---

shearing movements, the worst being rotational shearing, as occurs when a blow is delivered off centre. The result is axon damage and rupture of the small vessels, particularly serious in the brain stem. A severe rotational shearing force may be transmitted down along the axis of the brain, and such forces shearing through the brain stem are usually fatal.

Localized brain injury
Local brain damage occurs as the brain impacts against the skull.

Coup and contre-coup (Fig. 13.1)
The direct impact of the brain on the skull at the site of injury and the contre-coup injury as it rebounds against the opposite wall of the skull results in oedema and bruising at the sites of impact. Common sites of impaction are the frontal lobes in the anterior fossa and temporal lobes within the middle fossa, with contrecoup to the occipital lobes.

Laceration within the skull
The brain may impinge on sharp bony edges within the skull, such as the sphenoid ridge, and sustain a laceration.

COUP AND CONTRE-COUP

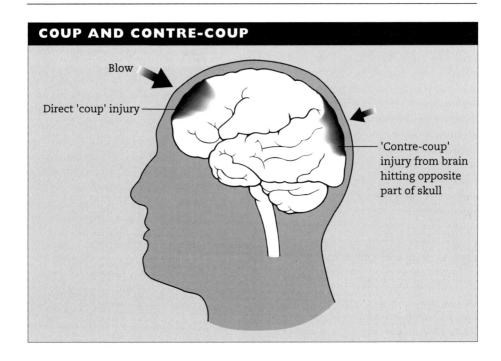

Blow

Direct 'coup' injury

'Contre-coup' injury from brain hitting opposite part of skull

Fig. 13.1 Coup and contre-coup injuries— mechanism.

Cerebral perfusion

Understanding the mechanisms underlying the regulation of cerebral perfusion, and how these may be affected in trauma, is important in the management of head-injury victims. The main regulatory factors are described below.

Systemic arterial pressure

Cerebral perfusion is normally autoregulated by the vasoactive cerebral arterioles to maintain constant cerebral blood flow over a wide range of systemic blood pressures. If systemic arterial pressure falls, cerebral vasodilatation occurs to compensate; a further fall may exceed the arterioles' ability to compensate, and cerebral ischaemia occurs.

Intracranial pressure

Since the skull is a closed compartment, a rise in intracranial pressure (ICP) will reduce the cerebral perfusion pressure.

Cerebral perfusion pressure $= BP - ICP$

where BP is blood pressure. The flow of blood to the brain is autoregulated until the perfusion pressure is around 40 mmHg. A rise in ICP coupled with hypotension in trauma victims with head injuries reduces cerebral blood flow, and the resultant ischaemia affecting the cardio-respiratory centres in the floor of the fourth ventricle leads to reflex increase in systemic pressure and bradycardia — the Cushing reflex.* Hence, hypotension in head-injury victims is seldom due to the head injury.

Cerebro-vascular resistance

The cerebral arterioles can compensate for alterations in systemic blood pressure by altering vascular tone. The arterioles are sensitive

*Harvey Cushing (1869–1939), Professor of Surgery, Harvard Medical School, Boston, USA. One of the founders of neurosurgery.

to the presence of vasoactive mediators, the most important being pH, and its proxy, $P\text{co}_2$. Increase in arterial $P\text{co}_2$ (hypercapnia) causes cerebral vasodilatation. If reduction in cerebral blood volume is required therapeutically, e.g. in the treatment of post-traumatic cerebral oedema, elective hyperventilation with its resultant hypocapnia is often performed. Conversely, hypercapnia in the presence of oedema may further raise intracranial pressure and result in exacerbation of the brain injury, one of the causative factors in *secondary brain injury*.

Management of the patient with a head injury

The management of a patient with a head injury can be divided into:
• initial assessment;
• immediate management;
• delayed management.
In practice, the initial assessment and immediate management frequently overlap according to clinical priorities.

Initial assessment
The initial assessment is an active process and not just a period of history taking. However, the history is most important, in particular the account of a witness, as most victims of major head injuries are unable to give an accurate history.

History
Important points to note in the history are:
• *The mechanism of the injury.* This may enable some prediction as to the likely injuries, both visible and within the cranium. The nature of the injurious force and its direction relative to the recipient are important.
• *The immediate condition of the injured person.* What was the patient like immediately after the injury? In particular, note the level of consciousness in terms of an accepted scale such as the Glasgow coma scale (see below), as well as other vital signs (pulse, respiration,

blood pressure), the size and reaction of the pupils, and recorded limb movements (was the patient moving his or her legs after the accident?).
• *Any change in the condition of the injured person.* As well as establishing the patient's condition when first seen after the injury, it is also important to establish whether the condition has changed at all. For example, if the patient was talking and moving all limbs and is now comatose it suggests an intracranial mass lesion such as an intracranial haemorrhage is developing.
• *The prior condition of the injured person.* As much history about the injured as possible should be obtained from relatives and friends. Was the patient drunk at the time? Is the patient diabetic and so could the coma be hypoglycaemic? Does the patient have a glass eye or is he or she on treatment for chronic glaucoma to account for the absence of pupillary responses?

Examination
Your examination should reassess the patient's conscious level to decide whether the condition has worsened or improved, and look for associated injuries, in particular major occult injuries such as a tension pneumothorax or fractured spine. In patients with major injuries, the priorities for examination are usually quoted in terms of the ABC of resuscitation, to which may be added an additional C.
• *Airway.* Is the airway clear without obstruction such as vomitus or blood? If the patient is not maintaining the airway, intubation with an endotracheal tube should be performed. Occasionally, this may not be possible and a tracheostomy may be required.
• *Breathing.* Is the patient breathing spontaneously, or should ventilation be instituted? Controlled hyperventilation may be desirable to reduce intracranial pressure (see p. 97). An arterial blood sample for estimation of oxygen carriage should be taken as soon as convenient, and the patient should be monitored by pulse oximeter to ensure adequate haemoglobin saturation.

• *Circulation.* The patient's pulse and blood pressure should be taken and monitored. Raised intracranial pressure results in bradycardia and hypertension (Cushing reflex, see p. 108). *Hypotension is rarely due to head injury* and an alternative cause should be sought (a ruptured spleen, a haemothorax or a fractured pelvis for example). Occasionally, extensive scalp bleeding may result in hypotension, as may a head injury in a child.

• *Cervical spine.* Every patient who sustains a head injury should be considered to have a cervical spine injury as well until proved otherwise by good-quality radiography or computed tomography (CT) scan. The neck should therefore be immobilized in a hard collar.

Following the initial ABC, a full central nervous system (CNS) examination should be performed as well as complete examination of the chest, abdomen and limbs. Particular atten-tion should be paid to the parts that are usually forgotten, including examining the back for evidence of trauma and integrity of the spine, and a rectal examination with particular attention to anal tone (or its absence in spinal injury), and the position of the prostate in the male (a ruptured urethra results in a displaced prostate).

Special investigations

With respect to the head injury there are three immediate investigations that may be indicated.

1 *Skull X-ray.* Indicated wherever a period of loss of consciousness occurred.

2 *Cervical spine X-ray* in all unconscious patients following head injury.

3 *CT scan.* With the wide availability of CT scanning, most patients with severe head injuries can undergo a CT scan on admission. The resulting images may then be viewed

---

INDICATIONS FOR ADMISSION FOLLOWING A HEAD INJURY

• Confusion or impaired conscious level (Glasgow coma scale <15) at the time of examination.
• Skull fracture.
• Neurological symptoms or signs, including headache and fits.
• Difficulty in assessing patient, particularly children and those under the influence of alcohol.
• Complicating medical condition other than head injury.

• Lack of responsible adult to supervise patient, or other adverse social conditions.

Notes
• Patients who are discharged home should be given written instructions about the possible complications and what action should be taken.
• Post-traumatic amnesia with full recovery is not considered an indication for admission.

INDICATIONS FOR CT/NEUROSURGICAL CONSULTATION

• Fractured skull with confusion, impaired conscious level, focal neurological signs, fits, any other neurological symptoms.
• Depressed skull fracture or suspected penetrating injury.
• Persisting confusion or impaired conscious level.

• Deteriorating conscious level.
• Compound fracture of skull.
• Basal fracture of skull (possibly indicated by cerebrospinal fluid rhinorrhoea or otorrhoea).

locally, or transmitted to a regional neurosurgical centre for specialist opinion.

Immediate management

Skull X-ray, admission to hospital, CT scanning and neurosurgical referral should all be considered. The immediate management of complicated cases will include correcting any problems identified in the initial assessment, such as draining a pneumothorax, instituting ventilation if the patient is unable to maintain the airway or to breathe, and performing a laparotomy and/or orthopaedic procedures where appropriate.

Following the initial brain injury, further deterioration may be due to:

- *increasing cerebral oedema* as the brain swells consequent upon the damage it sustained;
- *intracranial haemorrhage*, either extradural, subdural or intracerebral haemorrhage;
- *hypoxia*, due to impaired ventilation or ischaemia;
- *infection*, secondary to compound fractures including fractures involving the paranasal sinuses or petrous temporal bone;
- *hydrocephalus*, either communicating or non-communicating.

Delayed management

With respect to the head injury, there follows a period of observation, with attention paid to the following:

- *conscious level*, according to the Glasgow coma scale;
- *pupil size and responses*—dilatation of a pupil, loss of response to light or asymmetry are late signs of increasing intracranial pressure;
- *vital signs* — pulse, blood pressure, temperature, oxygen saturation.

The conscious level: the Glasgow coma scale

Vague terms such as comatose, semicomatose, unconscious, stuporose, etc., should be avoided; they may be of value to a psychiatrist but not to a surgeon. Instead, the conscious level is charted according to the patient's motor, verbal and eye-opening responses to stimuli; these are very much the reactions of a patient recovering from deep anaesthesia. The best recognized scale is the Glasgow coma scale in which the responses within each group are allotted a score, the normal being 15. In each group a higher score is given to a more appropriate response. A score of 15 is normal. A mild head injury may score 13, a severe injury 8 or less.

Pupil size and responses

If a cerebral hemisphere is pressed upon by an enlarging blood clot, the third cranial nerve on that side becomes compressed by descent of the hippocampal gyrus over the edge of the tentorium cerebelli. Paralysis of the third nerve (which transmits parasympathetic pupilloconstrictor fibres) results in dilatation of the corresponding pupil (due to the intact unopposed sympathetic supply) and failure of the pupil to respond to light. An important sign of cerebral compression is, therefore, dilatation and loss of light reaction of the pupil on the affected side, although occasionally pupillary dilatation will be a false localizing sign and will be on the side opposite the mass lesion. Because the optic nerve pathway is intact, a light shone into this unreacting pupil produces constriction in the opposite pupil (consensual reaction to light). As compression continues, the contralateral third nerve becomes compressed, and the opposite pupil in turn dilates and becomes fixed to light. Bilateral fixed dilated pupils in a patient with head injury indicates very great cerebral compression from which the patient rarely recovers. Occasionally, local trauma to the nerves from extensive skull-base fractures may produce the same findings.

Pulse, respiration and blood pressure

With increasing intracranial pressure, the pulse slows and the blood pressure rises (Cushing reflex, see p. 108), the respirations become stertorious and eventually Cheyne–Stokes* in nature.

*John Cheyne (1777–1836), an Edinburgh-trained Physician who migrated to Ireland. William Stokes (1804–78), Physician, Meath Hospital, Dublin, Ireland.

THE GLASGOW COMA SCALE (GCS)

Eye opening
4 Spontaneously.
3 To speech/command.
2 To pain.
1 None.

Best verbal response
5 Orientated—knows who he or she is and where he or she is.
4 Confused conversation—disorientated; gives confused answers to questions.
3 Inappropriate words—random words; no conversation.
2 Incomprehensible sounds.
1 None.

Best motor response
6 Obeys commands.
5 Localizes pain.
4 Flexes to pain—flexion withdrawal of limb to painful stimulus.
3 Abnormal (decorticate) flexion—upper limb adducts, flexes and internally rotates so that it lies across chest; lower limbs extend (Fig. 13.2).
2 Extends to pain (decerebrate)—painful stimulus causes extension of all limbs.
1 None.

When assessing the GCS it is very important that an adequate stimulus is applied.

BRAIN INJURY POSTURES

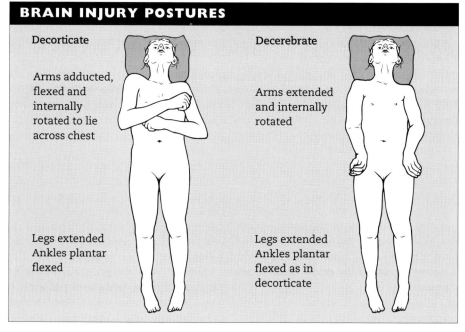

Decorticate

Arms adducted, flexed and internally rotated to lie across chest

Legs extended
Ankles plantar flexed

Decerebrate

Arms extended and internally rotated

Legs extended
Ankles plantar flexed as in decorticate

Fig. 13.2 Decerebrate and decorticate postures.

Nursing care of the unconscious patient
The airway
The most important single factor in the care of the deeply unconscious patient, whatever the cause, who has lost the cough reflex is the maintenance of the airway. The patient is transported and nursed in the recovery position, i.e. on one side with the body tilted head downwards, which allows the tongue to fall forward and bronchial secretions or vomit to drain from the mouth rather than be inhaled. Suction may be required to remove excessive secretions or vomit from the pharynx.

An endotracheal tube may be necessary if the airway is not satisfactory and if after some days it is still difficult to maintain an adequate airway tracheostomy may be required.

Restlessness
Opiates, particularly morphine, are generally contraindicated, as they will depress respiration, disguise the level of consciousness and will also produce constricted pupils, which may mask a valuable physical sign. Paracetamol, barbiturates or codeine preparations may be necessary but often all that is required is to protect the patient from self-injury by judicious restraint and padding.

A cause of restlessness may be a distended bladder; often if the retention is relieved the patient will then calm down.

Feeding
Many cases of head injury died in the past due to dehydration and starvation. Oro-gastric feeding is instituted if the patient remains unable to swallow. A naso-gastric tube is contraindicated in patients with cranio-facial injuries because of the danger of intracranial penetration.

Skin care
A deeply unconscious patient is liable to bed sores. Careful nursing care and the use of an intermittently inflatable mattress are required for their prevention.

Sphincters
The unconscious patient may be incontinent, and the resultant excoriation of the skin makes the patient still more liable to pressure sores. The use of Paul's tubing on the penis or of an indwelling catheter in the female patient will help in the nursing care. Retention of urine may require catheter relief.

Indications for surgery in head injuries
Early
- The excision and suture of scalp lacerations.
- Surgical toilet of a compound fracture.
- Cerebral decompression and evacuation of the haematoma for intracranial bleeding.

Delayed
- Repair of a dural tear with CSF rhinorrhoea.
- Late repair of skull defects.
- Late plastic surgery for deforming facial injuries.

Traumatic intracranial bleeding

Classification
Haemorrhage within the skull following injury may be classified as follows.
1 Extradural.
2 Subdural:
   (a) acute;
   (b) chronic.
3 Subarachnoid.
4 Intracerebral.
5 Intraventricular.

Extradural haemorrhage
This is sometimes wrongly named 'middle meningeal haemorrhage'. It may indeed arise from a tear of the middle meningeal artery, but an extradural collection of blood may also develop from a laceration of one of the other meningeal vessels, from the torn sagittal sinus or oozing from the diploë, bone and stripped dura mater on each side of any associated fracture (Fig. 13.3a).

Clinical features

The classic story is of a relatively minor head injury producing temporary concussion, recovery ('the lucid period') then, some hours later, the development of headache and progressively deeper coma due to cerebral compression by the extradural clot. This picture may give rise to the tragedies of the drunk who is put into the cells for the night and is found dead in the morning, or the cricketer who goes home to bed after being mildly concussed by a cricket ball and perishes during the evening. It is important to note, however, that this classic picture is *not* as common as is thought. Often there is no lucid period; the patient progressively passes into deeper coma from the time of the initial injury.

The physical signs are those of rapidly increasing intracranial pressure, which have already been discussed (p. 97).

In addition, there are certain localizing signs that may help the surgeon decide on which side to explore the skull. These are as follows.

Fig. 13.3 (a) Extradural haematoma and (b) acute subdural haematoma. The latter is usually associated with a severe brain injury.

- The pupils: a good neurosurgical aphorism is 'explore the side of the dilated pupil' (see p. 111). In 10% of patients the dilated pupil will be a false localizing sign.
- Hemiparesis or hemiplegia (common) or Jacksonian fits (uncommon) usually indicate contralateral compression.
- A boggy haematoma of the scalp usually overlies the extradural clot.

Special investigations

- *CT scan* is diagnostic and allows accurate localization of the position and of the size of the clot.
- *Skull X-ray* may be entirely normal. However, the clot tends to be on the side of the fracture, if one is visible. A calcified pineal gland may be seen to be pushed over from the midline in a good antero-posterior film.

Treatment

An extradural haemorrhage is one of the few surgical emergencies where minutes really can matter. If a neurosurgeon is available a bone flap will be turned over the clot. Alternatively, a burr-hole is made over the suspected site of the clot, the opening enlarged with nibbling forceps and the clot evacuated. The major

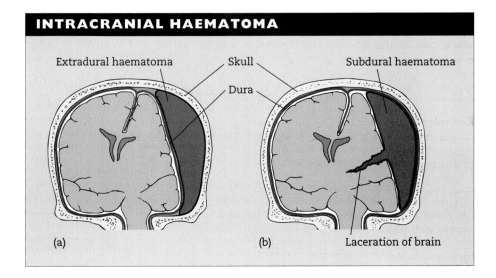

INTRACRANIAL HAEMATOMA

Extradural haematoma   Skull   Subdural haematoma

Dura

(a)   (b)   Laceration of brain

bleeding point on the dura is controlled either with diathermy, silver clips or by underrunning. Bleeding from the bone edges is plugged by means of bone wax.

Subdural haematoma (Fig. 13.3b)
Acute
This results from bleeding into the subdural space from lacerated brain or torn vessels. It is usually part of a severe head injury. The patient is frequently in deep coma from the moment of injury but the condition deteriorates still further.

Treatment
Release of the subdural clot through a craniotomy may give some improvement in the neurological state, but the outcome may be poor because of the severity of the underlying brain trauma.

Chronic subdural haematoma or hygroma
This follows a trivial (often forgotten) injury, usually in an elderly patient, sustained weeks or months before. There is a small tear in a cerebral vein as it traverses the subdural space. Whenever the patient coughs, strains or bends over a little blood extravasates. The resulting haematoma becomes encapsulated; as the clot breaks down, smaller molecules are formed with a rise in the osmotic pressure within the haematoma. Consequent absorption of tissue fluid produces gradual enlargement of the local collection, which may comprise liquid blood, clot or clear yellow fluid (hygroma).

Clinical features
Clinical features are those of a developing intracranial mass lesion. There is mental deterioration, headaches, vomiting and drowsiness, which progresses to coma. Moderate papilloedema is seen in about half the cases. The condition is indeed often confused with an intracerebral tumour but contrast-enhanced CT scanning will demonstrate the outline of the clot.

Treatment
Treatment comprises the evacuation of the clot through burr-holes.

Subarachnoid haemorrhage
Clinical features
Blood in the CSF after head injury is incidental, not surprisingly, to most severe head injuries and gives the clinical picture of meningeal irritability with headache, neck stiffness and a positive Kernig's sign. There may be a mild pyrexia.

Treatment
Analgesics and bed rest are required until the severe headache has subsided; rapid rehabilitation follows.

Intracerebral haemorrhage
Scattered small haemorrhages throughout the brain substance are a common post-mortem finding in severe head injuries and may be demonstrated at CT scanning in extensive cerebral injury. At other times a clot may develop within the brain substance often in the frontal or temporal lobes. If it is exerting mass effect and the intracranial pressure is high, the haematoma is evacuated and the injured lobe may have to be removed.

Intraventricular haemorrhage
Haemorrhage into a ventricle may occur from tearing of the choroid plexus at the time of injury or rupture of an intracerebral clot into the ventricle. It occurs particularly in childhood and is usually part of an overwhelming head injury.

Other complications

Meningitis
Infection of the meninges may complicate a fracture of the skull which is compound, either directly to the exterior or via a dural tear into the nasal or aural cavities (see p. 106).

Confirmation of the diagnosis of meningitis is the only positive indication for performing a lumbar puncture on a patient with a head injury.

Treatment

The treatment of established meningitis is antibiotic therapy. Infection via the nasal route is probably due to *Pneumococcus*; here penicillin should be the first drug of choice. For infection complicating a compound fracture, a second-generation cephalosporin (e.g. cefuroxime) should be used in the first instance, as this readily passes the blood–brain barrier. The antibiotic may have to be changed when the sensitivity of the organism obtained on lumbar puncture becomes known.

Hyperpyrexia

The temperature of a patient with severe brain-stem injury may soar to 40°C (105°F) or more as a result of injury to the heat-regulating centre. This is a serious complication and must be treated vigorously by means of cooling blankets.

Late complications

Post-concussional syndrome

Neurosis following a head injury is not uncommon. Unless reassured and rapidly rehabilitated, the patient who has had concussion is easily led to believe that the brain has been damaged and that he or she will never be fit to lead a normal life again.

Amnesia

Some idea of the severity of the injury is given by the period of amnesia, both the retrograde amnesia up to the time of the accident and the post-traumatic amnesia following injury. If the period of amnesia amounts to only minutes or a few hours the ultimate prognosis is good. Amnesia of several days or even weeks indicates a severe injury and poor prognosis for return of full mental function.

Epilepsy

Persistent epilepsy may complicate penetrating compound wounds with resultant cortical scarring. In such cases anticonvulsant therapy,

e.g. phenytoin, is given for at least 6 months following injury. Established post-traumatic epilepsy is treated medically by means of anti-convulsants. Occasionally, success may follow excision of a cortical scar.

Brain death

The medical and nursing care of patients with severe brain damage due to trauma, haemorrhage or intracranial tumour is now so good that the doctors and nurses are often faced with the sad case of a patient whose brain is completely and irreversibly destroyed, but whose heart and circulation are intact, provided the lungs are mechanically ventilated. This state of affairs may persist for some weeks with severe distress to the patient's relatives and to the ward staff.

The diagnosis of brain death depends on the demonstration of permanent and irreversible destruction of brain-stem function. The tests must be performed by two people with experience in the diagnosis of brain-stem death. *All brain-stem reflexes should be absent.* The following should first be excluded before tests for brain-stem death can be performed:

- hypothermia;
- intoxication;
- sedative drugs;
- neuromuscular blocking drugs;
- severe electrolyte and acid–base abnormalities.

In addition, there must be a clearly identified cause of death, which is usually obvious in the presence of head injury but may be less clear in other circumstances. The specific features of brain-stem death are as follows.

- The patient is in a coma and on a ventilator.
- The pupils are dilated and do not respond to direct or consensual light.
- There is no corneal reflex.
- Vestibulo-ocular (doll's eye) reflexes are absent, such that when the head is passively turned the eyes remained fixed relative to the head.

• Caloric reflexes are absent. These are tested by slow injection of 20 ml of ice-cold water into each external auditory meatus in turn, clear access to the tympanic membrane having been established by direct inspection. If no eye movement occurs during or after the test, it is considered positive.

• No motor responses within the cranial nerve distribution can be elicited by adequate stimulation of any somatic area.

• There is no gag reflex response to bronchial stimulation by a suction catheter passed down the trachea.

• No respiratory movements occur when the patient is disconnected from the mechanical ventilator for long enough to ensure that the arterial CO_2 tension rises above the threshold for stimulating respiration, i.e. the Pa_{CO_2} must normally reach 7 kPa (50 mmHg).

If this situation persists over a period of observation and is confirmed by a second practitioner, death can be certified. The period of observation depends upon the age of the patient (child or adult) and the cause of the coma.

The decision to stop mechanical ventilation rests on the above factors. Once this decision has been made, the possibility of the patient becoming an organ donor for transplantation should be considered. This should be discussed fully and sympathetically with available relatives so that their informed consent is obtained for the removal of organs.

CHAPTER 14

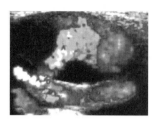

The Spine

Spina bifida

The neural tube develops by an infolding of the neural ectoderm to become the spinal cord. The surrounding meninges and vertebral column derive from mesodermal tissue. Failure of embryonic fusion may result in the following anomalies.

• *Spina bifida occulta*: failure of the vertebral arch fusion only; meninges and nervous tissue normal. It occurs in 10% of the population.
• *Meningocele*: a cystic protrusion of the meninges through a posterior vertebral defect without nervous tissue involvement.
• *Myelomeningocele*: neural tissue (the cord or spinal roots) protrudes into, and may be adherent to, the meningeal sac.
• *Myelocele (rachischisis)*: failure of fusion of the neural tube; an open spinal plate occupies the defect as a red, granular area weeping cerebrospinal fluid (CSF) from its centre.

Ante-natal screening (presence of high levels of α-fetoprotein in the amniotic fluid, and ultrasound) enables a high degree of accuracy in intra-uterine diagnosis of neural tube defects, and gives the opportunity for termination of the pregnancy. The number of infants born with severe spinal abnormalities has, in consequence, greatly declined. The incidence of open spina bifida (meningocele, myelomeningocele and myelocele) is 1 in 1000 births.

Clinical features

These defects are particularly common in the lumbo-sacral area, although any part of the spine may be involved. There may be an associated overlying lipoma, tuft of hair or skin dimple, which may be an important clue to the astute clinician of the underlying defect. Where nervous tissue is involved there may be paraparesis, paraplegia, sensory disturbances in the limbs and loss of sphincter control.

Hydrocephalus nearly always coexists with the myelomeningocele due to the *Arnold–Chiari malformation*,* in which the cerebellar tonsils descend below the foramen magnum with consequent obstruction of the CSF pathway.

As with any other congenital deformity there may be multiple developmental anomalies, e.g. congenital dislocation of the hip, talipes equinovarus, cleft lip or palate, cardiac lesions or supernumerary digits.

Spina bifida occulta is usually an incidental finding noted on X-ray. Where overlying skin changes (dimple, hair tuft, lipoma, sinus) are present, the cord beneath may be tethered to the skin by a fibrous band, and as the child grows weakness in the legs may occur with

---

*Julius Arnold (1835–1915), Professor of Pathology, Heidelberg, Germany. Hans von Chiari (1851–1916), Viennese pathologist successively Professor at Strasbourg and Prague.

sensory loss, pes cavus, or difficulty with bladder and bowel sphincters — 'the tethered cord syndrome'.

Treatment

Minor degrees of spina bifida are left alone unless there is a risk of tethering or infection. Skin-covered lesions require only cosmetic surgery. All cases with an exposed neural plate should be repaired within a few hours of birth to prevent meningitis. Associated hydrocephalus should be drained within the next 1 or 2 weeks provided there is no ascending meningitis. Surgery to improve bladder function and to correct orthopaedic limb problems arising as a result of spasticity or paralysis is often required as the child grows. The most grossly malformed are better left untreated.

Spinal injuries

Spinal injuries have two components — the bony injury and the neurological injury — both of which must be considered in all patients with spinal trauma.

The bony injury

The bony injury may comprise either a fracture or dislocation, or a combination (fracture dislocation). The most important consideration is the stability of the fracture. A *stable fracture* is one that is unlikely to undergo further displacement in contrast to an *unstable fracture*, which may undergo further displacement with the risk of further neurological damage.

Assessing stability

The assessment of stability is fundamental to the initial management of the patient. It depends upon the integrity of the structures that make up the normal spinal column, namely the vertebrae, intervertebral discs and ligaments. While it is relatively easy to determine stability in upper cervical fractures, it is less easy in lower fractures such as thoraco-lumbar

fractures. To overcome this, the concept of the three-column spine is useful (Fig. 14.1). The three columns are made up as follows.

The anterior column

The anterior longitudinal ligament, the anterior annulus fibrosus and the anterior part of the vertebral body.

The middle column

The posterior longitudinal ligament, posterior annulus fibrosus and the posterior part of the vertebral body.

The posterior column

The posterior arch and the intervening ligament complex, itself comprising supraspinous ligaments, interspinous ligaments and ligamentum flavium.

Disruption of two or all of these columns results in spinal instability. Disruption of a single column, such as in a wedge fracture, affects the anterior half of the vertebral body and so is a stable injury without risk of further displacement or further neurological damage.

Types of fractures

Most fractures are caused by a sudden hyperextension or hyperflexion, often combined with compression or distraction. The results of such forces may be considered in terms of five distinct levels in the spine.

1 *Upper cervical (C1, C2).* In the upper cervical spine, flexion/extension injuries may result in fracture of the dens (odontoid process) at its base, atlanto-axial dislocation or fracture of the atlas or axis (hangman's fracture). The spinal canal is wide in the upper cervical region and immediate spinal cord damage may be minor, although in more severe injuries fatal damage to the cord may occur.

2 *Lower cervical (C3 to C7). Hyperflexion* injuries may result in anterior dislocation of facet joints, with consequent narrowing of the spinal canal and neurological injury. A corresponding step may be seen on a lateral cervical spine X-ray. Either one or both facet joints may be

THE THREE-COLUMN SPINE

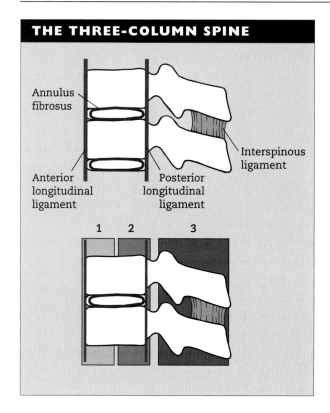

Annulus fibrosus

Interspinous ligament

Anterior longitudinal ligament

Posterior longitudinal ligament

1 2 3

Fig. 14.1 The three-column spine concept.

involved. Because of the much closer fit of the cervical cord within the vertebral canal compared with the wider lumbar region, the incidence of cord damage in these injuries is extremely high, with resultant tetraplegia or paraplegia. If the facet joints do not lock there may be spontaneous reduction and little to see on a lateral X-ray, although complete transection of the cord may have occurred. *Hyperextension* may result in rupture of the anterior longitudinal ligament and disc with backward displacement of the vertebral body to narrow the spinal canal and impinge on the cord, before springing back. *Compression*, when combined with flexion, may result in a wedge-shaped fracture of the vertebral body. Severe compression injuries may result in a comminuted fracture with fragments encroaching on the spinal canal.

3 *Thoracic.* The thoracic spine is relatively stable due to the splinting afforded by the rib cage and sternum. Pathological fractures, commonly a result of osteoporosis or secondary tumour, are more common in this region.

4 *Thoraco-lumbar.* The thoraco-lumbar junction is relatively unsupported, and liable to injuries caused by flexion, rotation and compression. Such injuries may follow a fall from a height landing on the feet or the buttocks, or forward flexion of the spine in a decelerating car crash, or a heavy weight falling on the shoulders.

5 *Lumbar. Compression* injuries may cause wedge-shaped fractures where the body of the vertebra collapses. *Burst fractures*, with comminution of the vertebral body and hence disruption of anterior and middle columns may occur following axial compression and result in an unstable fracture, often with cord or cauda equina damage if bone fragments encroach into the canal. Such fractures are often associated with crushing of the intervertebral disc.

In practice, the commonest fractures are those in the cervical and thoraco-lumbar regions.

Clinical features

There is the typical history of injury followed by localized pain, bruising, tenderness and often a kyphus. Careful neurological examination is imperative (see below).

It is obligatory to examine every head injury for suspected spinal fracture, as this is easily overlooked in the unconscious patient. Unskilled handling of such a case may produce an irreparable spinal injury.

Special investigations

• *Spine X-ray*. The exact type of fracture is usually shown. Lateral films are the most important. Cervical spine films should show all seven cervical vertebra *and* T1, with additional special views (such as a swimmer's view or an oblique view) to show the lower vertebrae, and an open-mouth view to show the dens.
• *Computed tomography (CT) scan* to confirm a fracture and demonstrate the extent of comminution.
• *Magnetic resonance imaging (MRI)* to assess injury to the intervertebral disc or cord.

The neurological injury
Mechanism of cord injury
Cord compression

The cord may be compressed by bone, intervertebral disc or haematoma. This is particularly common where a previous abnormality exists, such as congenital spinal stenosis or cervical spondylosis. Facet joint dislocation, where the cord is trapped in the narrow canal at the level of the dislocation, is another common example.

Direct injury

Open injuries, or shards of fractured bone may penetrate the neural canal and lacerate the cord.

Ischaemia

A vascular insult to the spinal vessels may result in cord damage, and may be delayed and exacerbated by cord oedema and haematoma.

Types of neurological injury
Spinal concussion

Nervous continuity is not lost, paraplegia is only partial and recovery commences within a few hours. Full return of function can be anticipated.

Cord transection

Loss of function due to anatomical division of the cord is irrecoverable, as the axons within the cord have no power of regeneration. There is an initial period of spinal shock with complete flaccid paralysis below the line of cord section, loss of tendon reflexes, atonicity of the bladder (which becomes distended), faecal retention and priapism. This phase generally lasts for a few days. The cord below the line of transection then recovers reflex function so that the paralysis becomes spastic with muscle spasms, the plantar responses become extensor and bladder and bowel commence to empty reflexly.

Cauda equina injury

This may complicate fractures below the level of termination of the spinal cord at the lower border of the first lumbar vertebra. There is saddle anaesthesia (over the buttocks, anus and perineum), weakness of the lower leg muscles, absent ankle reflexes and urinary retention. The cauda equina are the roots of peripheral nerves and therefore possess the power of regeneration providing that continuity of the nerve trunk is not lost. However, recovery is rarely complete if compression occurs for more than a few hours.

Combined cord and cauda equina injury

As many spinal injuries take place at the thoraco-lumbar junction, there is usually a combination of spinal cord and nerve-root injury. For example, a fracture dislocation at

EXAMINING NEUROLOGICAL INJURY

The examination of nerve injuries requires testing for sensation, power and reflexes. The components of sensation include light touch, vibration and joint position sense (dorsal columns), and temperature and pain (spino-thalamic tract). Abnormalities should be noted in relation to both dermatome and, in the case of peripheral nerve injuries, innervation.

Motor responses should be examined in relation to spinal level or peripheral nerve according to injury.

Movement	Muscle responsible	Innervation
Arm abduction	Deltoid	C5,6
Elbow flexion	Biceps	C5,6
Wrist extension	Forearm extensors	C6,7
Elbow extension	Triceps	C7,8
Finger abduction	Intrinsic muscles of hand	C8,T1
Hip flexion	Iliopsoas	L2,3
Knee extension	Quadriceps femoris	L2,3,4
Foot dorsiflexion	Tibialis anterior, extensor hallucis longus, extensor digitorum longus	L4,5
Knee flexion	Hamstrings	L5,S1
Hallux extension	Extensor hallucis longus	L5,S1
Foot plantar flexion	Gastrocnemius and soleus	S1,2
Anal tone	Anal sphincter	S2,3,4

Motor responses should be graded according to the MRC scale:
0 Total paralysis
1 Flicker of movement
2 Active movement with gravity eliminated
3 Normal movement against gravity but not against additional resistance
4 Movement against both gravity and resistance, but still overcome
5 Normal power.

The reflexes are innervated as follows:
Biceps jerk   C5,6
Triceps jerk   C7,8
Knee jerk   L3,4
Ankle jerk   S1,2

Plantar reflex. Extension is abnormal and indicates an upper motor neurone lesion.
Two other reflexes are useful in the assessment of patients with spinal cord injuries, the presence of which suggests an incomplete cord lesion:

Bulbocavernosus reflex. Contraction of the anal sphincter in response to pinching of the penile shaft.
Anal reflex. Contraction of the anus in response to stroking of the perianal skin.

the T12/L1 junction will divide the cord at the first sacral segment but clinical examination may reveal paralysis being due to damage to the spinal roots as they pass the site of the fracture dislocation (Fig. 14.2). In this instance, the roots may recover with return of knee and hip movement, although the sacral paralysis will be permanent.

COMPONENTS OF NEUROLOGICAL INJURY

The neurological injury following spinal cord damage can be divided into three components.

Sensory loss
Somatic and visceral sensation are lost below the level of section. Hyperaesthesia may be present at the level of section.

Motor loss
Spinal cord injuries result in an upper motor neurone spastic paralysis with hyperreflexia. Cauda equina injuries, being injuries of nerve roots, produce a lower motor neurone paralysis characterized by reduced tone and areflexia.

Autonomic loss
Loss of sympathetic outflow injuries below T5 results in hypotension as a result of loss of vasomotor tone. Thermoregulation, which also depends on vasomotor activity, is also impaired. Sphincter control is also autonomic. With injuries above the level of the sacral outflow the spinal reflex arc triggering micturition remains intact so the bladder empties automatically. Injuries below this level interrupt the reflex and an atonic bladder results.

Brown-Séquard syndrome*
A penetrating injury of the spinal cord, which is unilateral and results in spastic paralysis on the compressed side (involvement of the ipsilateral pyramidial tract), loss of position and vibration sense also on the affected side (posterior column involvement), and loss of pain and temperature sensation on the opposite side to the lesion (involvement of the spinothalamic tract). Such an injury is often partial, and rarely occurs after a closed injury.

Treatment of spinal injuries
The treatment of spinal injuries depends whether or not there has been neurological injury, and also upon the stability of the fracture.

Immediate management
Spinal injury should be suspected in anyone following severe trauma or who is unconscious following trauma. In addition, patients following minor trauma with sensory or motor

*Charles Edward Brown-Séquard (1817–94), born in Mauritius, trained in Paris. Neurologist at The National Hospital for Nervous Disease, Queen's Square, London, and later Professor of Medicine at Harvard and then the Collège de France in Paris.

symptoms should be treated as possessing a spinal injury until proved otherwise. Before such a patient is moved, the neck should be immobilized in a hard collar and the patient log rolled or 'scooped' onto a stretcher for transfer. Airway management is the immediate consideration. The principles are the same as those following head injury. In addition, following spinal cord injury, loss of sympathetic tone may lead to vasodilatation and hypotension, on top of any losses as a result of trauma, so replacing circulating volume is important to prevent ischaemia.

Treatment with no neurological injury
Stable fractures of the spine are treated by bed rest for 2–3 weeks, to allow the associated soft-tissue injury to subside, followed by early exercise and active mobilization. There is no need to reduce the fracture by hyperextension and prolonged fixation; often this results in permanent residual pain.

Unstable fractures require immobilization in order to secure bony stability and thus to protect the cord from later damage. Gross instability in the presence of an incomplete neurological injury is an indication for urgent operative stabilization.

NERVE ROOT LEVELS

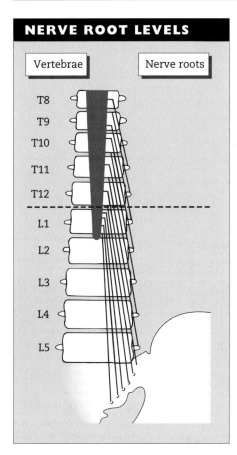

Vertebrae   Nerve roots

T8
T9
T10
T11
T12
- -
L1
L2
L3
L4
L5

Fig. 14.2 The relationship of the spinal cord and nerve roots to the vertebrae. Because of the disparity between the two, a fracture dislocation at the dorso-lumbar junction, shown here by the dotted line, will miss the lumbar cord but may transect the *sacral* segments of the cord together with injury to the *lumbar* nerve roots. (From Holdsworth.)

Unstable cervical fractures are immobilized by traction using tongs applied to the skull for 6 weeks, or are fixed by open reduction and plating. This is followed by a cervical collar for a further month. Traction may also be used to try to reduce facet joint dislocation, although open reduction may be necessary.

Unstable thoraco-lumbar fractures may be treated by operative reduction and internal fixation, or by conservative measures.

Treatment with paraplegia or tetraplegia

The patient is transported in a neutral position (so that flexion and extension are not possible), to a spinal or neurosurgical centre, the spine being supported by suitably arranged pillows and the patient being moved frequently from side to side to prevent bed-sore formation. The distended bladder is best left alone until catheterization can be carried out under full aseptic precautions to prevent infection. Methyl prednisolone should be given as early as possible and continued for 24 hours, as it has been shown to improve recovery of motor function.

The following are the main principles of treatment.

The management of the fracture. Two techniques of management may be employed. The conservative approach, favoured in most centres in the UK, comprises nursing the patient on a circo-electric bed or a Stryker frame.* This allows regular turning of the paraplegic (thus avoiding pressure sores), while keeping the fracture immobilized. This is continued for 6 weeks. Plaster casts or beds are avoided, as pressure sores are almost inevitable. Once the fracture has become stable, the patient can progress to the rehabilitation stage of treatment. The surgical approach, more often used on the Continent and in the USA, consists of open reduction and internal rod fixation of the unstable fracture.

Care of the skin. Pressure sores may develop with extraordinary rapidity in the first weeks because of the combination of anaesthesia and immobilization. Two-hourly turning, aided by use of the circo-electric bed or a Stryker frame, and meticulous skin care are required.

The bladder. In the initial phase of complete bladder paralysis, acute urinary retention is

*Homer Stryker (1894–1980), Orthopaedic Surgeon, Stryker Corporation, Kalamazoo, Michigan, USA.

common and continuous catheter drainage by means of a fine silastic urethral or suprapubic catheter is instituted. With recovery from spinal shock, the patient may develop an automatic (reflex) bladder wherein stroking the side of the thigh or abdominal compression may evoke reflex bladder emptying.

The bowels. Acute spinal injury results in paralytic ileus. Following recovery of motility, constipation is common and is best managed by regular enemata. Faecal impaction must be watched for and treated by digital evacuation.

Peptic ulceration prophylaxis. Prophylaxis with antacids, H_2-receptor antagonists, proton-pump inhibitors or sucralfate should be initiated since acute peptic ulceration is common in the early days following spinal cord injury.

Pulmonary embolism prophylaxis. Five per cent of patients with paralysis of the legs following spinal cord injury get pulmonary emboli. Prophylaxis with subcutaneous heparin should be instituted.

Rehabilitation. Active development of muscles with an intact or partial innervation by expert physiotherapy can restore mobility in 80% of paraplegic patients. However, they require callipers and crutches so that they can swing their paralysed legs by the use of abdominal, flank and shoulder muscles. At the same time vocational training can be commenced and a large percentage of these unfortunate patients can be restored to useful activity.

Degenerative spinal disorders

Degenerative spinal disorders may arise from degenerative changes in either the vertebral body, the intervertebral joints or the intervertebral discs. The resulting symptoms may arise from a combination of effects, so apophyseal joint degeneration may result in local back pain (lumbago), together with a radiculopathy

attributable to encroachment of osteophytes into the intervertebral foramen.

Neurological sequelae of spinal degeneration

- *Local pain* arises from osteoarthritis of the intervertebral joints. Backache (lumbago) in the lumbar spine, neck ache in the cervical spine.
- *Radiculopathy*, causing lower motor neurone symptoms, arises from compression and irritation of the nerve roots as they exit the intervertebral foramen. This may be due to disc or osteophyte encroachment into the intervertebral canal, and is compounded by loss of intervertebral joint space.
- *Myelopathy* causes upper motor neurone symptoms and results from compression of the spinal cord within the canal and arises from prolapse of an intervertebral disc or osteophyte encroachment into the spinal canal, and is exacerbated in the presence of a congenital narrowing of the spinal canal.
- *Claudication of the cauda equina* may arise as a result of lumbar canal stenosis. Symptoms are similar to those resulting from peripheral vascular disease, but more often occur at rest, are bilateral, and relieved by sitting rather than standing.

Prolapsed intervertebral disc

Disc herniation comprises a protrusion of the nucleus pulposus posteriorly, or more commonly postero-laterally, through a defect in the annulus fibrosus. It is probable that most ruptures are initiated by trauma, which may be severe but which is more often mild or repetitive. It is probably for this reason that the great majority of prolapsing discs occur in the active adult male.

By far the commonest sites are between L4 and L5 vertebrae, and L5 and the sacrum. Cervical disc protrusion most commonly occurs between C5 and C6 or between C6 and C7. The cervical lesion is often associated with degenerative changes in the spine and is therefore usually found in older patients than the lumbar disc prolapse.

Lumbar disc herniation

Clinical features

There is often lumbar pain early in the history, with exacerbations as a result of straining or heavy lifting. The majority of patients complain of *sciatica*, their pain being usually unilateral and radiating from the buttock along the back of the thigh and knee and then down the lateral side of the leg to the foot. This pain is aggravated by coughing, sneezing or straining (which raise the intrathecal pressure) or by straight leg raising (which stretches the sciatic nerve). Sometimes there is the complaint of weakness of ankle dorsiflexion (L5) or plantar flexion (S1). There may be paraesthesiae or numbness in the foot. A central prolapse of the lumbar disc is more devastating, producing bilateral sciatic pain, sphincter disturbance and complete or incomplete cauda equina compression.

Examination reveals flattening of the normal lumbar lordosis, scoliosis and limited spinal flexion. The erector spinae muscles are in spasm and straight leg raising is limited and painful. There may be weakness of plantar or dorsiflexion of the ankle and there may be disuse muscle wasting of the leg on the affected side. Sensory loss on the medial side of the dorsum of the foot and the great toe (L5 innervation) suggest an L4/5 disc lesion. Sensory loss on the lateral side of the foot (S1 innervation) may occur in L5/S1 disc lesions. The ankle jerk may be diminished in the latter cases.

Special investigations

- *X-rays of the spine* may or may not reveal narrowing of the affected disc space on the lateral view.
- *CT scanning* or *MRI* are the investigations of choice and may demonstrate a disc protrusion.
- *Erythrocyte sedimentation rate (ESR)* is normal, and is helpful in the differential diagnosis of tumour or abscess.

Differential diagnosis

This includes the other common spinal lesions: sacro-iliac strain, osteoarthritis, spondylolis-thesis, spinal tumours and tuberculosis. One should consider, particularly in the elderly patient, an intrapelvic tumour, e.g. of the prostate or rectum, involving the sacral plexus; never omit a rectal examination in any patient with sciatica, both to detect rectal and prostatic tumours and to assess anal tone. Intermittent claudication is readily differentiated by careful history and examination. An abdominal aortic aneurysm may cause low back pain, and upon rupture may cause sciatica.

Treatment

The majority of cases respond to conservative treatment. In the acute episode of pain, 7–10 days' bed rest on a hard bed is prescribed. In less severe cases, gentle mobilization and physiotherapy is advised. Operative removal of the prolapsed disc is indicated if conservative measures fail, if repeated attacks occur, if there are severe neurological disturbances and particularly if a large central protrusion is diagnosed. If bladder sphincter disturbance occurs, surgical decompression must be performed urgently.

Spinal stenosis

Narrowing of the spinal canal may be congenital, but more commonly follows degeneration of the spine with osteophyte formation. It generally extends over several segments, and occurs predominantly in the lumbar spine.

The clinical features have been likened to intermittent claudication, but in spinal claudication the patient presents with pain, numbness and weakness in the legs brought on by standing or walking, and, in contrast to vascular claudication, it is not relieved by standing still but by sitting down or otherwise flexing the spine. Neurological examination of the legs is most revealing after the patient has been walking for a few minutes.

The diagnosis is confirmed by MRI (or CT scan) of the spine, which shows evidence of bony and soft-tissue encroachment into the spinal canal. Treatment is usually conservative, although surgery with decompression and fusion may be required.

Cervical spondylosis

Cervical spondylosis refers to degenerative changes that occur in the neck, with similar pathological process as in the lumbar spine. In the cervical spine, coexistent myelopathy and radiculopathy is more common.

Clinical features

Local cervical pain is usually overshadowed by a more severe pain radiating into the arm and accompanied by numbness and tingling in the fingers. Patients with myelopathy also complain of leg stiffness and difficulty in walking. Sensory changes may be present in the legs or arms, and bladder sphincter control may be disturbed. Examination of the arms reveals a lower motor neurone weakness with wasting and decreased tendon reflexes. Sensation is reduced with a nerve-root distribution. Examination of the legs may reveal an upper motor neurone pattern with a spastic paraplegia, increased tone, leg weakness, brisk reflexes and extensor plantars.

Differential diagnosis

There is an extensive differential diagnosis, which includes spinal tumour, multiple sclerosis and motor neurone disease. When the radiculopathy alone is present with unilateral or bilateral arm pain, the differential diagnosis includes cervical rib, carpal tunnel syndrome and angina pectoris.

Treatment

Radiculopathy usually settles with conservative treatment. A severe episode may require a period of neck traction, otherwise the neck is supported in a plastic collar. Operative removal of the prolapsed cervical disc has the same indications as lumbar disc protrusions.

Extradural spinal abscess

An abscess in the extradural spinal compartment usually represents a metastatic infection as part of a *Staphylococcus aureus* septicaemia. Occasionally, it is secondary to an osteomyelitis of the spine.

Clinical features

Clinical features are local pain and tenderness, fever, malaise and anorexia, and a rapidly progressive paraplegia. The white-blood-cell count is raised and the ESR is elevated.

Treatment

Urgent: the abscess is drained via a laminectomy, and antibiotic therapy is commenced. Provided surgery is performed in the initial stages, the paraplegia recovers but delay carries with it the risk of permanent cord damage.

Spinal tumours

Spinal tumours are conveniently classified, both from the pathological and clinical points of view, into those which occur outside the spinal theca (extradural), those within the theca but outside the cord itself (intradural extramedullary) and those occurring within the cord (intramedullary).

The tumours most commonly encountered are the following.

1 *Extradural*:
   (a) secondary deposits in the spine—by far the commonest;
   (b) primary vertebral bony tumours (e.g. osteoclastoma, myeloma);
   (c) lymphomas (Hodgkin's disease, non-Hodgkin's lymphoma).
2 *Intradural extramedullary*:
   (a) meningioma;
   (b) neurofibroma.
3 *Intramedullary* (rare):
   (a) glioma;
   (b) ependymoma;
   (c) others, such as haemangioma.

Clinical features

The three groups of spinal tumours listed above tend each to have a fairly distinctive clinical picture.

The *extradural tumours* are usually fast growing and malignant; they therefore give a picture of rapidly progressive cord compression leading to paraplegia, although symptoms of root irritation (see below) may also be present.

The *intradural extramedullary tumours* are usually slow growing and benign. Initially there is irritation of the involved nerve roots; pain occurs in the localized area of nerve distribution, which is often aggravated by recumbency and by factors such as coughing, sneezing or straining which raise the CSF pressure. There may be hyperalgesia in the affected cutaneous segment. Motor symptoms due to anterior root pressure are not a feature if only one nerve segment is involved, as most major muscle groups are innervated from several segments; however, if more than one segment is affected there may be localized flaccid paralysis.

As the tumour increases in size, cord compression takes place. There may be features of the *Brown-Séquard syndrome* (see p. 123). Further compression results in complete paraplegia of the spastic type with increased tendon jerks and extensor plantar response, together with overflow retention of urine and severe constipation.

Cauda equina tumours produce a lower motor neurone lesion: flaccid paralysis with diminished reflexes and paralysis of the anal and bladder sphincters with incontinence.

The *intramedullary tumours* may be accompanied by pain, but much more frequently give a picture very similar to that of syringomyelia. Progressive destruction of the cord produces bilateral motor weakness below the lesion and, as the crossed spino-thalamic tracts are the first to be involved, there may be dissociation of sensory loss below the lesion, with abolition of pain and temperature but with persistence of vibration and position sense until late on in the progress of the disease.

Differential diagnosis

Spinal tumours are relatively uncommon and are great impersonators of other diseases; indeed a correct diagnosis made *ab initio* is

something of a rarity. The root pain, if it occurs in the thoracic or abdominal segments, is often mistaken for intrathoracic or intra-abdominal disease; if the pains radiate to the leg they may be at first diagnosed as a prolapsed disc or intermittent claudication. The intramedullary lesions closely simulate syringomyelia and it may be difficult at first to differentiate them from disseminated sclerosis or other intraspinal lesions.

Special investigations

• *MRI* has become the definitive investigation and gives almost anatomically perfect imaging of spinal tumours.

• *X-rays of the spine* may show obvious bony deposits within the vertebral bodies. In other cases, pressure erosion from the enlarging tumour may scallop the posterior aspect of the vertebral body, erode one or more vertebral pedicles or enlarge the intervertebral foramen. Occasionally, calcification is seen within a meningioma.

• *Lumbar puncture.* Cytological examination of the CSF, together with its protein content and CSF pressure measurement, may be useful. The protein in the CSF is nearly always raised above the normal 0.4 g/L and may indeed be grossly elevated with yellow (xanthochromic) fluid, which may actually clot in the container. Queckenstedt's test* may show either no rise or else a very slow rise and fall of the CSF pressure on jugular compression, indicating a complete or partial block within the spinal canal.

• *A radiculogram*, in which radio-opaque water-soluble contrast medium is injected into the theca, will confirm the presence of a space-occupying lesion and localize its position accurately.

Treatment

A laminectomy (or vertebral body excision and grafting) is required to confirm the pathologi-

*Hans Heinrich Queckenstedt (1876–1918), Physician, Leipzig. He described his test while serving in the German Army; he was accidentally killed two days before the Armistice.

cal nature of the tumour and also to decompress the cord. Wherever possible the tumour is completely excised; this is usually confined to the benign meningiomas and neurofibroma, in which case complete recovery can be anticipated. In the malignant tumours, radiotherapy is usually the only practical treatment and the prognosis is poor.

CHAPTER 15

Peripheral Nerve Injuries

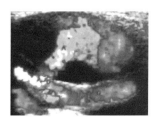

Although there is no regeneration of divided tracts in the central nervous system, injured peripheral nerve fibres may recover to a varying extent, depending on the severity of the trauma.

Classification

Nerve injuries are commonly the result of a laceration, stretching (traction) or compression (crush) injuries. There are three types of injury.

1 *Neurapraxia.* Damage to the nerve fibres without loss of continuity of the axis cylinder, and is analogous to concussion in the central nervous system. The conduction along the fibre is interrupted for only a short period of time. Recovery usually commences within a few days and is complete in 6–8 weeks.

2 *Axonotmesis.* Injury to the axon and myelin sheath without disruption of the continuity of its perineural sheath. The axon distal to the lesion degenerates (Wallerian degeneration) and regrowth of the axon occurs from the node of Ranvier proximal to the injury. As the sheath is intact, the correct axon will grow into its original nerve ending. The rate of regeneration is approximately 1 mm/day, therefore the time to recovery depends upon the distance between the injury and end organ.

3 *Neurotmesis.* Actual physical disruption of the peripheral nerve. Regeneration will take place provided the two nerve ends are not too far apart, but functional recovery will never be complete.

Following the complete disruption of neurotmesis, the distal part of the severed nerve undergoes Wallerian degeneration. The medullary sheath is depleted of myelin and the axon cylinders vanish; the empty endoneural sheaths remain as tubules composed of proliferating neurilemmal cells. The proximal end of the nerve degenerates up to the first uninjured node of Ranvier. New axis cylinders proliferate from this point and grow into the empty neurilemmal tubules. However, there is no selection of tubules for the appropriate axon; the distal growth is governed solely by the position of the nerve fibres. Thus, with most mixed nerves, there is likely to be considerable wastage due to regenerating fibres growing into endings which will be functionless, i.e. motor nerve fibres growing into sensory nerve endings, and vice versa. Even when a motor nerve grows into a motor nerve ending it may not supply the original muscle and the patient will have to relearn the affected movement.

Because a peripheral nerve contains a large number of individual fibres it is quite possible in a nerve injury for some fibres to suffer from neuropraxia, others axonotmesis and others neurotmesis. However, a distinction between the first two and the last may be quite clear in that if the nerve is found to be severed at surgical exploration, neurotmesis must have occurred.

Partial nerve injury may occur as the result of pressure or friction, for instance from a crutch, a tightly applied plaster cast or a tourniquet, as well as from closed injuries or open wounds.

Special investigation
• *Electromyography (EMG)* plays an important part in the diagnosis and assessment of nerve injuries. Serial studies are useful in demonstrating the amount and rate of regeneration. EMG is also useful in the diagnosis of nerve compression syndromes.

Treatment
Neuropraxia and axonotmesis
Those joints whose muscles have been paralysed are splinted in the position of function to avoid contractures. They are put through passive movements several times a day so that, when recovery of the nerve lesion occurs, the joints will be fully mobile.

Neurotmesis
Operative repair using an operating microscope is usually required. If a section of the nerve has been lost such that approximation is not possible, the nerve is freed proximally, or even moved from its original position to a new anatomical plane where more length will be available. For example, the ulnar nerve can be transposed from the posterior to the anterior aspect of the elbow joint to allow compensation for a distal loss of nerve substance.

After nerve suture, recovery cannot be expected to take place until the time for regeneration has been allowed for, at the rate already mentioned of 1 mm/day. Eventual recovery will seldom be full.

Nerve grafts
When important nerves are divided, sometimes useful function can be obtained by grafting sections of non-essential nerves such as the sural nerve to act as conduits for axon regrowth.

Tendon transfers
If restoration of nerve function cannot be achieved after injury, tendon transfers may allow the patient to perform movements that were otherwise impossible. Thus, wrist drop after a radial nerve lesion may be treated by transposing some of the flexor tendons into the extensor group.

It is outside the scope of this book to discuss lesions of all the individual nerves, but a few important peripheral nerve injuries will be mentioned.

Brachial plexus injuries

Upper trunk lesions (Erb's paralysis*)
These are the result of damage to the upper trunk when the head is forced away from the shoulder, a common injury in motor cyclists. It may also occur as an obstetric injury. C5 and C6 are damaged and there is paralysis of the biceps, brachialis, brachioradialis, supinator, supraspinatus, infraspinatus and deltoid. The limb will assume the 'waiter's tip' position, being internally rotated with the forearm pronated. The arm hangs vertically (deltoid paralysis) and the elbow cannot be flexed (biceps and brachialis). There will be an area of impaired sensation over the outer side of the upper arm.

T1 injury (Klumpke's paralysis†)
This may occur with a cervical rib or dislocation of the shoulder. The small muscles of the hand are wasted and there is loss of sensation on the inner side of the forearm and medial three and a half fingers. There may also be Horner's syndrome due to associated damage of sympathetic fibres passing to the inferior cervical ganglion (see p. 135).

*Wilhelm Erb (1840–1921), Professor of Neurology, Heidelberg.
†Auguska De Jerine-Klumpke (1859–1927), Neurologist, Paris.

Radial nerve injuries
(Fig. 15.1a)

Usually the radial nerve is injured by a fracture of the humerus involving the spiral groove where the nerve is closely applied to the bone. The nerve supply to the triceps comes off the radial nerve before it enters the spiral groove, and the lesions distal to that point will not affect extension of the elbow. However, there will be wrist drop due to paralysis of the wrist extensors and also loss of sensation over a small area on the dorsum of the hand at the base of the thumb and index finger. This surprisingly small sensory loss is due to considerable overlap from the median and ulnar nerves.

Median nerve injuries
(Fig. 15.1b)

This nerve may be damaged in fractures around the elbow joint or laceration of the forearm or wrist. In high lesions the pronators of the forearm and flexors of the wrist and fingers will be involved, with the exception of the flexor carpi ulnaris and the medial half of the flexor digitorum profundus, which are supplied by the ulnar nerve and which produce ulnar deviation of the wrist. When the patient clasps the two hands together, the index finger on the affected side remains extended — the 'pointing sign' of a high median nerve injury. Whether the injury is in the forearm or wrist, there will be paralysis of the small muscles of the thumb so that the thenar eminence is wasted. The patient is unable to abduct the thumb, i.e. lift it at right angles to the plane of the hand. The

Fig. 15.1 (a) Radial nerve injury: wrist drop, together with anaesthesia of a small area of the dorsal aspect of the hand at the base of the thumb and index finger. (b) Median nerve injury: thenar eminence paralysis with anaesthesia of the palmar aspect of the radial three and a half digits and corresponding palm.

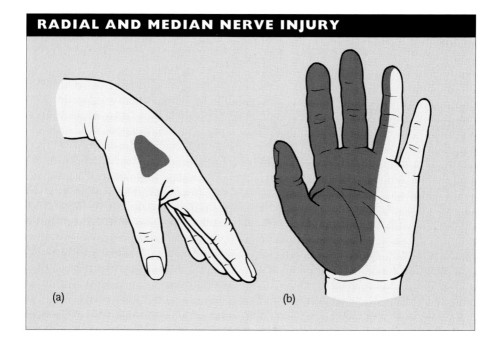

RADIAL AND MEDIAN NERVE INJURY

(a)   (b)

sensory loss with a median nerve lesion is serious. There is anaesthesia over the palmar aspects of the thumb and the lateral two and a half fingers, and the loss extends onto the dorsum of the distal phalanges of these digits. This sensory defect makes it difficult to perform fine and delicate tasks.

Median nerve compression at the wrist (carpal tunnel syndrome)

The median nerve is compressed as it passes through the carpal tunnel formed by flexor retinaculum stretching from the hook of the hamate and pisiform medially to the trapezium and scaphoid laterally. This results in wasting of the thenar eminence, diminished sensation, and most often unpleasant pain (characteristically at night), paraesthesia (numbness and tingling) in the thumb and radial two fingers and sometimes paraesthesia extending up into the arm. The reason for this latter symptom is not clear. Females are affected four times more commonly than males, and there is an association with pregnancy, rheumatoid arthritis, myxoedema and acromegaly. Wrist fractures also predispose to the syndrome.

EMG confirms the diagnosis. Treatment consists of dividing the flexor retinaculum at the wrist deep to which the median nerve is compressed, although conservative management using a wrist splint may also be effective.

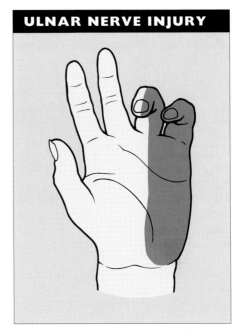

ULNAR NERVE INJURY

Fig. 15.2 Ulnar nerve injury: '*main en griffe*' with anaesthesia of the ulnar one and a half digits and ulnar border of the hand on both palmar and dorsal aspects.

Ulnar nerve injuries (Fig. 15.2)

Like the median, this nerve is also injured by fractures around the elbow joint and by lacerations of the forearm and wrist.

The ulnar nerve supplies all the intrinsic muscles of the hand apart from the three muscles of the thenar eminence (abductor pollicis brevis, opponens and flexor pollicis brevis) and the two radial lumbricals, all of which are supplied by the median nerve. The affected intrinsic muscles are the adductor pollicis, the muscles of the hypothenar eminence, the ulnar two lumbricals and the interossei, which are the abductors and adductors of the fingers and which also extend the interphalangeal joints. In the forearm the ulnar nerve supplies flexor carpi ulnaris and the medial half of flexor digitorum profundus.

Damage to the ulnar nerve produces the typical deformity of clawed hand or *main en griffe*. The clawed appearance results from the unopposed action of the long flexors and extensors of the fingers. The flexor profundus and sublimis, inserted into the bases of the distal and middle phalanges respectively, flex the interphalangeal joints, while the long extensors, inserted into the bases of the proximal phalanges, extend the metacarpophalangeal joints.

If the nerve is injured at the elbow, flexor digitorum profundus to the fourth and fifth finger is paralysed so that the clawing of these fingers, rather anomalously, is less intense than in injuries at the wrist. Paralysis of flexor carpi ulnaris produces a tendency to radial deviation at the wrist. In late cases, wasting of the intrinsic muscles is readily evident on inspecting the dorsum of the hand. Sensory loss occurs over the dorsal and palmar aspects of the ulnar one and a half digits and the ulnar border of the hand on both palmar and dorsal aspects. If the ulnar nerve is divided at the level of the wrist, the sensory loss is confined to the palmar surface, as the dorsal branch of the ulnar nerve, supplying the dorsal aspects of the ulnar one and a half fingers, is given off 5 cm above the wrist and thus escapes injury.

Division of the ulnar nerve leaves a surprisingly efficient hand. The long flexors enable a good grip to be taken; the thumb, apart from the loss of adductor pollicis, is intact, and the important sensation over the palm of the hand is largely maintained. Indeed, it may be difficult to be certain clinically that the nerve is injured. A reliable test is loss of the ability to abduct and adduct the fingers with the hand laid flat, palm downwards, on the table. This eliminates the trick movements of adduction and abduction of the fingers brought as part of their flexion and extension, respectively.

Differential diagnosis of flexion deformities of the fingers

Ulnar nerve lesion
This has been described above: there is hyperextension of the metacarpo-phalangeal joints and clawing of the hand, with sensory loss along the ulnar border of the hand and ulnar one and a half fingers.

Dupuytren's contracture*
This is a common condition in the elderly, usually male, subject in which there is fibrosis of the palmar aponeurosis. This produces a flexion deformity of the finger at the metacarpo-phalangeal and proximal interphalangeal joints, usually starting at the

ring finger and spreading to the little finger and sometimes the middle finger. As the aponeurosis only extends distally to the base of the middle phalanx, the distal interphalangeal joint escapes. The contracture is often bilateral and may occasionally affect the plantar fascia also.

Volkmann's contracture† due to ischaemic fibrosis of flexors of the fingers
The fingers will be curled up in the hand with metacarpo-phalangeal extension and wrist flexion. This deformity can to some extent be relieved by flexion of the wrist when the shortened tendons are no longer so taut and the fingers can be partially extended.

Congenital contracture
This usually affects the little finger and produces very little, if any, disability. The proximal interphalangeal joint is typically affected, the condition is usually bilateral and, of course, dates from birth.

Mallet finger
This follows trauma (common in cricketers) with flexion deformity of the distal interphalangeal joint due to avulsion of the extensor tendon insertion to the base of the distal phalanx.

Trauma
Scar formation following burns, injury or surgery to the fingers or the palm may produce gross flexion deformities wherever a scar crosses a joint line.

Sciatic nerve injuries

This nerve may be wounded in penetrating injuries or torn in posterior dislocation of the hip associated with fracture of the posterior lip of the acetabulum, to which the nerve is closely related. Injury is followed by paralysis of

---

*Baron Guillaume Dupuytren (1777–1835), Surgeon, Hôtel Dieu, Paris.

† Richard von Volkmann (1830–89), Professor of Surgery, Halle.

the hamstrings and all the muscles of the leg and foot; there is loss of all movement below the knee joint with foot drop deformity. Sensory loss is complete below the knee, except for an area extending along the medial side of the leg over the medial malleolus to the base of the hallux, which is innervated by the saphenous branch of the femoral nerve.

Common peroneal nerve injuries

The common peroneal nerve is in a particularly vulnerable position as it winds around the neck of the fibula. It may be injured at this site by direct trauma or compression, such as the pressure of a tight plaster cast, or in severe adduction injuries to the knee. Damage is followed by foot drop (due to paralysis of the ankle and foot extensors) and inversion of the foot (due to paralysis of the peroneal muscles with unopposed action of the foot flexors and invertors). There is anaesthesia over the anterior surface of the leg and foot. The medial side of the foot, innervated by the saphenous branch of the femoral nerve, and the lateral side of the foot, supplied by the sural branch of the tibial nerve, both escape.

Lateral cutaneous nerve of the thigh compression: meralgia paraesthetica

The lateral cutaneous nerve of the thigh may be trapped as it emerges beneath the inguinal ligament a finger's breadth medial to the anterior superior iliac spine. It commonly occurs in overweight middle-aged men and in athletes undergoing physical training. Symptoms comprise painful paraesthesiae over the anterolateral aspect of the thigh, worse on standing and relieved on sitting (hip flexion). Sensation in the distribution of the nerve is diminished.

Cervical sympathetic nerve injuries: Horner's syndrome*

If the T1 contribution to the cervical sympathetic chain is damaged, the result is known as Horner's syndrome, in which there is the following.
• *Meiosis*: paralysis of the dilator pupillae, resulting in constriction of the pupil.
• *Ptosis*: paralysis of the sympathetic muscle fibres transmitted via the oculomotor nerve to the levator palpebrae superioris results in drooping of the upper eyelid.
• *Anhidrosis*: loss of sweating on the affected side of the face and neck.

Horner's syndrome may follow operations on, or injuries to, the neck in which the cervical sympathetic trunk is damaged, malignant invasion from lymph nodes or adjacent tumour, or spinal cord lesions at the T1 segment (e.g. syringomyelia).

*Johann Horner (1831–86), Professor of Ophthalmology, Zurich, Switzerland.

CHAPTER 16

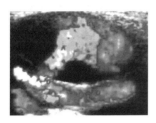

The Oral Cavity

It is a useful exercise (and a favourite examination topic) to consider what can be learned by examining a specific anatomical site such as the fingers, nails or eyes, in making a clinical diagnosis. The mouth and tongue can be conveniently used to illustrate how best to deal with this subject, which can be considered under three headings.

1 *Information about local disease.* Tumours of the mouth and tongue, congenital anomalies, etc., are obviously diagnosed by local examination.

2 *Local manifestations of diseases elsewhere.* The smooth tongue of pernicious anaemia, the ulcerated fauces of agranulocytosis or of severe glandular fever, the hemiatrophy of the tongue in hypoglossal nerve palsy, the pigmentation of Addison's disease, the pigmented spots of the Peutz–Jeghers syndrome and the gingivitis, swollen bleeding gums and loosened teeth of vitamin C deficiency, are examples of intrabuccal signs of more widespread diseases.

3 *Information given about the general condition and habits of the patient,* e.g. the dry tongue of dehydration, the brown dry tongue of uraemia, the coated tongue with foetor oris of acute appendicitis and the typical response of the hypochondriac to the command 'show me your tongue', upon which the patient opens his or her mouth to an extraordinary degree and enables the nethermost recesses of the oral cavity to become exposed.

The lips

Cleft lip and palate

These developmental abnormalities are very common. Cleft lip occurs in one in every 750 live births, cleft palate in one in every 2000. In half the cases, cleft lip and cleft palate coexist, in one-quarter the cleft of the lip is the only anomaly and in one-quarter the cleft of the palate occurs alone. It is important here, as in all congenital anomalies, to make a careful search for other developmental defects—10% of patients with clefts have some other malformation.

Embryology

These deformities can only be understood if the embryological development of the face and palate is revised (Fig. 16.1).

Around the primitive mouth or stomodaeum the following develop:

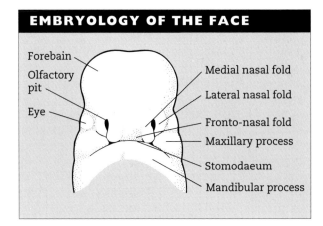

EMBRYOLOGY OF THE FACE

Forebain
Olfactory pit
Eye
Medial nasal fold
Lateral nasal fold
Fronto-nasal fold
Maxillary process
Stomodaeum
Mandibular process

Fig. 16.1 The ventral aspect of a fetal head showing the three processes—frontonasal, maxillary and mandibular—from which the face, nose and jaw are derived.

• The *fronto-nasal process*, which projects downwards from the cranium. Two olfactory pits develop in this process, then rupture into the pharynx to form the nostrils. The fronto-nasal process forms the nose, the nasal septum, the nostril, the philtrum of the upper lip and the premaxilla; this is the V-shaped anterior portion of the upper jaw, which usually bears the four incisor teeth.

• The *maxillary processes* on either side, which fuse with the fronto-nasal process to become the cheeks, the upper lip (exclusive of the philtrum), the upper jaw and the palate apart from the premaxilla.

• The *mandibular processes*, which meet in the midline to form the lower jaw.

Cleft lip (Fig. 16.2)

Once termed hare-lip, but only rarely is the cleft a median one, like the upper lip of a hare, although this may occur as a failure of development of the philtrum from the fronto-nasal process. Much more commonly the cleft is on one side of the philtrum as a result of failure of fusion of the maxillary and fronto-nasal process. In 15% of cases the cleft is bilateral. The cleft may be a small defect in the lip or may extend into the nostril, split the alveolus or even extend along the side of the nose as far as the orbit as a very rare anomaly. Associated with the deformity is invariably a flattening and widening of the nostril on the same side.

Cleft of the lower lip occurs very rarely but may be associated with a cleft of the tongue and of the mandible.

Cleft palate

A failure of fusion of the segments of the palate. The following stages may occur (Fig. 16.3).

• *Bifid uvula*, which is of no clinical importance.

• *Partial cleft*, which may involve the soft palate alone or the posterior part of the hard palate also.

• *Complete cleft.* This may be unilateral, running the full length of the maxilla and then alongside one face of the premaxilla, or bilateral in which the palate is cleft with an anterior V which separates the premaxilla completely. The premaxilla floats forward to produce a hideous deformity.

Principles of management

The details of surgical repair belong to the realms of the specialist plastic surgeon, but the principles underlying management are of importance to the paediatrician and the general practitioner.

Cleft lip alone presents no feeding or nursing problems. Repair is required at an early stage so that normal moulding of the bones of the

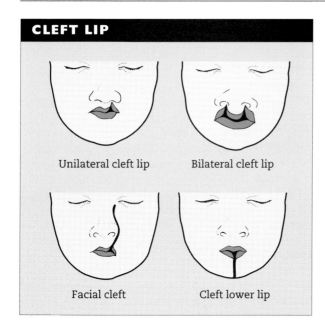

Fig. 16.2 Types of cleft lip.

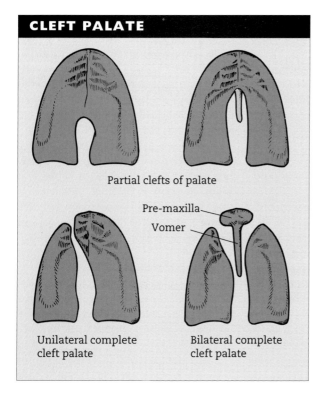

Fig. 16.3 Types of cleft palate.

face may occur during growth. Early repair within a few days of birth is now preferred to the previous practice of waiting 3–6 months.

Cleft palate interferes with the normal suckling mechanism. The infant is fed either by using a spoon or by dripping milk into the mouth from a bottle provided with a large hole in the teat. The defect is repaired at between 6 months and 1 year in order to allow normal speech to develop. If delayed beyond this time the child will develop bad speech, which will require considerable rehabilitation to restore to normal.

Where both defects coexist, the lip is repaired early (before 10 weeks) and the palate then operated upon at a second stage at the age of about 6 months.

Lesions on the lip
Angular stomatitis
Superficial ulceration at the corners of the mouth. Causes range from iron deficiency anaemia to habitual licking in children.

Retention cyst
A mucous retention cyst appears as a blue, domed, translucent swelling of the buccal aspect of the lower lip. It represents an obstructed mucous gland.

Herpes simplex (cold sores)
Painful ulceration, which starts as a crop of vesicles near the vermilion border and develops into a crusting ulcer before resolving. The cause is a herpes virus (herpes simplex types I and II), which remains latent in the nerve ganglion and recurs when triggered by trauma, sunburn or endogenous factors such as menstruation. Recurrence starts with a pricking sensation, followed by the appearance of a cluster of vesicles, which breaks down to produce painful ulcers. Early topical treatment with aciclovir may curtail the infection and reduce symptoms.

Carcinoma
Ulcerating squamous carcinomas have characteristic raised edges. Evidence of regional lymph-node involvement should be sought (see p. 141).

Less common lesions include Peutz–Jehgers circumoral pigmentation,* which is associated with intestinal hamartomatous polyps, and telangiectasia typical of hereditary haemorrhagic telangiectasia (Osler–Rendu–Weber syndrome†), which is associated with intestinal telangiectasia and bleeding.

Ulcers in the mouth

Traumatic
Usually due to a sharp edge of a tooth or a denture, and usually present on the tongue. Healing rapidly takes place when the cause is removed. Rarely seen nowadays is the ulcer produced on the under-aspect of the tongue as this is rubbed against the lower incisor teeth in whooping cough.

Aphthous ulcer
Recurrent, small, round, white, painful ulcers, which may occur singly or in crops anywhere in the mouth but particularly on the edge of the tongue. The ulcers have a sloughy base and a rim of erythema surrounding them. The cause is unknown. They are particularly common around puberty and occasionally they are associated with inflammatory bowel disease. The ulcer will usually heal rapidly if a hydrocortisone tablet is held against it.

Herpes simplex
Can be extensive in the oropharynx, nose, oesophagus and larynx in patients on immuno-

*John Law Augustine Peutz (1886–1957), Physician, The Hague, Holland. Harold Jos Jeghers (Contemporary), Professor of Medicine, New Jersey College of Medicine, Jersey City, USA.
† Sir William Osler (1849–1919), Professor of Medicine successively at McGill, Montreal, Johns Hopkins and Oxford. Henri Rendu (1844–1902), Physician, Necker Hospital, Paris. Louis Vaquez (1860–1936), Physician, Paris.

suppressive drugs or infected with human immunodeficiency virus (HIV).

Carcinoma

Carcinoma (see p. 141) and lymphoma may cause intra-oral ulceration.

Syphilitic ulcers

Now rarely seen, ulcers were features of the first, second and third stages of syphilis. A chancre in the first, a 'snail-track' ulcer in the second and a midline punched-out gumma in the third. In addition, tertiary syphilis may produce leukoplakia or diffuse fibrosis of the tongue. All these conditions are extremely rare now that early syphilis is efficiently treated.

Rarer causes of ulceration

Other causes of oral ulcers include neutropenia and agranulocytosis, Behçet's syndrome, Reiter's syndrome, Wegener's granulomatosis and tuberculosis

Other lesions within the mouth

Leukoplakia

Leukoplakia refers to thickened white patches of mucosa. In contrast to *Candida* infection, the lesions cannot be rubbed off. This condition may occur anywhere within the mouth, particularly on the tongue. Other sites are the larynx, the anus and the vulva. The affected area may show cracks or fissures.

Microscopically, there is hyperplasia of the squamous epithelium with hyperkeratosis. It is usually found in middle-aged or elderly subjects and may result from chronic irritation. One invokes the well-known S list — smoking, syphilis, sepsis, spices, sore tooth and spirits — but it must be confessed than often no cause at all can be found.

The importance of the condition is that it is often pre-malignant. Malignant change especially occurs within the fissures and should be suspected if there is local thickening, pain or bleeding, or areas of erythema.

Treatment

Remove any underlying irritant cause. Any area suspicious of malignancy should be biopsied. Superficial areas of leukoplakia are usually satisfactorily treated by excision, with skin grafting if the area is large.

Mucous retention cysts

These result from leakage of mucus due to minor trauma of the mucous glands and are better termed extravasation cysts. They are commonly found on the inside of the lips and inner aspects of the cheek. They are blue in appearance and contain glairy mucoid fluid. Their nuisance value is that they tend to be chewed upon by the patient.

Ranula

A large mucous extravasation cyst on one or other side of the floor of the mouth arising from a sublingual salivary gland. Often the submandibular duct can be seen passing over the cyst. The word ranula means a small frog and the lesion is so-called because it resembles a frog's belly. Small cysts may be excised, larger cysts are marsupialized.

Midline dermoid

This occupies the floor of the mouth and may project below the chin. It represents a congenital seeding of ectoderm during the process of fusion of the two mandibular processes. Similar inclusion dermoid cysts occur at the outer and inner margins of the orbit (external and internal angular dermoids). Treatment is excision.

Epulis

Epulis is a non-specific term applied to a localized swelling of the gum. This may be:
• *Fibrous*: a nodule of dense fibrous tissue covered by epithelium, which arises from the submucosa of the gum.
• *Giant cell*: with the histological appearance of an osteoclastoma.
• *Granulomatous*: peculiarly likely to occur in

pregnancy and probably arises as a result of minor trauma followed by chronic infection.
• *Denture granuloma*: originates from the persistent irritation of an ill-fitting denture.
• *Dental abscess*: while not a true epulis, it initially presents as an acute inflammatory swelling of the mucosa adjacent to the diseased tooth.

Malignant disease of the mouth and pharynx

General features
In broad principles, the pathology, diagnosis and treatment of malignant disease of lips, tongue, floor of mouth, gums, inner aspects of the cheek, the hard and soft palate, tonsils, fauces and the pharynx can be considered as one. Specific features of each site are given in the next section. Common hiding places for oral tumours include the base of tongue, sulci lateral to base of tongue, tonsillar fossa (is one tonsil bigger than the other?) and nasopharynx.

Pathology
Sex distribution
For the most part, oral tumours are more common in males than in females, but in tumours of the hard palate and posterior one-third of the tongue the sex distribution is equal and in the post-cricoid region females are more often affected than males.

Predisposing factors
These can be divided into three groups.
1 *Chronic irritation*: there is the well-known S list: smoking, syphilis, sepsis, spices, sore tooth and spirits. Certainly mouth cancer is particularly seen amongst old men of poor social class with gross dental caries and heavy smoking habits. Especially at risk is the heavy smoker who is also a heavy drinker. In India, betel nut chewing is associated with a high incidence of mouth cancer.
2 *Leukoplakia*: a definite pre-cancerous condition (see p. 140).

3 *Iron deficiency*: the Plummer–Vinson* syndrome with smooth tongue, cracks at the angles of the mouth (cheilosis), koilonychia, dysphagia and an iron deficiency anaemia is often present in oral and pharyngeal cancer in females.

Macroscopic appearance
Macroscopically, malignant tumours of the mouth present as one of three types:
1 a nodule;
2 an ulcer or fissure, usually feels hard to the palpating finger;
3 a warty or papilliferous growth.

Microscopic appearance
Microscopically, by far the commonest tumours are keratinizing squamous cell carcinomas. In addition, two other types may be seen, particularly in the posterior third of the tongue, the tonsil and the nasopharynx. These are:
1 *transitional cell carcinoma*, made up of undifferentiated epithelial cells, which simulate the transitional carcinomas of the urinary tract;
2 *lymphoepithelioma*, comprising sheets of rather anaplastic epithelial cells pervaded with a diffuse lymphocytic infiltration.
Probably both these variations are merely examples of undifferentiated squamous cell tumours. Tumours may also arise in the minor salivary glands, which are abundantly distributed over the mucous membrane of the mouth.

Spread
Occurs by local infiltration, which often transgresses nearby anatomical boundaries. Thus, a carcinoma of the tongue may invade the floor of the mouth, the gum and the fauces. Cervical lymph-node involvement is common and is often the presenting feature. Thirty per cent of patients have cervical node involvement at the time of diagnosis. Distant blood-borne spread

*Henry Plummer (1874–1957) and Porter Paisley Vinson (1890–1959), Physicians, Mayo Clinic, Rochester, Minnesota.

(e.g. to the lung and liver) is late and relatively uncommon.

Causes of death

Tumours of the mouth and pharynx are particularly horrible in their late stages. The patient becomes cachectic due to difficulty in swallowing and anorexia resulting from the infected, foul-smelling, fungating ulcer within the mouth. As a result of this sepsis, inhalation bronchopneumonia is a common termination. Fatal haemorrhage may occur, either from the primary ulcerating growth or from the breaking down of cervical lymph nodes, which may erode the internal jugular vein or carotid artery.

Special investigations

- *Endoscopy* and examination under anaesthetic to look at the larynx and exclude second primaries, or diagnose the primary in patients presenting with cervical lymphadenopathy
- *Orthopantomogram (OPG)* may demonstrate bone invasion in tumours arising close to the mandible.
- *Computed tomography (CT) scan* may demonstrate local disease including bone invasion and involvement of the maxillary sinus, and may demonstrate cervical nodal involvement.
- *Magnetic resonance imaging (MRI)* has a slightly better resolution than CT.

Principles of treatment

The diagnosis is first confirmed by biopsy. The search for predisposing factors includes syphilis serology and haemoglobin estimation. A chest X-ray is taken to exclude the rare pulmonary secondary spread. Where relevant, X-rays of the skull and mandible and a CT scan may be required to estimate bony invasion. In every case, treatment must be considered with respect: (i) to the primary tumour, and (ii) to the regional lymph nodes.

Management of the primary tumour

The treatment of choice is radiotherapy. Where the tumour is readily accessible, e.g.

the lip, the anterior part of the tongue and the buccal mucosa, this is conveniently carried out by implantation of radium needles. More posteriorly placed tumours are treated by external beam radiotherapy.

With conventional radiotherapy, invasion of the mandible or maxilla by the tumour was a contra-indication to treatment because bone necrosis almost invariably took place. In such circumstances only radical surgery could be offered. Fortunately, modern external beam radiotherapy only infrequently causes radionecrosis so that jaw involvement is no longer a bar to treatment.

Irradiation is abandoned under two circumstances; first if the tumour proves to be radio-resistant and second if recurrence takes place subsequent to satisfactory regression. In these circumstances it may be necessary to consider radical surgical excision, e.g. a hemiglossectomy or mandibulectomy and block dissection of the cervical nodes in continuity.

Management of the regional lymph nodes

If the lymph nodes are not enlarged, the patient is kept under close regular observation.

If the lymph nodes are enlarged but mobile and obviously operable, block dissection is performed providing the primary tumour is controllable; clearly there is little point in carrying out a radical block dissection of the neck in the presence of a hopelessly inoperable carcinomatous mass within the mouth.

If the lymph nodes are enlarged but are fixed and clinically irremovable, palliative deep X-ray therapy is given and may be combined with cytotoxic treatment.

Prognosis

Prognosis becomes increasingly worse as we pass backwards into the mouth; the outlook is best in tumours of the lip, then of the anterior two-thirds of the tongue, but it is usually grave in tumours of the pharynx, tonsil, etc. As with tumours elsewhere, the prognosis also depends on the degree of differentiation of the tumour on histological examination and on the extent of spread, particularly whether or not the lymph nodes are involved.

Specific features

The local pathological and clinical features at specific sites can now be considered. In every case the management of the tumour and the regional lymph nodes are as described in the above scheme.

Carcinoma of the lip
Clinical features

This disease commonly affects men (90%); nearly always elderly, and those exposed to a weather-beaten outdoor life associated with sunlight exposure. The lower lip is by far the commonest site, accounting for 93% of the tumours. Five per cent occur on the upper lip and 2% at the angle of the mouth — these last have a particularly bad prognosis. The lesion appears either as a fissure, a typical malignant ulcer or a warty papilliferous tumour. The majority are slow growing, and spread to the regional lymph nodes is comparatively late, first to the submental, then the submandibular and finally the internal jugular chain of nodes. Distant metastasis is rare.

Differential diagnosis

The differential diagnosis of carcinoma of the lip conveniently sums up the other swellings that may be found in this situation. They are:
• simple papilliferous wart, which may itself be premalignant;
• keratoacanthoma (molluscum sebaceum), see page 38;
• haemangioma;
• lymphangioma;
• herpes simplex;
• mucous cyst — this is probably the commonest swelling to be found upon the lip (see p. 140);
• chancre — the lip is the commonest extragenital site for a chancre. Usually the upper lip is affected; it is accompanied by considerable local oedema and exuberant enlargement of the regional lymph nodes.

Carcinoma of the tongue

Carcinoma of the tongue occurs more commonly in men than women, affecting older men who drink and smoke excessively. The tumours are conveniently divided into those of the anterior two-thirds and those of the posterior one-third of the tongue.

Clinical features

The tumour itself tends to occur on the lateral border of the tongue, and rarely affects the dorsum. The anterior tumour commences as a nodule, fissure or ulcer, although occasionally a widely infiltrating type of tumour is seen. At first the lesion is painless but becomes painful as it invades and becomes grossly septic. The pain often radiates to the ear, being referred from the lingual branch of the trigeminal nerve, supplying the tongue, along its auriculo-temporal branch. Ulceration is accompanied by bleeding. The typical picture of late disease is an old man sitting in the out-patient department spitting blood into his handkerchief, with a plug of cotton wool in his ear. As the tumour extends onto the floor of the mouth and the alveolus, speech and swallowing become difficult because of fixation of the tongue (ankyloglossia). Palpation is especially valuable. Malignant ulcers in the mouth, as in the rectum, feel hard with surrounding induration.

Lymphatic spread occurs to the submental, submandibular and deep cervical nodes. Unless the primary tumour is situated far laterally on the margin of the tongue, this lymphatic spread may be bilateral.

Tumours of the posterior third of the tongue are rapidly growing and of the lympho-epitheliomatous type with early spread bilaterally to the cervical nodes.

Any nodule or chronic ulcer of the tongue must be regarded with great suspicion of malignant disease, particularly if there is any predisposing factor such as leukoplakia.

Differential diagnosis

This is to be made from the other ulcers of the tongue discussed on page 139, from the comparatively rare benign tumours of the tongue (papilloma, haemangioma, lymphangioma and fibroma) and from the still rarer lingual thyroid which occurs as a midline nodule. More commonly, the nervous patient may suddenly discover a circumvallate papilla seen on the tongue in the mirror, and presents to the surgeon having decided it is a cancer of the tongue.

Carcinoma of the soft palate and fauces

These tumours usually resemble those of the posterior third of the tongue in their behaviour.

Carcinoma of the hard palate

Tumours in this region are usually warty, spread over the palate and later invade the bone. Differential diagnosis must be made from secondary involvement of the palate from an antral tumour and from mixed salivary tumours, which arise from the small accessory salivary glands scattered over the hard palate.

Floor of mouth, alveolus and cheek

Here the tumour is commonly an ulcerating carcinoma, which often involves more than one of these structures; thus, an ulcer is often found wedged in the floor of the mouth extending upwards onto the gum and backwards to involve the root of the tongue. There is early spread to the regional nodes.

In addition, adenomas or adenocarcinomas occasionally arise in the mucous and salivary accessory glands of this region.

Tonsil

About 85% of the tumours of the tonsil are squamous carcinomas, about 10% are lymphomas arising from the lymphoid tissue of the tonsil and 5% are lympho-epitheliomas, which show rapid lymph-node spread.

Carcinoma of the nasopharynx

As elsewhere, the predominant tumour is a squamous carcinoma. In addition, a rapidly growing lympho-epithelioma occurs in younger subjects and for some unexplained reason is particularly common amongst the Chinese, with a high incidence of raised antibody titres to the Epstein–Barr virus; indeed, in this race it is second in frequency only to uterine cancer. Rarely, a fibrosarcoma of the nasopharynx arises from the periosteum of the basiocciput.

These tumours may present with nasal obstruction and bleeding, Eustachian tube blockage with deafness, involvement of one or more of the cranial nerves and severe deeply situated headache. Tumours at this site are notoriously difficult to locate even on careful inspection and palpation under anaesthesia. One-third present first as a cervical node mass.

Carcinoma of the oro- and laryngo-pharynx

Carcinomas at these sites present first with discomfort in the throat, excessive salivation and expectoration of blood-stained mucus, which then becomes foetid. Later, there may be alteration of the voice progressing to hoarseness and then dysphagia. Often, however, these tumours present with enlarged cervical lymph nodes. The hypopharyngeal tumours (post-cricoid carcinoma) are almost always confined to women, many of whom present features of the Plummer–Vinson syndrome (see p. 155). Diagnosis is confirmed by oesophagoscopic examination and biopsy.

Tumours of the jaw

Tumours of the jaw are of extremely wide pathological variety because they may arise from the bone of the jaw itself, from the tissues over the surface of the jaw or, in the case of the maxilla, from the mucosa lining the maxillary antrum.

Tumours of the bone

These may originate from any of the histological structures forming the bone, e.g. osteogenic sarcoma or osteoma from the bone itself, chondroma and chondrosarcoma from the cartilage, osteoclastoma from the osteoclasts, myeloma from the marrow cells, haemangioma from the blood vessels and fibrosarcoma from the periosteum. In addition to this, the jaw is the occasional site for secondary deposits, the common sources of which are lung, breast, prostate, thyroid and kidney.

Ameloblastoma (adamantinoma)

This is an interesting benign tumour, which is derived from the epithelial cells of the enamel organ. Its histological appearance resembles these cells arranged in clumps within a fibrous stroma. Gradual destruction of the jaw takes place but the tumour metastasizes only rarely. It is multilocular, and usually involves the lower jaw towards its angle. Any age may be affected, but the majority present in the second and third decades with equal sex distribution.

Surface tumours

Carcinoma, mixed salivary tumour, or rarely melanoma of the palate, gum, cheek or floor of the mouth may invade the underlying bone.

Antral tumours

Probably the commonest tumour of the upper jaw is the squamous carcinoma arising from the mucous membrane of the maxillary antrum.

The antral carcinoma occurs in middle-aged and elderly subjects with equal sex distribution.

Clinical features

Symptoms and signs are late in manifesting themselves, indeed the tumour must burst through the bony walls of the antrum before it becomes obvious. Presentation then depends on the direction of growth of the tumour and can be deduced by the application of some knowledge of the anatomy of the region.

Medial extension

Blockage of the ostium of the maxillary antrum with consequent infection of the sinus, or with nasal obstruction and epistaxis.

Lateral extension

Swelling of the face, which often has an inflammatory appearance and may well be mistaken for an acute infection.

Upward extension

Orbital invasion with proptosis, diplopia and lacrimation due to blockage of the tear duct. Anaesthesia of the cheek may result from invasion of the maxillary branch of the trigeminal nerve.

Inferior extension

Bulging and ulceration into the palate. Metastases to the upper jugular lymph nodes occur at a relatively late stage.

Special investigations

• *Skull X-rays* usually reveal decalcification and erosion of the maxilla. There may be opacification of the normally translucent maxillary antrum.

• *CT scan and MRI* are valuable in indicating the exact spread of the tumours.

Treatment

• *Benign tumours* are treated by local excision, in the case of the lower jaw this may require bone graft to the resected portion of the mandible.

• *Malignant tumours* of the mandible and of the maxillary antrum are treated initially by radiotherapy, followed by hemi-mandibulectomy or maxillectomy.

CHAPTER 17

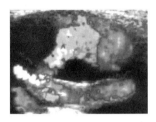

The Salivary Glands

The salivary glands comprise three paired glands — the parotid, submandibular and sublingual — together with tiny accessory salivary glands scattered over the walls of the buccal cavity. The parotid gland secretes a serous saliva, in contrast to the mucus product of the sublingual glands. The submandibular saliva is sero-mucus, and represents 75% of the total saliva produced. The parotid and submandibular gland drain into the mouth via long ducts, the parotid (Stensen's*) duct opening adjacent the second upper molar tooth, while the submandibular (Wharton's†) duct opens on the floor of the mouth through a papilla at the base of the frenulum of the tongue. The sublingual gland's mucus secretion drains by a series of very short ducts into the floor of the mouth.

The two principal surgical conditions of the salivary glands are inflammation, with or without calculus, and neoplasm. The different cells within the gland, and the different composition of the saliva account for the different incidence of these conditions in the different salivary glands.

*Niels Stensen (1638–86), Professor of Anatomy, University of Copenhagen, Denmark. Gave up his Chair in 1669 to become a Bishop.
†T. Wharton (1614–73), Physician, St Thomas's Hospital, London.

Inflammation

Aetiology
• *Associated with calculus*: usually submandibular gland (see below).
• *Mumps*: usually parotid; rarely submandibular.
• *Acute bacterial infection*: usually occurs postoperatively involving parotid.
• *Chronic recurrent sialadenitis*: usually occurs in the parotid.
• *Mikulicz's syndrome*: involving all the salivary and the lacrimal glands.

Mumps
A viral infection (incubation period 17–21 days), which is common in children and affects the parotid glands, and is usually bilateral. Rarely the submandibular or sublingual glands may be involved.

Mumps is of interest to the surgeon for the following reasons:
• As an occasional puzzling cause of painful parotid swelling in an adult.
• As an occassional cause of acute orchitis, especially when mumps occurs in adolescents or young adults (orchitis complicating this condition is rare before puberty). Pain and swelling in the testicle occur 7–10 days after the onset of the parotitis and may lead to testicular atrophy. If bilateral orchitis occurs, there may be sterility or eunuchoidism. Very

rarely the orchitis occurs without prodromal parotitis.

- As a rare cause of pancreatitis, mastitis, thyroiditis or oöphoritis.

Most children are now vaccinated against mumps before starting school.

Acute bacterial parotitis

Ascending infection of the parotid gland via its duct may occur after major surgical procedures. Aetiological factors include dental sepsis, dehydration, the presence of a nasogastric tube for a prolonged period and poor oral hygiene. This complication may also occur in any severe debilitating illness and in uraemia. The infection is usually streptococcal (*viridans* or *Pneumococcus*) and occasionally staphylococcal.

Clinical features

Clinically, there is swelling and intense pain in one or both parotid glands, which are hard, enlarged and tender, often with associated trismus (masseter spasm). There may be a purulent discharge from the duct. Abscess formation occasionally occurs.

Treatment

Prophylaxis is important. Adequate hydration with elimination of the above aetiological factors has rendered this complication rare nowadays. In the established case, the patient must be kept fully hydrated and the flow of saliva encouraged by sucking sweets or chewing gum. Parenteral antibiotic therapy is commenced. Occasionally, surgical drainage is required.

Chronic recurrent parotid sialadenitis

Repeated episodes of pain and swelling in one or both parotids is not uncommon and is caused by a combination of obstruction and infection of the gland. There may be an associated dilatation of the duct system and alveoli of the gland, termed sialectasia (which resembles bronchiectasis in the lung), associated with a stricture of the duct or a stone. These changes are best demonstrated by performing a *sialogram.*

Treatment

An associated stricture is treated by dilatation or plastic enlargement, and if stones are present these must be removed. Massage of the gland several times a day, and the use of sialogogues (such as acid drops) encourage drainage. Occasionally, in severe and refractory cases, excision of the gland with preservation of the facial nerve is required.

Mikulicz's syndrome*

Mikulicz's syndrome is characterized by enlargement of the salivary and lacrimal glands, and is associated with dry eyes, leading to conjunctivo-keratitis, and dry mouth (xerostomia). It may occur in the following conditions:

- sarcoid (commonest);
- lymphoma, particularly non-Hodgkin's lymphoma;
- tuberculosis;
- Sjögren's syndrome,† principally affecting middle-aged females and associated with connective tissue disorders such as rheumatoid arthritis and systemic lupus erythematosus.

Calculi

Stone formation is common in the submandibular gland and its duct, rare in the parotid and unknown in the sublingual. The different composition of the saliva from each gland probably explains this difference. Stasis of the more viscid secretion of the submandibular gland in its long duct, changes in composition of the saliva, trauma to the duct, infection, stricture and several metabolic diseases such as hyperparathyroidism may predispose to stone formation. The stones

*Johann von Mikulicz-Radecki (1850–1905), Professor of Surgery successively at Cracow, Konigsberg and Breslau, Poland. One of the first surgeons to use rubber gloves and to wear a face mask.
†Henrik Sjögren (1899–1986), Ophthalmologist, Gothenburg, Sweden.

themselves consist of calcium phosphate and calcium carbonate, and are therefore radio-opaque.

Clinical features

There is painful swelling of the affected gland, aggravated by food (classically by sucking a lemon) and there may be an unpleasant taste in the mouth due to the purulent discharge. On examination, the obstructed gland is enlarged and tender. The submandibular duct, visible in the floor of the mouth, is red and swollen and the calculus may be visible or palpable on bimanual examination of the duct. Gentle pressure on the gland may produce a purulent exudate from the orifice of the duct.

Special investigations

• *X-rays* invariably confirm the presence of the stone.

• *Sialogram*, where contrast material is injected into the duct, may be necessary if no stone is visible. This may reveal stenosis of the ostium of the duct, which mimics a stone, or sialectasis.

Treatment

If the stone lies within the submandibular duct, it can be removed from within the mouth, with the duct being marsupialized at the site of extraction. If one or more stones are impacted in the gland substance, excision of the whole gland is required.

Salivary tumours

Classification

Benign

• Pleomorphic adenoma (mixed salivary tumour).

• Adenolymphoma.

Malignant

• *Primary*: carcinoma.

• *Secondary*: direct invasion from skin or from secondarily involved lymph nodes.

PAROTID SWELLING: DIFFERENTIAL DIAGNOSIS

A swelling in the parotid region may be one of the following.

Swelling of the parotid gland itself
• Parotitis.
• Mixed salivary tumour or adenolymphoma.
• Carcinoma.

Swelling in other anatomical structures in the vicinity
• Sebaceous cyst.
• Lipoma.
• Enlarged pre-auricular or parotid lymph nodes.
• Neuroma of facial nerve.
• Ameloblastoma (adamantinoma) and other tumours of the mandible.

Pleomorphic adenoma

Ninety per cent occur in the parotid, although occasionally they are found in the submandibular, sublingual or accessory salivary glands. Ninety per cent present before the age of 50 years, although any age may be affected. Sex distribution is equal.

Pathology

Macroscopic appearance

The tumour is lobulated and lies within a false capsule of compressed salivary tissue. The cut surface is glistening and translucent; the consistency is crumbly.

Microscopic appearance

The tumours vary in a spectrum from a typical adenoma to a frank carcinoma. The majority show glandular acini within a blue-staining stroma, which gives the appearance of a cartilage but which is, in fact, mucus. The appearance of epithelial cells and 'cartilage' gave rise to the older concept of a 'mixed tumour'.

Surgical considerations

If treated by enucleation, at least 25% of the tumours recur, because:

• the capsule surrounding the tumour is a false one, which itself is incomplete and may contain tumour cells;

• serial sections show that the tumour often has 'amoeboid' processes, which may be left behind;

• implantation of tumour cells may occur into the wound.

Although slow growing, these tumours *cannot* be considered benign because of the lack of encapsulation, the occasional wide infiltration of surrounding tissues and the tendency to recur. Moreover, the less differentiated tumours, which are extremely difficult to distinguish from frank carcinoma, may metastasize to the regional lymph nodes and distantly via the blood stream.

Clinical features

The patient presents with a slow-growing swelling anywhere within the parotid gland, but usually in the lower pole and in the region of the angle of the jaw. The lump is well defined, usually firm or hard but sometimes cystic in consistency. It is usually placed in the superficial part of the gland but may occasionally be in its deep prolongation and indeed may project into the pharynx. The facial nerve is never involved, except by frankly malignant tumours. Its integrity should be confirmed.

Treatment

Wide excision of the tumour and the surrounding parotid tissue, with careful preservation of the fibres of the facial nerve (superficial parotidectomy). Some centres advise local excision followed by radiotherapy, especially in elderly patients.

Where the tumour involves one of the other salivary glands, complete excision of the gland is performed.

Prognosis

Providing the tumour is completely excised, the prognosis is excellent but inadequate surgery is followed by a recurrence in a high percentage of cases.

PAROTID SWELLING: EXAMINATION

The following should always be performed, in addition to examination of the gland itself.

• *Inspection of the parotid duct*: redness, oedema of the duct or exudation of pus indicate parotitis.

• *Testing the integrity of the facial nerve*: it is invariably intact in benign swelling, but may be paralysed in malignant disease.

• *Inspection and palpation of the fauces*: a parotid tumour may plunge into the pharynx.

• *Palpation of the regional lymph nodes*: they may be involved with secondary deposits from a parotid carcinoma.

Adenolymphoma

Adenolymphoma (Warthin's tumour[*]) accounts for about 10% of parotid tumours, and is very rare elsewhere. Adenolymphomas usually occur in men over the age of 50 years, and are occasionally bilateral.

Macroscopically, the tumour is soft and cystic. Microscopically, it consists of columnar cells forming papillary fringes, which project into cystic spaces and which are supported by a lymphoid stroma. These tumours probably arise from the salivary duct epithelium, the lymphoid tissue originating from the lymphoid aggregates which are present in the normal parotid gland. Presence of the lymphoid tissue may lead to confusion with lymphoproliferative disorders. Prognosis is excellent after local removal.

Carcinoma
Clinical features

Again this usually affects the parotid. Sex distribution is equal, and the patients are usually over the age of 50 years. The tumour is hard and infiltrating. Clinically, the diagnosis is based on rapid growth, pain, involvement of the facial nerve and of the regional lymph nodes. Eventually, surrounding tissues are infiltrated and the overlying skin becomes ulcerated.

*Aldred Scott Warthin (1866–1931), Professor of Pathology, University of Michigan, USA.

Microscopically, most tumours are adeno-carcinomas, rapidly progressive with a high incidence of metastasis to regional lymph nodes. A small proportion represent malignant change in slow-growing pleomorphic adenomas.

Treatment

When the tumour lies in the parotid, radical parotidectomy is performed with sacrifice of the facial nerve. This is combined if necessary with block dissection of the regional lymph nodes if these are involved, and is followed by radiotherapy. When the tumour arises in the other sites of salivary tissue, wide local excision is performed, again with block dissection if this is indicated by the presence of enlarged but mobile lymph nodes.

The prognosis is not good for this tumour, particularly when the submandibular gland is the site of origin.

CHAPTER 18

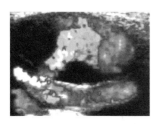

The Oesophagus

Dysphagia

Dysphagia is difficulty in swallowing. The causes may be local or general. The local causes of obstruction of any tube in the body are subdivided into those in the lumen, those in the wall and those outside the wall.

Local causes
In the lumen
• Foreign body.

In the wall
• Congenital atresia.
• Inflammatory stricture, secondary to reflux oesophagitis.
• Caustic stricture.
• Achalasia.
• Plummer–Vinson syndrome with oesophageal web.
• Pharyngeal pouch.
• Tumour of oesophagus or cardia.

Outside the wall
• Pressure of enlarged lymph nodes (malignant or one of the lymphomas).
• Thoracic aortic aneurysm.
• Bronchial carcinoma.
• Retrosternal goitre.

General causes
• Myasthenia gravis.
• Bulbar palsy.
• Bulbar poliomyelitis.
• Diphtheria.
• Hysteria.

Investigation
History
The subjective site of obstruction is not always exact; the patient often merely points vaguely to behind the sternum. The diagnosis may be given by a history of swallowed caustic in the past. A previous story of reflux oesophagitis suggests peptic stricture. Patients with achalasia tend to be young and the history is often long, usually without loss of weight.

Malignant stricture has a short history, occurs usually in elderly people and is associated with severe weight loss.

Examination
Often this is negative, but search is made for clinical evidence of Plummer–Vinson syndrome (a smooth tongue, anaemia and koilonychia) (see p. 155), secondary nodes from a carcinoma of the oesophagus may be felt in the neck and supraclavicular fossae, and the upper abdomen is carefully palpated, as a carcinoma

of the cardia is a common cause of dysphagia in elderly patients and indeed is commoner in this country than carcinoma of the oesophagus.

Special investigations

• *Barium swallow*, with cine-radiography, may demonstrate the characteristic appearances of a cervical web, extrinsic compression and the dilated oesophagus of achalasia, amongst others (Fig. 18.1).
• *Oesophagoscopy*. Fibre-optic oesophagoscopy enables biopsies to be taken to confirm

malignancy, and permits therapeutic dilatation or intubation if indicated.

The investigations are complementary and both may be indicated.

Swallowed foreign bodies

Foreign bodies are swallowed either accidentally, usually in children, or deliberately by mentally disturbed people, prison inmates and circus side-show performers. Obstruction of the oropharynx and tracheal opening by a large

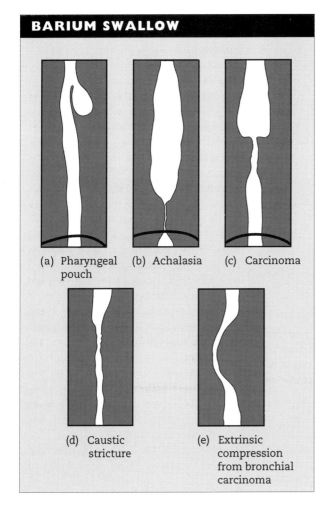

BARIUM SWALLOW

(a) Pharyngeal pouch

(b) Achalasia

(c) Carcinoma

(d) Caustic stricture

(e) Extrinsic compression from bronchial carcinoma

Fig. 18.1 Barium swallow appearances of common causes of dysphagia.

portion of meat can rapidly become fatal. A sharp blow just below the xiphoid, Heimlich's manoeuvre,* causing a sudden rise in intra-abdominal pressure may dislodge the plug and save the patient's life.

Unless they are sharp or irregular, amazingly large foreign bodies will pass into the stomach. If a smooth object, such as a bolus of food, impacts in the oesophagus, one must suspect the presence of a stricture. Occasionally, for example, a carcinoma of the oesophagus presents as an acute dysphagia when a morsel of food lodges above it. Absolute dysphagia, with failure to swallow even saliva, is then characteristic.

The presenting feature is painful dysphagia. The danger depends on the nature of the body. Perforation may occur with resultant mediastinitis; rarely perforation of the aorta occurs with fatal haematemesis. The diagnosis may be confirmed by a plain X-ray if the foreign body is radio-opaque, otherwise it may be shown up on a barium swallow.

Treatment

Oesophagoscopic removal is indicated where the foreign body is stuck. Occasionally, oeso-phagotomy is required. The great majority of foreign bodies, once they have passed into the stomach, proceed uneventfully along the alimentary canal and are passed per rectum. Occasionally, a sharp foreign body penetrates the wall of the bowel (there is a particular tendency for it to lodge in, and pierce, a Meckel's diverticulum).

The treatment of a foreign body that has passed the cardia is initially conservative. The patient is watched and serial X-rays taken to observe its progress if it is radio-opaque. Operation is performed if a sharp object fails to progress or if abdominal pain or tenderness develop.

Where the foreign body is potentially toxic when ingested, emetics or laxatives may be indicated.

---

*H. J. Heimlich (Contemporary), Physician, Xavier University, Cincinnati, Ohio, USA.

Perforations of the oesophagus

Classification
From within
• Swallowed foreign body — may occur anywhere in the oesophagus.
• Rupture at oesophagoscopy — usually at the level of crico-pharyngeus.
• Rupture during dilatation or biopsy — usually at the lower end of the oesophagus and especially likely in the presence of oesophageal disease (carcinoma or stricture)

From without
• Perforating wounds (rare).

Spontaneous
• Lower thoracic oesophagus (Boerhaave's syndrome†).

Clinical features
After instrumentation, perforation is suspected if the patient complains of pain in the neck, chest or upper abdomen, together with dysphagia and pyrexia. Diagnosis is certain if surgical emphysema is felt in the supraclavicular area.

Spontaneous rupture of the oesophagus occurs rarely and is associated with vomiting after a large meal (Boerhaave's syndrome). There is severe pain in the chest, the dorsal region of the spine or the upper abdomen (acute mediastinitis). The patient is collapsed and cyanosed. The abdomen may be rigid and often a false diagnosis of perforated peptic ulcer or myocardial infarction is made. However, there is usually surgical emphysema in the neck due to gas escaping into the mediastinum.

Special investigations
• *Chest X-ray* shows gas in the neck and

---

†Hermann Boerhaave (1668–1738), Physician, Leiden, Holland. Diagnosed spontaneous rupture of the oesophagus at post-mortem on the Grand Admiral of the Dutch Fleet.

mediastinum and there may be fluid and gas in the pleural cavity.

• *Gastrograffin swallow* (a water-soluble contrast fluid) will confirm the perforation and define its position.

Treatment

Cervical perforation is managed conservatively with parenteral antibiotics, nil by mouth and intravenous drip. Abscess formation in the superior mediastinum requires drainage via a supraclavicular incision.

Thoracic rupture is treated by immediate suture (or resection if a carcinoma is instrumentally perforated). The prognosis from spontaneous rupture is inversely related to the time to surgery, and after 12 hours is very poor.

Caustic stricture of the oesophagus

This follows accidental or suicidal ingestion of strong acids or alkalis (particularly caustic soda and ammonia). It often occurs in children.

In the acute phase there are associated burns of the mouth and pharynx. The mid and lower oesophagus are usually affected, as these are the sites of temporary hold-up of the caustic material where the oesophagus is crossed by the aortic arch and at the cardiac sphincter.

Treatment

In the acute phase this is to neutralize the alkali with vinegar, or acid with bicarbonate of soda. The damaged oesophagus is rested by instituting feeding via a gastrostomy, nil being given by mouth. Systemic steroids are given to reduce scar formation. If a stricture develops, gentle dilatation with bougies is commenced after 3 or 4 weeks. An established, impassable stricture is treated by a bypass operation, a loop of colon or small bowel being brought up on its vascular pedicle between the stomach below and the upper oesophagus above.

Achalasia of the cardia (cardiospasm)

This is a neuromuscular failure of relaxation at the lower end of the oesophagus with progressive dilatation, tortuosity, incoordination of peristalsis and often hypertrophy of the oesophagus above.

Clinical features

Achalasia may occur at any age but particularly in the third decade. The ratio of female to male is 3:2. It is indistinguishable from Chagas' disease,* which occurs in South America secondary to *Trypanosoma cruzi* infection.

There is progressive dysphagia over months to years. Regurgitation of fluids from the dilated oesophageal sac may be followed by an aspiration pneumonia. Occasionally, malignant change occurs in the dilated oesophagus.

Special investigations

• *Chest X-ray* may reveal the dilated oesophagus as a mediastinal mass, with an air–fluid level, and pneumonitis from aspiration of oesophageal contents. (Note that there are three other 'pseudo-tumours': scoliosis, tuberculous paravertebral abscess and thoracic aortic aneurysm, all of which may simulate a mediastinal tumour on a chest X-ray (see p. 58).)

• *Barium swallow* shows gross dilatation and tortuosity of the oesophagus leading to an unrelaxing narrowed segment at the lower end (said to resemble a bird's beak) (see Fig. 18.1).

• *Oesophagoscopy* demonstrates an enormous sac of oesophagus containing a pond of stagnant food and fluid.

Treatment

Satisfactory results are obtained by Heller's operation,† which is a cardiomyotomy dividing the muscle of the lower end of the oesophagus and the upper stomach down to the mucosa in

---

*Carlos Chagas (1879–1934), Brazilian Physician.
†Ernst Heller (1877–1964), Surgeon, Leipzig, Germany.

a similar manner to Ramstedt's operation for congenital pyloric hypertrophy. This procedure may now be performed thoracoscopically, reducing morbidity.

The same effect may be achieved by forcible dilatation of the oesophago-gastric junction by means of a hydrostatic bag. Although this avoids open operation, it is accompanied by the risk of rupture of the oesophagus.

Plummer–Vinson syndrome*

A syndrome actually described by Paterson and Kelly before Plummer and Vinson, and which sometimes rejoices in all four names, comprising dysphagia and iron-deficiency anaemia (with its associated smooth tongue and koilonychia) usually in middle-aged or elderly females.

The dysphagia is associated with hyperkeratinization of the oesophagus and often with the formation of a web in the upper part of the oesophagus. The condition is premalignant and is associated with the development of a carcinoma in the crico-pharyngeal region.

Treatment

The dysphagia responds to treatment with iron, although the web may require dilatation through an oesophagoscope.

Oesophageal diverticula

The only common diverticulum of the gullet is the pharyngeal pouch.

---

*Henry Strong Plummer (1874–1957), Physician, Mayo Clinic, Rochester, Minnesota, USA. Porter Paisley Vinson (1890–1959), Physician, Mayo Clinic, Rochester, Minnesota, USA. Donald Rose Paterson (1862–1939), ENT Surgeon, Royal Infirmary, Cardiff, Wales. Adam Brown Kelly (1865–1914), ENT Surgeon, Victoria Infirmary, Glasgow, Scotland.

Pharyngeal pouch

This is a mucosal protrusion between the two parts of the inferior pharyngeal constrictor — the thyro-pharyngeus and crico-pharyngeus (Fig. 18.2). The weak area between these portions of the muscle is situated posteriorly (Killian's dehiscence†). The pouch is believed to originate above the spasm of crico-pharyngeus; it develops first posteriorly but cannot then expand in this direction and protrudes to one or other side, usually the left. As the pouch enlarges it displaces the oesophagus laterally. It is an example of a pulsion diverticulum, forming as a result of increased intraluminal pressure.

Clinical features

It occurs more often in men and usually in the elderly. There is dysphagia, regurgitation of food, which collects in the pouch, and often a palpable swelling in the neck, which gurgles. Food retained in the pouch leads to a foetor, and late regurgitation may lead to aspiration pneumonia and lung abscess. Diagnosis is confirmed by a barium swallow.

Treatment

Excision of the pouch combined with a posterior myotomy of the crico-pharyngeus.

Other oesophageal diverticula

Other oesophageal diverticula are very rare.

- *Traction diverticula* may occur in association with fixation to tuberculous nodes or to pleural adhesions.
- *Pulsion diverticula* may be associated with cardiospasm and occur at the lower end of the oesophagus.
- *Congenital diverticula* are occasionally found. These are usually X-ray findings only, although they may occasionally produce dysphagia.

Reflux oesophagitis

See page 160.

---

† Gustav Killian (1860–1921), Professor of Otorhinolaryngology, Freiburg and Berlin.

PHARYNGEAL POUCH

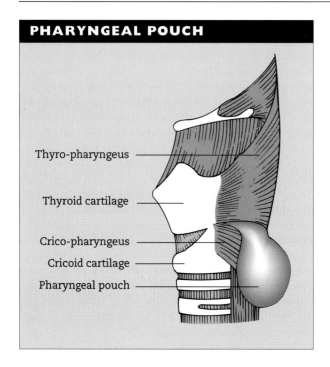

Thyro-pharyngeus

Thyroid cartilage

Crico-pharyngeus

Cricoid cartilage

Pharyngeal pouch

Fig. 18.2 A pharyngeal pouch emerging between the two components of the inferior constrictor muscle.

Tumours of the oesophagus

Classification
Benign
• Leiomyoma.

Malignant
1 Primary:
   (a) carcinoma;
   (b) leiomyosarcoma.
2 Secondary: direct invasion from lung or stomach.

Carcinoma
Post-cricoid carcinoma usually occurs in females and is associated with the Plummer–Vinson syndrome (see above). The remaining oesophageal growths occur more often in males, usually elderly. The commonest site is the mid-oesophagus, then the lower, then the upper oesophagus. Carcinoma of the oesophagus is a relatively common tumour (12 per 100 000 incidence) in the UK, but is 20 times more common in China, and up to 10 times more common in France. Overall prognosis is less than 10% at 3 years.

Predisposing factors include achalasia of the cardia, caustic stricture, Barrett's oesophagus, excessive intake of alcohol and cigarettes, and coeliac disease.

Pathology
The tumour commences as a nodule, which then develops into either an ulcer, a papilliferous mass or an annular constriction.

Microscopically, the majority are squamous carcinomas, but adenocarcinoma may occur at the lower end of the oesophagus, either arising in gastric metaplasia or as a result of an invasion of the oesophagus from a tumour developing at the cardiac end of the stomach.

Spread
• *Local*: into the mediastinal structures — the trachea, aorta, mediastinal pleura and lung.

- *Lymphatic*: to para-oesophageal, tracheo-bronchial, supraclavicular and sub-diaphragmatic nodes.
- *Blood stream*: to liver and lungs (relatively late).

Clinical features

Carcinoma of the oesophagus may present:
- with local symptoms—dysphagia;
- as a result of secondary deposits—enlarged neck nodes, occasionally jaundice and/or hepatomegaly;
- with general manifestations of malignant disease—loss of weight, anorexia, anaemia.

Dysphagia in an elderly male with a short history is almost invariably due to carcinoma of the oesophagus or the upper end of the stomach. Progression is from dysphagia for solids to dysphagia for liquids. Hoarseness and a bovine cough suggest invasion of the left recurrent laryngeal nerve by an upper oesophageal tumour.

Special investigations

- *Barium swallow* shows an irregular filling defect.
- *Oesophagoscopy* enables the tumour to be inspected and a biopsy taken. This may be combined with endoluminal ultrasound to evaluate local invasion.
- *Computed tomography (CT) scan of thorax and liver* assess the primary growth, local invasion, and secondary spread to the liver and lymph nodes.
- *Chest X-ray*, together with bronchoscopy, will exclude a primary tumour of the lung invading the oesophagus or oesophageal invasion of the mediastinum.
- *Liver ultrasound* screens for hepatic deposits, useful in staging the tumour.

Differential diagnosis

Other causes of dysphagia (p. 151).

Treatment

The two treatment aims are to cure the cancer where possible, and to palliate the dysphagia.

The treatment options are curative resection and palliative intubation or laser.

Resection

Where cure is possible, resection is undertaken. The growth is removed and the defect is usually bridged by mobilizing the stomach up into the chest, with anastomosis to residual oesophagus or to the pharynx in the neck.

Intubation

If the tumour is inoperable, dysphagia may be relieved by intubation with a stent.

Laser

Endoscopic laser therapy to vaporize growth and restore lumen. Repeated courses may be necessary, but disease progression rapidly overtakes the patient.

Radiotherapy

This may be used for squamous tumours.

The average expectation of life is in the region of 3 months with a maximum survival of about a year, but at least the patient is spared the misery of total dysphagia.

Barrett's oesophagus[*] and adenocarcinoma

The normal oesophagus is lined by stratified squamous epithelium. In patients with long-standing reflux of gastric contents, the lower oesophageal epithelium undergoes metaplasia to a gastric-type columnar epithelium. Continued inflammation may lead to dysplasia and subsequently to malignant change. Carcinomas in such cases are adenocarcinomas, and most occur in the lower third of the oesophagus.

As metaplasia to a Barrett-type oesophagus is pre-malignant, such patients should undergo annual endoscopic surveillance, with biopsies to look for dysplasia. Severe dysplasia (carcinoma-*in-situ*) is an indication for resection.

[*]Norman Barrett (1903–79), Surgeon, St Thomas's Hospital, London.

CHAPTER 19

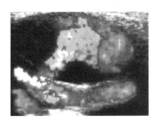

The Diaphragm

This is of principal importance as the site of herniae.

Classification of diaphragmatic herniae
1 *Congenital.*
2 *Acquired:*
   (a) traumatic;
   (b) hiatal.

Congenital diaphragmatic hernias

Embryology
These hernias can best be understood by reference to the embryology of the diaphragm (Fig. 19.1). The diaphragm is developed by fusion of the following:
• *The septum transversum*, which forms the central tendon, and which develops from mesoderm lying in front of the head of the embryo. With the folding of the head, this mesodermal mass is carried ventrally and caudally to lie in its definitive position at the anterior part of the diaphragm. During this migration, the cervical myotomes and cervical nerves contribute muscle and nerve supply respectively, thus accounting for the long course of the phrenic nerve (C3, 4, 5) from the neck to the diaphragm.
• *The dorsal oesophageal mesentery.*
• *The pleuro-peritoneal membranes*, which close the primitive communication between the pleural and peritoneal cavities.
• *A peripheral rim* derived from the body wall.
   In spite of this complex story, congenital abnormalities of the diaphragm are unusual. They may be:
• hernia through the foramen of Morgagni,* between the xiphoid and costal origins;
• hernia through the foramen of Bochdalek,† a defect in the pleuro-peritoneal canal;
• hernia through a deficiency of the whole central tendon;
• hernia through a congenitally large oesophageal hiatus.

Clinical features
Hernias through the foramen of Morgagni are usually small and unimportant. Those through the foramen of Bochdalek or through the central tendon are large and present as respiratory distress shortly after birth. Urgent surgical repair is required.
   The congenital hiatal hernias present with regurgitation, vomiting, dysphagia and progressive loss of weight in small children; they usually respond to conservative treatment, nursing the child in a sitting position. If this fails, surgical repair is necessary.

Traumatic diaphragmatic hernias

These are comparatively rare and follow blunt (crush) injuries to the chest or abdomen, or

* Giovanni Battista Morgagni (1682–1771), Professor of Anatomy, Padua, Italy.
† Victor Bochdalek (1801–83), Professor of Anatomy, Prague, Czechoslovakia.

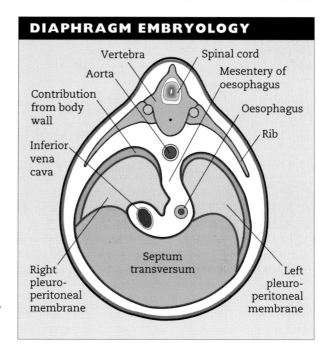

DIAPHRAGM EMBRYOLOGY

Vertebra

Aorta

Spinal cord

Mesentery of oesophagus

Contribution from body wall

Oesophagus

Inferior vena cava

Rib

Septum transversum

Right pleuro-peritoneal membrane

Left pleuro-peritoneal membrane

Fig. 19.1 The development of the diaphragm. The drawing shows the four contributory elements: septum transversum, dorsal mesentery of oesophagus, body wall and pleuro-peritoneal membrane.

penetrating injuries such as stab wounds, which implicate the diaphragm. The left diaphragm is far more often affected than the right (which is protected by the liver) and is accompanied by herniation of the stomach and spleen into the thoracic cavity. The gas-filled stomach lying in the left chest after a crush injury may be mistaken for a tension pneumothorax on chest X-ray. Passage of a naso-gastric tube or ingestion of a small amount of contrast material confirm the diagnosis.

Treatment comprises urgent surgical repair, through either the chest or abdomen.

Acquired hiatal hernias

Classification
These are divided into:
- sliding (90%);
- rolling (10%).

In the *sliding* variety, the stomach slides through the hiatus and is covered in its anterior aspect with a peritoneal sac while the pos-

terior part is extraperitoneal. It thus resembles an inguinal hernia *en glissade* (Fig. 19.2a). This type of hernia produces both the effects of a space-occupying lesion in the chest and disturbances of the cardio-oesophageal sphincter mechanism.

In the *rolling* (or para-oesophageal) hernia the cardia remains in position but the stomach rolls up anteriorly through the hiatus, producing a partial volvulus. Because the cardio-oesophageal mechanism is intact, there are no symptoms of regurgitation (Fig. 19.2b).

These hernias probably represent a progressive weakening of the muscles of the hiatus. They occur in the obese, middle-aged and elderly, and are four times commoner in women than men.

Clinical features
Most are symptomless, but when they occur symptoms fall into three groups.

1 *Mechanical*, produced by the presence of the hernia within the thoracic cavity: cough, dyspnoea, palpitations, hiccough.

HIATUS HERNIA

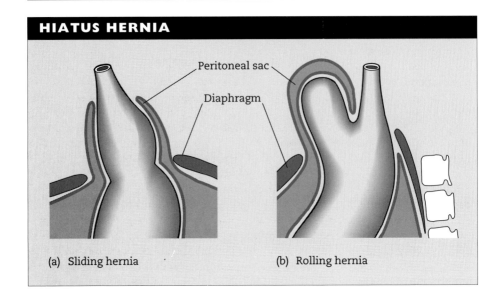

Peritoneal sac

Diaphragm

(a) Sliding hernia   (b) Rolling hernia

Fig. 19.2 (a) Sliding hiatus hernia: the stomach and lower oesophagus slide into the chest through a patulous oesophageal hiatus.
(b) Rolling hiatus hernia: the stomach rolls up through the hiatus alongside the lower oesophagus (para-oesophageal hernia).

2 *Reflux*, resulting from incompetence of the cardiac sphincter: burning retrosternal or epigastric pain aggravated by lying down or stooping, and which may be referred to the jaw, or arms, thus simulating cardiac ischaemia. Alkalis provide relief. In severe cases, spill-over into the trachea may cause pneumonitis.
3 *The effects of oesophagitis*: stricture formation with dysphagia and bleeding, which may be acute or occult.

Treatment

Sliding hiatus hernias are treated symptomatically. Para-oesophageal (rolling) hernias are usually asymptomatic, but potentially more serious with the risk of complete gastric volvulus into the chest. Should this occur, urgent surgical repair is indicated.

Reflux oesophagitis

This is produced by the reflux of peptic juice through the incompetent cardiac sphincter into the lower oesophagus, resulting in ulceration and inflammation and eventually to stricture formation. The exact mechanism of the cardio-oesophageal sphincter is not understood; it is sufficient to prevent regurgitation into the oesophagus when standing on one's head or in forced inspiration, when there is a pressure difference of some 80 mmHg between the intragastric and intra-oesophageal pressure, yet it can relax readily to allow vomiting or belching to occur. The mechanism is probably a complex affair comprising:
• positive intra-abdominal pressure acting on the lower (intra-abdominal) oesophagus, maintaining a high-pressure zone at the cardia;
• physiological muscle sphincter at the lower end of the oesophagus;
• valve-like effect of the obliquity of the oesophago-gastric angle;
• pinch-cock effect on the lower oesophagus of the diaphragmatic sling when the diaphragm contracts in full inspiration;
• plug-like action of the mucosal folds at the cardia.

The diaphragm is an important but not essential part of the cardiac sphincter mechanism, as sliding hiatus hernias are not necessarily accompanied by regurgitation. Similarly, free regurgitation occurs in some subjects with a normal oesophageal hiatus, presumably because of some defect in the function of the physiological sphincter.

Reflux oesophagitis may also occur in association with:

- repeated vomiting, especially in the presence of a duodenal ulcer with high acid content of gastric juice;
- long-standing naso-gastric intubation;
- resections of the cardia with gastro-oesophageal anastomosis;
- the presence of ectopic acid-secreting gastric mucosa within the oesophagus ('Barrett's oesophagus').

Special investigations

- *Fibre-optic oesophagoscopy* demonstrates the presence of oesophagitis, and facilitates biopsy to exclude carcinoma, or the presence of gastric-type epithelium.
- *24-hour oesophageal pH studies*: a probe in the oesophagus will demonstrate reflux of gastric acid and its temporal relation to pain.
- *Acid infusion test*: infusion of a dilute solution (0.1 mol/L) of hydrochloric acid will trigger pain similar to that complained of with reflux. The pain should resolve when the infusion is switched to saline.
- *Barium swallow*: this will demonstrate the outline of a hernia and the presence of any associated stricture. Tilting the patient's head down will demonstrate reflux, but does not necessarily confirm that the pain is due to reflux.

Differential diagnosis

The pain of hiatus hernia may be confused with cholecystitis, peptic ulcer or angina pectoris — indeed, these conditions often coexist.

The obstructive symptoms of an associated stricture must be differentiated from carcinoma of the oesophagus or of the cardia.

Treatment

This may be medical or surgical.

Medical treatment comprises weight loss, stopping smoking, dietary manipulation and the abandonment of corsets. Regurgitation is discouraged by avoiding stooping or lying and by sleeping propped up in bed. Alginate antacids (e.g. gaviscon) taken after meals reduce the acidity as well as line the gullet. H_2-receptor antagonist drugs (e.g. cimetidine or ranitidine) and proton-pump inhibitors (e.g. omeprazole) provide more complete reduction in gastric acidity. Prokinetic drugs to increase gastric emptying, such as metoclopramide or cisapride, may also be useful. Many patients with mild symptoms obtain considerable relief from such regimens.

Surgical repair of the hernia through a transthoracic or abdominal approach is undertaken when medical treatment fails. This may be supplemented by fundoplication in which the fundus of the stomach is sutured around the lower oesophagus in an ink-well fashion in order to produce an anti-reflux valve. This may be done open or via a laparoscope.

Stricture. In the presence of stricture, surgical treatment is indicated. In a mild case, continuous acid reduction treatment with a proton-pump inhibitor (e.g. omeprazole) and endoscopic dilatation will provide good palliation, with repeat dilatation every year or so. Anti-reflux surgery to repair the hernia in younger patients combined with pre-operative dilatation may also give good long-term palliation. In the advanced case, where frequent dilatation is required or is unsuccessful, resection of the stricture may be necessary.

CHAPTER 20

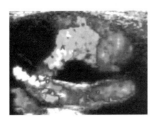

The Stomach and Duodenum

Congenital hypertrophic pyloric stenosis

Aetiology
The aetiology of the pyloric muscle 'tumour' in pyloric obstruction in infants is unknown. It may result from an abnormality of the ganglion cells of the myenteric plexus; failure of the pyloric sphincter to relax may then produce an intense work hypertrophy of the adjacent circular pyloric muscle.

It is a familial condition. Eighty per cent occur in male infants, 50% are first-born and the condition often occurs in siblings.

Clinical features
The child usually presents at 3–4 weeks of age, although symptoms may be present rarely at or soon after birth. It is extremely uncommon for a previously healthy infant to develop this condition after 12 weeks of age.

The presenting symptom is projectile vomiting. The vomit does not contain bile and the child takes food avidly immediately after vomiting, i.e. it is always hungry. There is failure to gain weight and, as a result of dehydration, the baby is constipated (the stools resembling the faecal pellets of a rabbit).

The infant may be dehydrated and visible peristalsis of the dilated stomach may be seen in the epigastrium. Ninety-five per cent have a palpable pyloric tumour, which is felt as a firm 'bobbin' in the right upper abdomen, especially after vomiting a feed.

Differential diagnosis
• *Enteritis*: diarrhoea accompanies this.
• *Neonatal intestinal obstruction* from duodenal atresia, volvulus neonatorum or intestinal atresia: symptoms commence within a day or two of birth and the vomit contains bile.
• *Intracranial birth injury*.
• *Overfeeding*: here there are no other features to suggest pyloric stenosis apart from vomiting.

Special investigations
If the clinical features are characteristic and a pyloric mass is palpable, no further investigations are necessary.
• *Ultrasound* scan demonstrates the thickened pylorus and large stomach.
• *Abdominal X-ray* reveals a dilated stomach with minimal gas in the bowel, in contrast to dilated coils of bowel in intestinal obstruction.
• *Barium meal* reveals the pyloric obstruction with characteristic shouldering of the pyloric antrum due to the impression made on it by the hypertrophied pyloric muscle.

Treatment
This is anomalous in that the more seriously ill

RAMSTEDT'S PYLOROMYOTOMY

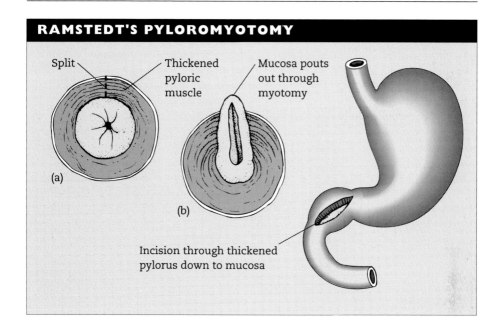

Split

Thickened pyloric muscle

Mucosa pouts out through myotomy

(a)

(b)

Incision through thickened pylorus down to mucosa

Fig. 20.1 Ramstedt's pyloromyotomy. The thickened muscle at the pylorus is split down to the mucosa. (a) and (b) show the pathology and the operative procedure in transverse section.

the child, the less urgent is the operation. With prolonged vomiting the infant becomes dehydrated with a hypochloraemic metabolic alkalosis. In such cases a day or two must be spent in gastric lavage and fluid replacement (saline with added potassium chloride), either by the subcutaneous or intravenous route. The otherwise healthy child can be submitted to operation soon after admission.

Surgical treatment
*Ramstedt's pyloromyotomy.** A longitudinal incision is made through the hypertrophied muscle of the pylorus down to mucosa and the cut edges are separated (Fig. 20.1).

The infant is given glucose water 3 hours after the operation and this is followed by 3-hourly milk feeds, which are steadily increased in amount.

*Conrad Ramstedt (1867–1963), Surgeon, Munster, Germany.

Results are excellent and the mortality is extremely low.

Duodenal atresia

Duodenal atresia may be partial or complete, and principally affects the second part of the duodenum near the ampulla of Vater. An annular pancreas may be present (p. 265).

Clinical features
Antenatally the diagnosis is suggested by the presence of polyhydramnios and ultrasound appearances. Vomiting occurs from birth and the stomach may be visibly distended. As the common bile duct usually enters above the obstruction, the vomit usually contains bile.

There is a strong association between duodenal atresia and Down's syndrome, 30% of whom are affected.

Differential diagnosis
• *Oesophageal atresia*: there is choking rather than vomiting.
• *Pyloric stenosis*: bile is absent from the vomit,

there is a palpable pyloric tumour and onset is later.

• *Congenital intestinal obstruction*: there is abdominal distension and X-rays show multiple distended loops of bowel with fluid levels (see p. 182).

Plain X-ray of the abdomen is diagnostic and shows distension of the stomach and proximal duodenum with absence of gas throughout the rest of the bowel (the 'double bubble' sign).

Treatment

Duodeno-jejunostomy or gastro-jejunostomy is performed after rehydration and gastric aspiration.

Peptic ulcer

Pathology

The pathogenesis of peptic ulcer involves a disturbance in the balance between the secretion of acid and pepsin by the stomach on the one hand and mucosal barrier (a thick layer of mucus) on the other. The normal stomach mucosa is adapted to contain the acid produced by the parietal (oxyntic) cells. Where the mucosal defence is compromised, or non-existent, the acid causes mucosal ulceration. Ulcers also occur where acid attacks mucosa not specialized to deal with it.

Sites of ulceration

Typical sites for peptic ulcers are the oesophagus (peptic oesophagitis), stomach and duodenum, at the stoma of a gastro-jejunal anastomosis or in a Meckel's diverticulum when ectopic parietal cells are present.

Aetiology
Historical background

The vast majority of peptic ulcers are now known to be caused by infection with *Helicobacter pylori*. Until the discovery of this organism in the 1970s, the majority of peptic ulcers were thought to be due to over-activity of parietal cells. The stimuli to parietal cell function are neural (via the vagus nerve) and humoral (gastrin and histamine). Earlier treatments were therefore directed at reducing acid secretion by surgical denervation of the stomach (vagotomy) or removal of the parietal cells (partial gastrectomy). More recently, pharmacological control has been possible with histamine H_2-receptor antagonists (e.g. cimetidine and ranitidine), and proton-pump inhibitors (e.g. omeprazole). With hindsight we now realize that none of these treatments dealt with the primary cause of the peptic ulceration, *H. pylori*.

H. pylori

H. pylori (previously called *Campylobacter pyloridis*) is a spiral-shaped, Gram-negative, motile rod, which is able to penetrate the viscid mucus layer lining the stomach. Its potent urease activity splits any urea in the vicinity producing ammonia, thus neutralizing the pH in the local milieu surrounding the organism. Many *H. pylori* strains also produce cytotoxins that possess protease and phospholipase activity, allowing them to attack and damage mucosal membranes. This direct damage, together with the resultant inflammation, impair the gastric mucosal barrier and allow further damage by gastric acid. Non-cytotoxin-producing strains explain asymptomatic carriage of the organism.

Evidence identifying *H. pylori* as a causative agent in peptic ulceration includes the following observations.

• Ingestion of *H. pylori* results in chronic gastritis (as demonstrated by the discoverers of the organism).

• Animal inoculation with *H. pylori* mimics human gastritis.

• Antimicrobial treatment which eradicates *H. pylori* also eliminates gastritis.

• *H. pylori* can be identified in almost all patients with duodenal ulcers, and most patients with gastric ulcers.

Zollinger–Ellison syndrome*

This is a syndrome in which a non-insulin-secreting islet-cell tumour of the pancreas produces a potent gastrin-like hormone (see p. 271). It is an uncommon cause of peptic ulceration. In this syndrome the ulcers are often multiple, and ulceration may be more widespread within the small bowel.

Other factors in the aetiology of peptic ulceration

A number of other factors decrease the effectiveness of the mucosal defences against gastric juice. In particular, non-steroidal anti-inflammatory drugs (NSAIDs) inhibit the production of protective prostaglandins in the mucosa. Steroids also predispose to ulceration, as do smoking and stress, which are thought to have an effect on both acid secretion and mucosal defences.

The acute peptic ulcer

This may be single or multiple (multiple erosions), may occur without apparent cause, or may be associated with ingestion of alcohol, NSAIDs (aspirin, indomethacin and butazolidine are common culprits), steroid therapy, acute stress, a major operation, head injury (Cushing's ulcer†) or severe burns (Curling's ulcer‡). It may present with sudden pain, haemorrhage or perforation. A proportion of acute ulcers probably go on to become chronic.

The chronic peptic ulcer

The prevalence of peptic ulceration in the adult population is up to 13%. At least 80% occur in the duodenum. Duodenal ulcers may occur at any age but especially in the thirties to forties;

*Robert Milton Zollinger (1903–92), Professor of Surgery, Ohio State University, Columbus, USA. Edward Horner Ellison (1918–1970), Associate Professor at the same institution.
†Harvey Cushing (1869–1939), Professor of Surgery, Harvard Medical School, Boston, USA.
‡Thomas Blizzard Curling (1811–88), Surgeon, The London Hospital, London.

about 80% occur in males. Females are relatively immune to duodenal ulceration before the menopause and especially during pregnancy.

Gastric ulcers occur predominantly in males, but the sex preponderance is less marked, about 3 : 1 male to female. Any age may be affected but especially the forties to fifties (i.e. a decade later than the peak for duodenal ulceration).

Duodenal ulcers particularly occur among the executive and business classes in the UK, whereas there is a higher incidence of gastric ulcer among poorer patients.

Clinical features

Physical signs in the uncomplicated case are absent or confined to epigastric tenderness. Clinical diagnosis depends on the careful history.

The pain is typically epigastric, occurs in attacks that last for days or weeks and is interspersed with periods of relief. Pain that radiates into the back suggests a posterior penetrating ulcer. Peptic ulcer pain may come on immediately after a meal but more typically commences about 2 hours after food so that the patient says it precedes a meal ('hunger pain'). Characteristically, it wakes the patient at 0200 hours, so much so that the patient may adopt the habit of taking a glass of milk or an alkali preparation to bed. However, it is a myth to say that one can differentiate between a gastric and a duodenal ulcer merely on the time relationship of the pain. The pain is aggravated by spicy foods and relieved by milk and alkalis, although the relief is lost in deep and penetrating ulcers. There may be associated heartburn, nausea and vomiting. The patient may lose weight because of the pain produced by food but often may gain weight because of the high intake of milk.

Special investigations

1 *Fibre-optic gastroscopy*: enables the oesophagus, stomach and duodenum to be

examined. The ulcer can be identified and, particularly in the case of a gastric lesion, biopsy material obtained to enable differentiation between a benign and malignant ulcer.

2 *H. pylori detection.*

(a) *Endoscopic biopsy.* Histological examination will confirm the presence of the organism and identify mucosal damage. Culture of biopsy samples is difficult (low sensitivity) but is specific for the organism. A urease test, where a biopsy sample is placed in a solution of urea together with a pH indicator, is highly specific and sensitive for the organism. *H. pylori* splits urea, releasing ammonia, which changes the pH of the solution.

(b) *Breath test.* The patient ingests a normal meal together with labelled urea, either ^{13}C-urea (non-radioactive) or ^{14}C-urea (radioactive). The urease from the organism cleaves the urea load and bicarbonate (HCO_3^-) is released into the blood, and expired as labelled CO_2. Measurement of labelled CO_2 in breath samples confirms the diagnosis, and serial tests can be used to confirm eradication of the organism.

(c) *Antibody testing.* Infection with *H. pylori* results in generation of antibodies, which may be detected. Antibody titre falls slowly after eradication.

3 *Barium meal.*

(a) *Gastric ulcers* show the following features: a niche along the otherwise smooth line of the lesser curvature, usually in the typical position above the incisura, often associated with a notch of spasm immediately opposite on the greater curvature. A blob of barium may be left behind in the ulcer crater when the stomach empties. Normal peristaltic waves are seen, but there is distortion of adjacent mucosal folds around the ulcer.

(b) *Duodenal ulcers* are often associated with a large hypermotile stomach with thick mucosal folds. The duodenal cap is deformed and tender to palpation; an ulcer crater may be visualized. If there is stenosis there is excess of resting juice, dilatation of the stomach, gross narrowing of the first part of the duodenum and delay of 6 hours or more in gastric emptying.

4 *Occult blood* examination of the stools is often positive.

Treatment

Treatment of a peptic ulcer is medical in the first instance; surgery is indicated when complications supervene. The complications are *chronicity, perforation, stenosis, haemorrhage* and, in the case of gastric ulcer, *malignant change.* They are considered in detail later in this chapter.

Principles of medical treatment

The main principles of treatment are to eradicate *H. pylori* and to reduce and neutralize (using alkalis and milk) acid secretion. Failure to eradicate *H. pylori* by giving antacid therapy alone results in high relapse rates.

Acid reduction. Acid secretion can be reduced by histamine H_2-receptor antagonists (e.g. cimetidine and ranitidine) or a proton-pump inhibitor (e.g. omeprazole), which blocks the enzyme that occurs almost exclusively in the gastric parietal cell and which mediates the final stage of gastric acid secretion. All these drugs result in rapid reduction in acid secretion and the majority of ulcers heal within 1–2 months, but will recur if *H. pylori* has not been eradicated.

H. pylori eradication. A short course of antimicrobial therapy will eradicate *H. pylori*, and combined acid reduction therapy results in rapid ulcer healing. Initial protocols consisted of triple therapy with metronidazole, amoxycillin (or tetracycline) and bismuth combined with acid reduction therapy (e.g. ranitidine). It is now clear that double therapy combining amoxycillin or clarithromycin with omeprazole, given for 2 weeks will eradicate *H. pylori* in most cases. However, due to a high incidence of antibiotic resistance, combinations of two antibiotics are recommended (e.g. clarithromycin *and* amoxycillin, plus omeprazole for 10 days). The optimal protocol remains to be proven.

Other agents. Synthetic prostaglandins (e.g. misoprostol) have been shown to have ulcer-healing properties. The main use of this type of therapy is in the prevention of peptic ulceration in patients taking NSAIDs, especially in those who give a past history of peptic ulcer or of bleeding while previously taking these preparations.

Violent gastric acid stimulants such as alcohol should be avoided. Rest, sedation, avoidance of smoking and dealing with underlying anxiety states are helpful. Aspirin and other NSAIDs should be avoided wherever possible.

Results of medical treatment. The uncomplicated duodenal ulcer can be cured in the majority of cases, with over 90% eradication of H. pylori. Relapse rates in those in whom eradication is successful is low.

In gastric ulceration there is, in addition, a small, but definite risk of treating a gastric carcinoma under the mistaken diagnosis of benign gastric ulcer.

Principles of surgical treatment

Surgical treatment is now reserved for those cases where complications of ulceration occur. In the emergency situation, minimal surgery is practised with the confidence that medical cure of the underlying disease may be effected. The commonest indications for emergency surgery are bleeding or perforation (see below).

Gastric ulcers are treated by removing the ulcer together with the gastrin-secreting zone of the antrum; this is effected by the Billroth I gastrectomy.* The results are 90% satisfactory with a mortality in the region of 1%.

Duodenal ulcers will heal providing the high acid production of the stomach is abolished. This can be effected either by removing the

bulk of the acid-secreting area of the stomach (the body and the lesser curve), i.e. a partial (Polya†) gastrectomy, or by dividing the vagi. As total vagotomy interferes with the mechanism of gastric emptying, this operation must be accompanied by a drainage procedure, either gastro-jejunostomy or pyloroplasty. If the branches of the vagus that supply the pyloric sphincter (the nerves of Latarjet†) are left intact, the remaining vagal fibres can be divided without the necessity of gastric drainage (highly selective vagotomy) but nevertheless the goal of reduction in the vagal phase of acid secretion is achieved.

Post-gastrectomy syndromes. Even though about 85% of patients are well following Polya partial gastrectomy for peptic ulcer, a large number of unpleasant sequelae may occur. These may be classified into the following.
• The 'small stomach' syndrome: a feeling of fullness after a moderate sized meal.
• Bilious vomiting due to emptying of the afferent loop of a Polya gastrectomy into the stomach remnant.
• Anaemia due usually to iron deficiency (HCl is required for adequate iron absorption) or occasionally vitamin B_{12} deficiency due to loss of intrinsic factor with extensive gastric resection.
• The 'dumping syndrome': comprises attacks of fainting, vertigo and sweating after food, rather like a hypoglycaemic attack. This is probably an osmotic effect due to gastric contents of high osmolarity passing rapidly into the jejunum, absorbing fluid into the gut lumen and producing a temporary reduction in circulating blood volume.
• Steatorrhoea. In the presence of a long afferent loop, food passing into the jejunum traverses the bowel without mixing adequately with pancreatic and biliary secretions. Calcium deficiency and osteomalacia may occur.
• Stomal ulceration complicates about 2% of

---

*Theodor Billroth (1829–94), Professor of Surgery, Vienna. He performed the first successful gastrectomy for cancer at the pyloric end of the stomach in 1881.

†Eugen Alexander Polya (1876–1944), Surgeon, St Stephen's Hospital, Budapest, Hungary.
‡André Latarget (1876–1947), Professor of Anatomy, Lyon, France.

gastrectomies for duodenal ulcer; it is extremely rare after resection for gastric ulcer. It may be due to inadequate removal of the acid-secreting area of the stomach, or, rarely, because of the Zollinger–Ellison syndrome (p. 271). A stomal ulcer, like any other peptic ulcer, may perforate, stenose, invade surrounding structures or bleed. It is treated either by vagotomy or higher gastric resection.

Post-vagotomy syndromes. The following sequelae may occur after vagotomy.
• *Steatorrhoea and diarrhoea.* Frequently transient or episodic, they may be severe and persistent in about 2% of patients. The incidence is reduced in patients subjected to highly selective vagotomy without drainage.
• *Stomal ulceration* may occur if vagotomy is incomplete.

Complications of peptic ulceration

Peptic ulcer at any site may undergo the following complications.
• *Chronicity* due to formation of fibrous tissue in the ulcer base.
• *Perforation* either into the general peritoneal cavity or into adjacent structures, e.g. the pancreas, liver or colon.
• *Stenosis.*
• *Haemorrhage.*
• *Malignant change* does not occur in duodenal ulcers but may rarely take place in a gastric ulcer; a long history does not necessarily mean that the ulcer was not malignant *de novo*. Both gastric ulcer and gastric carcinoma are common conditions and there may merely be a chance association between the two. It would seem that about 1% of all gastric carcinomas arise in a gastric ulcer.

Perforated peptic ulcer
Pathology
Perforation of a peptic ulcer is still a relatively

common and important emergency. The incidence of perforation fell steadily from the 1950s (i.e. before the introduction of the H_2-receptor antagonists), but has been relatively constant for the past 10 years. Male preponderance, once very high, is now about 2:1. Until recently, perforation occurred particularly in young adults, but now the shift is towards the older age groups, especially in patients who are either on steroids or NSAIDs (aspirin, indomethacin, etc.).

Gastric carcinomas may occasionally present with perforation.

Clinical features
A previous history of peptic ulceration is obtained in about half the cases, although this may be forgotten by the patient in agony. Typically, the pain is of sudden onset and of extreme severity, indeed the patient can often recall the exact moment of the onset of the pain. Subphrenic irritation may be indicated by referred pain to one or both shoulders, usually the right. The pain is aggravated by movement and the patient lies rigidly still. There is nausea, but only occasionally vomiting. Sometimes there is accompanying haematemesis or melaena.

Examination reveals a patient in severe pain, cold and sweating with rapid, shallow respirations. In the early stages (hours), there may be no clinical evidence of true shock: the pulse is steady and the blood pressure normal; the temperature is either normal or a little depressed. The abdomen is rigid and silent, although in some instances an occasional bowel sound may be heard. Liver dullness is diminished in about half the cases due to escape of gas into the peritoneal cavity. Rectal examination may reveal pelvic tenderness.

In the delayed case, after 12 hours or more, the features of generalized peritonitis with paralytic ileus become manifest; the abdomen is distended, effortless vomiting occurs and the patient is extremely toxic and in oligaemic shock.

X-ray of the chest with the patient erect

shows free gas below the diaphragm in 70% of cases.

Differential diagnosis

The four conditions with which perforated ulcer is most commonly confused are:

1 perforated appendicitis;
2 acute cholecystitis;
3 acute pancreatitis;
4 myocardial infarction.

Treatment

A naso-gastric tube is passed to empty the stomach and diminish further leakage. It is essential as a pre-anaesthetic measure. Opiate analgesia is given to relieve pain and an intravenous infusion is started. Antibiotics are given to contend with the peritoneal infection, and an H_2-blocker or proton-pump inhibitor commenced. Most surgeons are in favour of immediate operative repair of the perforation.

Surgery involves suturing an omental plug to seal the perforation, together with lavage of the peritoneal cavity. In addition a gastric ulcer is biopsied at all four quadrants to exclude malignancy. An obviously malignant gastric ulcer is removed by partial gastrectomy (see p. 167). Definitive ulcer treatment at the time of emergency surgery is now uncommon, and medical control of acid secretion together with *H. pylori* eradication is undertaken post-operatively. A definitive procedure may be indicated where medical therapy has failed.

Prognosis

The mortality for perforated peptic ulcer lies between 5 and 10%. Most deaths are in patients incorrectly diagnosed, with consequent delay in correct treatment, or too ill for operation. The subjects who die are typically either over the age of 70 years or reach hospital 12 hours or more from the time of perforation.

The late prognosis following perforation depends on whether or not the ulcer is chronic, and whether a treatable cause, such as *H. pylori* or NSAIDs, is present. Some patients may come to further surgery.

Pyloric stenosis

This is an inaccurate term when applied to duodenal ulceration, as the obstruction is in the first part of the duodenum.

Pathology

At first, fibrotic scarring is compensated by dilatation and hypertrophy of the stomach muscle. Eventually, failure of compensation occurs, much like the failure of a hypertrophied ventricle of the heart with valvular stenosis.

Clinical features

During the phase of compensation there is nothing in the history to suggest stenosis. Once failure occurs, there is characteristic profuse vomiting, which is free from bile. The vomitus may contain food eaten 1 or 2 days previously and appear faeculent. Because of copious vomiting there is associated loss of weight, constipation (because of dehydration) and weakness due to electrolyte disturbance.

On examination the patient may appear dehydrated and wasted. The progressive dilatation and hypertrophy of the stomach can be summed up as 'the stomach you can hear, the stomach you can hear and see, and the stomach you can hear, see and feel'. At first, a gastric splash (*succussion splash*) can be elicited by shaking the patient's abdomen several hours after a meal. As the stomach enlarges, visible peristalsis can be seen also, passing from left to right across the upper abdomen. Finally, the grossly dilated, hypertrophied stomach, full of stale food and fluid, can actually be palpated.

Gastric aspiration yields a morning resting juice of over 100 ml. In advanced cases it may amount to a litre or more of foul-smelling gastric contents.

Special investigations
• *Barium meal* shows dilatation of the stomach, a narrow outlet and considerable delay in emptying.
• *Arterial blood gases and electrolyte estimation* show a hypochloraemic alkalosis, with hypokalaemia, and uraemia (see below).

Biochemical disturbances
Patients with a duodenal ulcer have a high gastric acidity. Pyloric obstruction with copious vomiting therefore results not only in dehydration from fluid loss, but also alkalosis due to loss of hydrogen ions. The alkalotic tendency is compensated by the renal excretion of sodium bicarbonate, which may keep the blood pH within normal limits. At this phase, the dehydration results in diminished volume and increased concentration of the urine, whose chloride content is first diminished and then disappears and whose reaction is alkaline. If vomiting continues, a large sodium deficit becomes manifest. This loss of sodium is partly accounted for by loss in the vomitus but it is mainly due to urinary excretion consequent upon the bicarbonate lost in the urine as sodium bicarbonate. As the body's sodium reserves become depleted, hydrogen and potassium ions are substituted for sodium as the cations that are excreted with the bicarbonate. This results in the paradox that the patient with advanced alkalosis now excretes an acid urine. The blood urea rises, partly as a result of dehydration and partly because of renal impairment secondary to the electrolyte disturbances. Eventually, the patient may develop tetany as a result of a shift of the ionized, weakly alkaline calcium phosphate to its un-ionized state, in attempted compensation for the alkalosis. The concentration of calcium ions in the plasma therefore falls, although the total calcium concentration is not affected.

The metabolic disturbances may be summarized as follows.
• The patient is dehydrated and the haematocrit level is raised.
• The urine is scanty, concentrated, initially

alkaline, but later acid; its chloride content is reduced or absent.
• Serum chloride, sodium and potassium are lowered and the plasma bicarbonate and urea are raised.

Differential diagnosis
• Carcinoma of the pylorus. Other causes of pyloric obstruction are unusual in the adult.
• Scarring associated with a benign gastric ulcer near the pylorus.
• Carcinoma of the head of the pancreas infiltrating the duodenum and pylorus.
• Chronic pancreatitis.
• Invasion of the pylorus by malignant nodes.
• Adult hypertrophy of the pylorus (see p. 162).

The differential diagnosis from a pyloric carcinoma cannot always be established until laparotomy, but a reasonable attempt can be made on the following points.
• *Length of history:* a history of several years of characteristic peptic ulcer pain is in favour of benign ulcer. Cancer usually has a history of only months and indeed may be painless.
• *Gross dilatation of the stomach* favours a benign lesion, as it may take several years for this to develop.
• *The presence of a mass* at the pylorus indicates malignant disease, although rarely a palpable inflammatory mass in association with a large duodenal ulcer can be detected.

Treatment
The treatment of established pyloric obstruction is invariably surgical. Before operation, dehydration and electrolyte depletion are corrected by intravenous replacement of saline together with potassium. Daily gastric lavage is performed to remove the debris from the stomach. In addition, this often restores function to the stomach and allows fluid absorption to take place by mouth. Vitamin C is given, as the patient with a chronic duodenal ulcer is often deficient in ascorbic acid. This may be a direct effect of *H. pylori*.

Surgical correction is carried out after a few days of pre-operative preparation. The choice of treatment lies between a partial gastrectomy of the Polya type and a vagotomy with drainage (pyloroplasty or gastro-enterostomy); the latter is to be preferred.

Gastrointestinal haemorrhage

Management

The management of patients presenting with haematemesis and/or melaena is threefold:

1 assessment and replacement of the blood loss;

2 diagnosis of the source of the bleeding;

3 treatment and control of the source of bleeding.

Blood loss assessment

The indications for blood transfusion are the general condition of the patient (i.e. whether the patient demonstrates features of shock with pallor, sweating, etc.), a pulse rate above 100 and a blood pressure that has a systolic below 100. The last two are general rules that may be varied with the general condition of the patient, e.g. if the patient is a known hypertensive then obviously a systolic pressure well above 100 may still be a strong indication for transfusion. Additional evidence of significant bleeding is a marked difference between lying and standing blood pressure, and a low central venous pressure. Every patient presenting with gastrointestinal haemorrhage has blood taken for grouping and cross-matching.

Direct inspection of the amount of blood vomited and melaena passed will generally underestimate losses; however, it may help to distinguish old from recent bleeding. The haemoglobin estimation on admission is of only limited value, as it may be more than 24 hours before haemodilution will reduce the haemoglobin level from its normal value.

Aetiology

Bleeding may be from some local source or result from a general bleeding diathesis.

General causes include haemophilia, leukaemia, anticoagulant therapy and thrombocytopenia, as well as conditions such as hereditary haemorrhagic telangiectasia.

Local causes are best considered anatomically, as follows.

1 *Oesophagus*:
   (a) peptic oesophagitis (associated with hiatus hernia);
   (b) oesophageal varices (associated with portal hypertension, see p. 250).

2 *Stomach*:
   (a) gastric ulcer;
   (b) acute erosions (associated with aspirin, other NSAIDs and corticosteroids);
   (c) Mallory–Weiss syndrome (p. 172);
   (d) tumours (benign and malignant).

3 *Duodenum*:
   (a) duodenal ulcer;
   (b) erosion of the duodenum by a pancreatic tumour.

4 *Small intestine*:
   (a) tumours;
   (b) Meckel's diverticulum.

5 *Large bowel*:
   (a) tumours (benign and malignant, commonly adenocarcinomas);
   (b) diverticulitis;
   (c) angiodysplasia;
   (d) colitis (ulcerative colitis, ischaemic colitis and infective colitis).

About 85% of patients with gastrointestinal bleeding of an acute form in this country have a peptic ulcer or erosion of the stomach or duodenum; chronic duodenal ulcer heads the list. About 5% of patients have oesophageal varices and the remainder are accounted for by the other causes listed above.

Diagnosis is made on history, examination and special investigations.

History

There may be a typical story of peptic ulceration and perhaps the patient has had a positive endoscopy or barium swallow in the past. It is important to take a history of drug habits, as many obscure bleeds are found to be due to recent ingestion of aspirin, anticoagulants, steroids, indomethacin, etc. A story of alcoholism or previous viral hepatitis may suggest cirrhosis and an alcoholic binge may also have precipitated an acute gastric erosion. Repeated violent vomits after a large meal or alcohol followed by a bright red haematemesis is typical of the Mallory–Weiss syndrome,* in which a stress mucosal tear in the upper part of the stomach may result in brisk haemorrhage.

Clinical examination

This is usually negative apart from the clinical features that enable assessment of blood loss. However, a bleeding tendency may be suggested by purpura, oesophageal varices due to cirrhosis by enlargement of the liver and spleen, the presence of spider naevi and liver palms, and hereditary haemorrhagic telangiectasia by circumoral telangiectasia.

Special investigations

• *Haemoglobin estimation*. This is useful as a baseline, but will not reflect acute blood loss until the circulating volume is restored. Until then the haemoglobin concentration is unchanged.

• *Upper gastrointestinal fibreoptic endoscopy*, viewing the oesophagus, stomach and duodenum, is the most valuable investigation, and can be carried out as an emergency as soon as possible after admission. It will usually identify the exact site of the bleeding in upper gastrointestinal haemorrhage. Some actively bleeding peptic ulcers may be treated endoscopically by injection of adrenaline or alcohol into the ulcer bed or by laser photocoagulation.

• *Barium meal* can be performed as soon as active bleeding has ceased.

If the above tests fail to detect a source for the blood loss, the following may be considered.

• *Colonoscopy* is performed to identify colonic sources of bleeding, particularly the presence of angiodysplasia in the right colon.

---

*George Kenneth Mallory (Contemporary), Professor of Pathology, Boston University, USA. Soma Weiss (1899–1942), Professor of Medicine, Harvard University, Boston, USA.

• *Technetium scan*, in a child or young adult, will identify the presence of ectopic gastric mucosa in a Meckel's diverticulum. Gastric mucosa takes up technetium, which is then detected by scintigraphy.

• *Selective visceral angiography* using a catheter inserted via the femoral artery into the mesenteric arteries may localize the source of haemorrhage in an obscure case, but usually only in the presence of active bleeding.

• *Laparotomy and on-table enteroscopy* is required rarely when bleeding continues and upper and lower gastrointestinal endoscopy are unproductive. An enterotomy is made at laparotomy through which a colonoscope is passed and guided throughout the entire small bowel seeking an obscure cause of bleeding such as an arterio-venous malformation.

Treatment

In the first instance this is on medical lines.

1 The patient is reassured, and reassurance is supplemented with morphine if the patient is restless.

2 A careful watch is kept on the general condition, pulse and blood pressure.

3 Shock is treated, if present, by blood transfusion. A central venous line is established to measure central venous pressure and assist in fluid replacement, and a urinary catheter is passed to monitor urine output.

4 Intravenous cimetidine (or ranitidine) is commenced to reduce acid secretion to a minimum.

5 As soon as active bleeding ceases, milk is allowed by mouth in the form of regular hourly or 2-hourly milk drinks. Oral anti-ulcer therapy is commenced as soon as possible, and the patient is transferred to a semi-solid gastric diet.

On this regimen three out of four patients with gastrointestinal haemorrhage settle down.

Indications for surgery

The mortality of gastrointestinal haemorrhage is in the region of 10%. This is almost confined to patients over the age of 45 years, especially the elderly, who continue to bleed, or in whom bleeding recurs, while in hospital on the above regimen. It is common sense therefore that surgery is advised in the presence of the following poor prognostic features.

1 Clinical features suggesting poor prognosis:
  (a) aged over 60 years;
  (b) chronic history;
  (c) relapse on full medical treatment;
  (d) serious coexisting medical conditions;
  (e) continued melaena or haematemesis;
  (f) more than four units of blood transfusion required during resuscitation.

2 Endoscopic features suggesting poor prognosis:
  (a) active bleeding;
  (b) visible vessel in ulcer base;
  (c) clot adherent to ulcer;
  (d) blood in stomach but source not identifiable.

In poor prognostic cases, blood transfusion is continued and urgent preparation made for laparotomy. At operation, the source of bleeding is found and controlled. This usually takes the form of a partial gastrectomy or simple ulcer excision for a chronic gastric ulcer, and vagotomy, pyloroplasty and undersewing of the gastro-duodenal artery at the base of the ulcer for duodenal ulceration. In other cases it may be possible to undersew an acute erosion or bleeding ulcer, particularly in the desperately ill patient who is unfit for gastrectomy.

In most cases, preoperative endoscopy will identify the cause of the haemorrhage. If blood is present in the stomach but the source of haemorrhage is not immediately obvious, the stomach is opened by a gastrotomy, the blood clot evacuated and the bleeding point sought by direct inspection of the gastric and duodenal mucosa. Endoscopic therapy with diathermy or laser coagulation, or adrenaline injection, may be possible for short-term control of bleeding during resuscitation and until other therapies are instituted.

In the patients who are treated medically and who settle down, careful assessment is made in the convalescent period. If the presence of a chronic duodenal or gastric ulcer is established, in the absence of *H. pylori*, surgery is usually advised as an elective procedure; once a chronic ulcer has bled, subsequent haemorrhages are likely to occur. *H. pylori* eradication therapy should be attempted first when it is found.

The management of haemorrhage from oesophageal varices

This is considered on page 252.

Tumours of the stomach

Classification
Benign
1 *Epithelial.*
  (a) Adenoma: (i) single; (ii) multiple (gastric polyposis).
  (b) Leiomyoma.

2 *Connective tissue:*
  (a) fibroma;
  (b) neurofibroma.

3 *Vascular:* haemangioma.

Malignant
1 *Primary:*
  (a) adenocarcinoma;
  (b) leiomyosarcoma;
  (c) lymphoma;
  (d) Hodgkin's disease.

2 *Secondary:* invasion from adjacent tumours (pancreas or colon).

Benign tumours: leiomyomas

These are rare, but the leiomyomas are an occasional cause of brisk haematemesis. Leiomyomas arise from the muscle of the gastric wall, project into the stomach lumen and ulcerate at their apex, producing a characteristic crater on a dome-like projection. On cut section, they have a fibroid-like whorled appearance. Occasionally, large leiomyomas may undergo malignant change.

Carcinoma
Pathology
This is a common (incidence 21 per 100 000 in

the UK) and important tumour, although its incidence is falling, both in Europe and the USA. It is the fifth biggest cancer killer in the UK, headed only by lung, colo-rectal, breast and prostate cancer. Distribution is worldwide, although it is particularly frequent in some races, especially the Japanese. Any age may be involved but it especially affects the 50–70 year age group.

Risk factors

There is no absolute association with diet, alcohol or tobacco, although these have been implicated. The incidence is raised in patients with pernicious anaemia and atrophic gastritis, conditions where achlorhydria is present. It is also more common in patients who have previously undergone gastric resection. There is also a definite link with subjects having blood group A, which suggests a genetic factor.

Around 1% of gastric carcinomas arise in a previous chronic gastric ulcer. Patients with *H. pylori* infection (detected by the presence of antibody) have a six- to ninefold risk of gastric cancer, with a disproportionate risk of mucosa-associated lymphoid malignancy. However, fewer than 1% of those infected with *H. pylori* will go on to develop gastric cancer.

Macroscopic pathology

One-third diffusely involve the stomach, one-quarter arise in the pyloric region and the remainder are distributed fairly evenly throughout the rest of the organ.

There are four macroscopic appearances.
1 A *malignant ulcer* with raised, everted edges.
2 A *polypoid tumour* proliferating into the stomach lumen.
3 A *colloid tumour*: a massive, gelatinous growth.
4 The *leather-bottle stomach (linitis plastica)* caused by submucous infiltration of tumour with marked fibrous reaction. This produces a small, thickened, contracted stomach without, or with only superficial, ulceration, hence occult bleeding is rare in this group.

Microscopic appearances

These tumours are all adenocarcinomas with varying degrees of differentiation. The leather-bottle stomach consists of anaplastic cells arranged in clumps with surrounding fibrosis.

Malignant change in a benign ulcer is suggested when a chronic ulcer, with characteristic complete destruction of the whole muscle coat and its replacement by fibrous tissue and chronic inflammatory cells, has a carcinoma developing in its edge.

Spread

Local. Spread is often well beyond the naked-eye limits of the tumour and the oesophagus or the first part of the duodenum may be infiltrated. Adjacent organs (pancreas, abdominal wall, liver, transverse mesocolon and transverse colon) may be directly invaded. A gastro-colic fistula may develop.

Lymphatic. Lymph nodes along the lesser and greater curves are commonly involved. Lymph drainage from the cardiac end of the stomach may invade the mediastinal nodes and thence the supraclavicular nodes of Virchow[*] on the left side (Troissier's sign[†]). At the pyloric end, involvement of the subpyloric and hepatic nodes may occur.

Blood stream. Dissemination occurs via the portal vein to the liver and thence occasionally to the lungs and the skeletal system.

Trans-coelomic spread. May produce peritoneal seedlings and bilateral Krukenberg[‡] tumours due to implantation in both ovaries.

Clinical features

Symptoms may be produced by the local

---

[*] R. L. K. Virchow (1821–1902), Professor of Pathology, Würzburg.
[†] Charles Émile Troisier (1844–1919), Professor of Anatomy, Wittenberg, Germany.
[‡] Friedrich Krukenberg (1871–1946), Pathologist, Halle, Germany.

effects of the tumour, by secondary deposits or by the general features of malignant disease.

Local symptoms

These are epigastric pain and discomfort, pain radiating into the back (suggesting pancreatic involvement), vomiting, especially with a pyloric or antral tumour producing pyloric obstruction (see p. 169), or dysphagia in tumours of the cardia. Occasionally, carcinoma of the stomach may present with perforation or haemorrhage.

Secondaries

The patient may first report with jaundice due to liver involvement or abdominal distension due to ascites.

General features

Anorexia (an extremely common presenting symptom), loss of weight and anaemia.

Examination may reveal features corresponding to these three headings. Local examination may reveal a mass in the upper abdomen. A search for secondaries may show enlargement of the liver with or without jaundice, ascites, enlarged, hard left supraclavicular nodes, or a palpable mass on pelvic examination due to secondary deposits in the pouch of Douglas. There may be obvious signs of loss of weight or anaemia.

Special investigations

1 *Gastroscopy* enables direct inspection and multiple biopsies of any lesion. The detection rate is related to the number of biopsies taken.
2 *Barium meal* may reveal the following are important radiological features.

(a) A space-occupying lesion, e.g. an irregular stricture at the pylorus or at the cardia, or evidence of complete involvement of the stomach (leather-bottle stomach).

(b) The presence of an ulcer with raised edges and surrounding infiltration.

(c) The size of the lesion: any ulcer over 2 cm in diameter is suspect, although giant benign ulcers of 5 cm or more are found, especially in elderly people.

3 *CT scan* may show nodal and metastatic spread, and is important before attempts at curative gastric resection.

It is important to know that considerable pain relief and 'healing' may occur when a gastric carcinoma is treated with H_2-antagonists, due to diminution in the adjacent oedema and may lead to a false diagnosis of benign ulcer.

Differential diagnosis

There are five common diseases that give a very similar clinical picture, of a patient with slight lemon-yellow tinge, anaemia and loss of weight:
1 carcinoma of stomach;
2 carcinoma of the caecum;
3 carcinoma of the pancreas;
4 pernicious anaemia;
5 uraemia.
They form an important quintet, and should always be considered together.

The principal differential diagnosis of gastric carcinoma is a benign gastric ulcer. If in doubt, resection should be advised, but it may be difficult, even at operation, to decide between the two, and a per-operative frozen-section microscopic examination is then useful in planning treatment.

Treatment

• *Curative*: partial or total gastrectomy, with extensive lymph-node clearance, depending on the extent of the tumour.
• *Palliative*: palliative gastrectomy may be carried out even in the presence of small secondary deposits elsewhere. A gastroenterostomy may be performed for an irremovable obstructive lesion of the pylorus. A carcinoma of the cardiac end that is irremovable and producing dysphagia can be intubated by means of a plastic Mousseau–Barbin tube. Irradiation and cytotoxic drugs are of limited value.

Prognosis

This depends on the extent of spread and degree of differentiation of the tumour. Microscopic spread is much further than apparent at operation, and lymph-node spread has a poor prognosis. Early gastric carcinomas confined to the stomach wall (stage 1) have a 72% 5-year survival with resection. Perigastric lymph-node involvement (stage 2) reduces survival to 32%, while more distant nodal involvement more than 3 cm away from the tumour (stage 3) has a survival rate of only 10% at 5 years. The presence of metastases (stage 4) is associated with death before 5 years.

CHAPTER 21

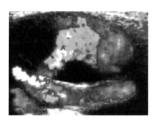

Mechanical Intestinal Obstruction

Classification

Intestinal obstruction is a restriction to the normal passage of intestinal contents. It may be divided into two main groups: paralytic and mechanical. Paralytic obstruction (paralytic or adynamic ileus) is discussed in Chapter 28.

Mechanical intestinal obstruction is further classified according to:
- *speed of onset*: acute, chronic, acute on chronic;
- *site*;
- *nature*: simple versus strangulating;
- *aetiology*.

Speed of onset

The speed of onset determines whether the obstruction is acute, chronic or acute on chronic. In acute obstruction the onset is rapid and the symptoms severe. In chronic obstruction the symptoms are insidious and slowly progressive (as, for example, in most cases of carcinoma of the large bowel). A chronic obstruction may develop acute symptoms as the obstruction suddenly becomes complete, e.g. when a narrowed lumen becomes totally occluded by inspissated bowel contents. This is termed acute-on-chronic obstruction.

Site

The site of the obstruction is classified into high or low, which is roughly synonymous with small or large bowel obstruction.

Nature

The nature of the obstruction is divided into simple or strangulated. Simple obstruction occurs when the bowel is occluded without damage to its blood supply. In strangulating obstruction the blood supply of the involved segment of intestine is cut off (as may occur, for example, in strangulated hernia, volvulus, intussusception or where a loop of intestine is occluded by a band), and, untreated, gangrene of the strangulated bowel is inevitable.

Aetiology (see also Chapter 182)

Whenever one considers obstruction of a tube anywhere in the body, this should be classified into:
- causes in the lumen;
- causes in the wall;
- causes outside the wall.

This can be applied to intestinal obstruction.
- *In the lumen*: faecal impaction, gall-stone 'ileus', food bolus, pedunculated tumour, etc.
- *In the wall*: congenital atresia, Crohn's disease, tumours, diverticulitis of the colon, etc.
- *Outside the wall*: strangulated hernia (external or internal), volvulus, obstruction due to adhesions or bands and intussusception.

It is also useful to think of the common intestinal obstructions that may occur at each age group.
- *Neonatal*: congenital atresia and stenosis (e.g. duodenal atresia), imperforate anus, volvulus

neonatorum, Hirschsprung's disease and meconium ileus.

• *Infants*: intussusception, Hirschsprung's disease, strangulated hernia and obstructions due to Meckel's diverticulum.

• *Young adults and middle age*: strangulated hernia, adhesions and bands, Crohn's disease.

• *The elderly*: strangulated hernia, carcinoma of the bowel, colonic diverticulitis, impacted faeces.

A strangulated hernia is an important cause of intestinal obstruction from infancy to old age. The hernial orifices must therefore be carefully examined in every case.

Pathology

When the bowel is obstructed by a simple occlusion, the intestine distal to the obstruction rapidly empties and becomes collapsed. The bowel above the obstruction becomes dilated, partly with gas (most of which is swallowed air), and partly with fluid poured out by the intestinal wall together with the gastric, biliary and pancreatic secretions. There is increased peristalsis in an attempt to overcome the obstruction, which results in intestinal colic. As the bowel distends, the blood supply to the tensely distended intestinal wall becomes impaired and in extreme cases there may be mucosal ulceration and eventually perforation. Perforation may also occur from the pressure of a band or the edge of the hernia neck on the bowel wall, producing local ischaemic necrosis, or from pressure from within the gut lumen, for example, by a faecal mass (stercoral ulceration).

In strangulating obstruction, the integrity of the mucosal barrier is lost as ischaemia progresses, so bacteria and their toxins can no longer be contained within the lumen. Transudation of organisms into the peritoneal cavity rapidly takes place, with secondary peritonitis. Unrelieved strangulation is followed by gangrene of the ischaemic bowel with perforation.

The lethal effects of intestinal obstruction result from fluid and electrolyte depletion due to the copious vomiting and loss into the bowel lumen, protein loss into the gut and toxaemia due to migration of toxins and intestinal bacteria into the peritoneal cavity, either through the intact but ischaemic bowel wall or through a perforation.

Clinical features

The four cardinal symptoms of intestinal obstruction are:

1 colicky abdominal pain;
2 distension;
3 absolute constipation;
4 vomiting.

It is important to note that not all of these four features need necessarily be present in a case of intestinal obstruction. The sequence of onset of symptoms will help

---

INTESTINAL OBSTRUCTION

There are three important points to remember about intestinal obstruction. First, it is diagnosed by the presence of:
• colicky abdominal pain;
• distension;
• absolute constipation;
• vomiting.
Second, examination should always include a search for herniae.
  Third, having made the diagnosis, the next question to ask yourself is whether there is evidence of strangulation. Features suggesting strangulation are:
• change in character of pain from colicky to continuous;
• tachycardia;
• pyrexia;
• peritonism;
• bowel sounds absent or reduced;
• leucocytosis.

localize the obstruction to the upper or lower intestine.

Pain

This is usually the first symptom of intestinal obstruction and is colicky in nature. In small-bowel obstruction it is peri-umbilical; in distal colonic obstruction it may be more suprapubic in location. In post-operative obstruction the colic may be disguised by the general discomfort of the operation and by opiates that the patient may be receiving.

Distension

This is particularly marked in chronic large-bowel obstruction and also in volvulus of the sigmoid colon. In a high intestinal obstruction, there may only be a short segment of bowel proximal to the obstruction, and distension will not then be marked.

Absolute constipation

Absolute constipation is the failure to pass either flatus or faeces. Although it is a usual feature of acute obstruction, a partial or chronic obstruction may be accompanied by the passage of small amounts of flatus. Absolute constipation is an early feature of large-bowel obstruction, but a late feature of small-bowel obstruction, as, even when the obstruction is complete, the patient may pass one or two normal stools as the lower bowel empties after the onset of the obstruction.

Vomiting

This usually occurs early in high obstruction, but is often late or even entirely absent in chronic or in low (large-bowel) obstruction. In the late stages of intestinal obstruction the vomiting becomes *faeculent* but not *faecal*. The faeculent vomiting is due to bacterial decomposition of the stagnant contents of the obstructed small intestine and of the altered blood that may transude into the bowel lumen. True vomiting of faeces only occurs in patients with gastro-colic fistula (e.g. due to a carcinoma of the stomach, carcinoma of the colon or ulceration of a stomal ulcer into the colon), or in coprophagists.

Clinical examination

The patient may be obviously dehydrated if vomiting has been copious. He or she is in pain and may be rolling about with colic. The pulse is usually elevated, but the temperature frequently is normal. A raised temperature and a very rapid pulse suggest strangulation. The abdomen is distended and visible peristalsis may be present. Visible peristalsis itself is not diagnostic of intestinal obstruction, as it may be seen in the normal subject if the abdominal wall is very thin.

During inspection it is important to look carefully for two features: the presence of a strangulated external hernia, which may require a careful search in the case of a small strangulated femoral hernia in a very obese and distended patient, and the presence of an abdominal scar. Intestinal obstruction in the presence of this evidence of a previous operation immediately suggests adhesions or a band as the cause.

Palpation reveals generalized abdominal tenderness. A mass may be present (e.g. in intussusception or carcinoma of the bowel).

Bowel sounds are usually accentuated and tinkling. Rectal examination must, of course, never be omitted. It may reveal an obstructing mass in the pouch of Douglas, the apex of an intussusception or faecal impaction.

Simple obstruction versus strangulating obstruction

Clinically, it is extremely difficult to distinguish with any certainty between simple obstruction and strangulation. The distinction is important, as strangulating obstruction with ensuing peritonitis has a mortality up to 15%. Features suggesting strangulation include:

• toxic appearance, with a rapid pulse and some elevation of temperature;
• colicky pain, becoming continuous as peritonitis develops;
• tenderness and abdominal rigidity are more marked;

• bowel sounds become reduced or absent, reflecting peritonism;
• a raised white-cell count, mostly neutrophils, is usual with infarcted bowel.

Special investigations
• *Abdominal X-rays* (erect and supine) are valuable in diagnosis of intestinal obstruction and in attempting to localize the site of the obstruction. A loop or loops of distended bowel are usually seen, together with fluid levels on an erect film.

Small-bowel obstruction is suggested by a ladder pattern of dilated loops, their central position and by striations that pass completely across the width of the distended loop produced by the circular mucosal folds.

Distended large bowel tends to lie peripherally and to show the haustrations of the taenia coli, which do not extend across the whole width of the bowel. A small percentage, perhaps 5% of intestinal obstructions, show no abnormality on plain X-rays. This is due to the bowel being completely distended with fluid in a closed loop and without the fluid levels produced by coexistent gas.
• *Barium follow-through.* A series of X-rays taken following ingestion of barium sulphate suspension may be used in suspected cases of small-bowel obstruction. Because of the considerable fluid accumulation above the block, the barium is rapidly diluted and there is little danger of impaction.
• *Barium enema.* An emergency contrast enema is helpful in the demonstration of a suspected large-bowel obstruction due to carcinoma or diverticular disease. Unlike a normal barium enema, no pre-examination laxative is given due to the risk of exacerbating the obstruction, and causing perforation if a closed loop exists.
• *Computed tomography (CT) scanning* is useful to detect colonic tumours, and may diagnose obturator hernias.

Treatment
Although the treatment of specific causes of intestinal obstruction is considered under the appropriate headings, certain general principles can be enunciated here.

Chronic large-bowel obstruction, slowly progressive and incomplete, can be investigated at some leisure (including sigmoidoscopy and barium enema) and treated electively.

Acute obstruction, of sudden onset, complete and with risk of strangulation, is invariably an urgent problem requiring emergency surgical intervention.

Pre-operative preparation in acute obstruction
This comprises the following.
1 *Gastric aspiration* by means of naso-gastric suction. This helps to decompress the bowel and to remove the risk of inhalation of gastric contents during induction of anaesthesia.
2 *Intravenous fluid replacement.* The large amount of fluid is sequestered into the gut and, together with losses due to vomiting, means that a lot of fluid may be required. Normal saline is given, with potassium if this is low and renal function satisfactory. If the patient is shocked, blood or plasma may be required.
3 *Antibiotic therapy* is commenced if there is the possibility of intestinal strangulation (or if this is found at operation).

Operative treatment
The affected bowel is carefully inspected to determine its viability, either at the site of the obstruction (e.g. where a band or the margins of a hernial orifice has pressed against the bowel) or of the whole segment of bowel involved in a closed loop obstruction. Non-viability is determined by four signs:
1 loss of peristalsis;
2 loss of normal sheen;
3 colour (greenish or black bowel is non-viable, purple bowel may still recover);
4 loss of pulsation of vessels in the supplying mesentery.

Doubtful bowel may recover after relieving the obstruction. It should be reassessed after it has been left for a few minutes wrapped up in a warm wet pack.

The general principle is that small bowel in intestinal obstruction can be resected and primary anastomosis performed with safety because of its excellent blood supply. Large-bowel obstruction must first be relieved, either by caecostomy or proximal colostomy, and a later resection performed. If resection is essential (as in strangulation), the affected segment is excised and the two loops of colon brought out as a temporary colostomy. If the distal end will not reach the surface it is closed (Hartmann's procedure*). This is because the blood supply of the large bowel is much less efficient and a colonic primary anastomosis is very liable to leak in the presence of obstruction.

Conservative treatment

Conservative treatment of obstruction by means of intravenous fluid and naso-gastric aspiration ('drip and suck') is only indicated under the following conditions.

• Where distinction from post-operative paralytic ileus is uncertain (see p. 229) and where a period of careful observation is indicated.

• Where the obstruction is one of repeated episodes due to massive intra-abdominal adhesions, rendering surgery hazardous, and where once again a short period of observation with conservative treatment is indicated. Increase in distension, aggravation of pain, increase in abdominal tenderness or rise in pulse are indications to abandon conservative treatment and to re-explore the abdomen.

*Henri Hartmann (1860–1952), Professor of Surgery, Faculty of Medicine, Paris, France.

• Where chronic obstruction of the large bowel has occurred. Here it is reasonable to attempt to remove the obturating faeces by enema, prepare the bowel and to carry out a subsequent elective operation.

Closed loop obstruction

This is a specific form of mechanical obstruction. It is characterized by increasing distension of a loop of bowel due to a combination of complete obstruction distally and a valve-like mechanism proximally allowing the bowel to fill, but preventing reflux back. It is most commonly seen with a left-sided colonic obstruction, in the presence of a competent ileo-caecal valve. The caecum, the most distensible part of the large bowel, blows up like a balloon, and perforation of the caecum, with faecal peritonitis, may occur if the obstruction is not rapidly relieved. Diagnosis is made on X-ray showing characteristic dilatation of the caecum. Other examples of closed loop obstruction include volvulus (gastric, caecal, sigmoid) and stomal obstruction of the afferent loop following Polya partial gastrectomy.

Adhesive obstruction

Adhesive obstruction is a common diagnosis in patients presenting with obstruction. It can only be safely diagnosed in patients who have had previous abdominal surgery. In the absence of peritonitis and signs of toxicity (rising tachycardia, pyrexia) it is initially managed conservatively by naso-gastric aspiration and intravenous fluid replacement. However, surgery is indicated if there are features to suggest strangulation, or if there is no history of previous abdominal surgery.

CHAPTER 22

Specific and Special Forms of Obstruction

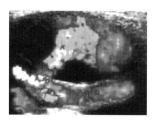

Neonatal intestinal obstruction

Classification
- Intestinal atresia.
- Volvulus neonatorum.
- Meconium ileus.
- Hirschsprung's disease.
- Ano-rectal atresias.

Continuous vomiting in the newborn suggests intracranial injury, infection or obstruction. Bile vomiting in the neonate indicates, almost without exception, intestinal obstruction.

In addition to vomiting there may be constipation, abdominal distension and visible peristalsis.

Plain X-ray of the abdomen shows distended loops of intestine with fluid levels.

Intestinal atresia
This may be a septum, complete or partial, or a complete gap, which may be associated with a corresponding defect in the mesentery. Multiple segments may be involved.

Treatment
Resection of the stricture and anastomosis. The operation is difficult and the mortality is high.

Volvulus neonatorum
This is due to a congenital malrotation of the bowel. The caecum remains high and the mid-gut mesentery is narrow, and drags across the duodenum, which may thus also be obstructed. Because of the narrow attachment of mesentery it readily undergoes volvulus. Untreated, the whole of the mid-gut becomes gangrenous.

Treatment
Laparotomy is performed as soon as possible. The operative procedure comprises untwisting the volvulus, and widening the narrow mesenteric attachment to the retroperitoneum. Adhesions between caecum and duodenum (Ladd's bands*) are divided, and the caecum and ascending colon are placed on the *left* side. An appendicectomy is performed if practical, as its unusual position may cause diagnostic difficulty in the future.

Meconium ileus
Eighty per cent of infants with meconium ileus have cystic fibrosis (mucoviscidosis), which is a generalized defect of mucus secretion of the intestine, pancreas (fibrocystic pancreatic

*William Edwards Ladd (1880–1967), Professor of Paediatric Surgery, Harvard Medical School, Boston, USA.

disease) and the bronchial tree. Because of the loss of intestinal mucus and a blockage of pancreatic ducts with loss of tryptic digestion, the lower ileum of the fetus becomes blocked with inspissated, viscous meconium. Perforation of the bowel may occur in intra-uterine life (meconium peritonitis).

Clinical features
The infant presents with acute obstruction in the first days of life, with gross abdominal distension and vomiting. The loop of ileum impacted with meconium may be palpable. X-ray of the abdomen shows, in addition to distended coils of bowel, the typical mottled 'ground glass' appearance of meconium.

Treatment
It may be possible to clear the meconium by installation of gastrograffin per rectum under X-ray control. This material is radio-opaque, hyper-osmolar (drawing fluid into the bowel lumen) and contains an emulsifying agent (Tween), which facilitates evacuation of the meconium. If this fails, or if the bowel has perforated, surgery is indicated. This comprises enterotomy and removal of the inspissated meconium by lavage. Occasionally, the impacted segment of ileum may show areas of gangrene and require resection. Postoperatively the infant is given pancreatic enzyme supplements by mouth.

The prognosis is poor, as, due to the lack of mucus secretion of the bronchi, recurrent chest infection is almost inevitable.

Necrotizing enterocolitis
This is a condition seen in premature infants and is due to mesenteric ischaemia, which permits bacterial invasion of the mucosa. Terminal ileum, caecum and distal colon are commonly affected. The condition probably represents the culmination of a number of disorders, such as hypoxia, hypotension and hyperviscosity, which reduce distal perfusion, together with sepsis and the presence of an umbilical artery cannula.

Clinical features
The infant shows signs of generalized sepsis with vomiting and listlessness. The abdomen is distended and tense. Blood and mucus are passed per rectum in over half the cases. The affected bowel may perforate or the condition resolve with stricture formation.

X-rays of the abdomen show distended loops of intestine, and gas bubbles may be seen in the bowel wall. Pneumoperitoneum signifies intestinal perforation.

Treatment
Initially this is medical. The infant is resuscitated and commenced on total parenteral nutrition and broad-spectrum antibiotics. Indications for surgery are failure to respond, profuse intestinal haemorrhage, evidence of perforation, or obstruction due to stricture formation. It comprises resection of the frankly gangrenous or perforated segment or segments of intestine with primary anastomosis where possible to avoid ileostomies, which are difficult to manage in neonates. Mortality remains around 25%.

Hirschsprung's disease*
This may present as acute obstruction in the neonate, with an incidence of 1 in 5000. Eighty per cent of the patients are male.

Pathology
This condition, also termed congenital or aganglionic megacolon, is produced by faulty development of the parasympathetic innervation of the distal bowel. There is an absence of ganglion cells in the submucosal plexus of Auerbach† and intermyenteric plexus of Meissner‡ affecting the rectum, which sometimes extends into the lower colon and, rarely, affects the whole of the large bowel. The involved segment is spastic, causing a functional

*Harald Hirschsprung (1830–1917), Paediatrician, Copenhagen, Denmark.
†Leopold Auerbach (1828–97), Neuropathologist, Breslau, Germany.
‡Georg Meissner (1829–1905), Professor of Physiology, Göttingen, Germany.

obstruction with gross proximal distension of the colon.

Until the true nature of the disease was determined, surgical treatment was directed, quite fruitlessly, to resection of the dilated, normally innervated portion of the colon.

Clinical features

In the most severe cases, obstructive symptoms commence in the first few days of life with failure to pass meconium; death results if untreated. Less marked examples present with extraordinarily stubborn constipation in infancy and these children survive into adult life with gross abdominal distension and stunted growth. Many untreated infants develop severe, life-threatening enterocolitis within the first 3 months of life.

Rectal examination reveals a narrow, empty rectum above which faecal impaction may be felt; this examination is usually followed by a gush of flatus and faeces.

Special investigations

• *Abdominal X-ray* shows dilated gas-filled loops of bowel throughout the abdomen except in the pelvis.
• *Barium enema* demonstrates the characteristic narrow rectal segment, above which the colon is dilated and full of faeces.
• *Rectal wall biopsy*, deep enough to include the submucosa, shows complete absence of ganglion cells. In difficult cases, a longitudinal full-thickness biopsy is required.

Differential diagnosis

The differential diagnosis is acquired megacolon, a condition of severe constipation commencing usually at the age of 1–2 years, often in a mentally defective child. Rectal examination in these cases is typical; impacted faeces being present right up to the anal verge. Biopsy of the rectal wall shows normal ganglion cells. This condition is relieved by regular enemas and aperients.

Treatment

If the child is obstructed in the neonatal period,

colostomy is performed. Elective surgery is carried out when the infant is 6–9 months old, or until at least 3 months have elapsed after a colostomy has been established. The aganglionic segment is resected and an abdomino-perineal pull-through anastomosis performed between normal colon and the anal canal.

It is important at operation to ensure by frozen-section histological examination that ganglion cells are present in the remaining colon.

Ano-rectal atresias

Ano-rectal atresias are a spectrum of abnormalities from imperforate anus to complete absence of anus and rectum. Fifty per cent are associated with fistula; in the female into the vagina, in the male into the bladder or urethra. Twenty-five per cent are associated with congenital anomalies elsewhere.

Clinical features

The anus may be entirely absent or represented by a dimple or by a blind canal. The extent of the defect is judged by X-raying the child, held upside down, with a metal marker such as a small coin at the site of the anus: the distance between the gas bubble in the distal colon and the marker can then be measured.

Treatment

• If the septum is thin, it is divided with suture of the edges of the defect to the skin.
• If there is an extensive gap between the blind end and the anal verge, a colostomy is fashioned with later attempt at a pull-through operation at about 2 years of age. Some surgeons perform an immediate pull-through procedure in the neonate.
• If a vaginal fistula is present, operation is not urgent, as the bowel decompresses through the vagina. Elective surgery is performed when the girl is older.
• If a recto-urethral or vesical fistula is present (meconium escaping in the urine) the fistula must be closed urgently, either with colostomy

or reconstruction of the anus in order to prevent ascending infection of the urinary tract.

Intussusception

Definition
An intussusception is the prolapse of one portion of the intestine into the lumen of the immediately adjoining bowel. The prolapsing, or invaginating bowel is called the intussusceptum.

Terminology
Different portions of intestine may form the apex of the intussusception.
• *Ileo-ileal*: the ileum is invaginated into the adjacent ileum.
• *Ileo-colic*: the ileo-ileal intussusception extends throuth the ileo-caecal valve into the colon. This is the commonest sort (75%).
• *Ileo-caecal*: the ileo-caecal valve is the apex of the intussusception.
• *Colo-colic*: the colon invaginates into adjacent colon (usually due to a protruding tumour of the bowel wall).

Aetiology
Ninety-five per cent occur in infants or young children, where there is usually no obvious cause. The mesenteric lymph nodes in these cases are invariably enlarged. It is postulated that the lymphoid tissue in Peyer's patches* in the bowel wall undergoes hyperplasia due to an adenovirus; the swollen lymphoid tissue protrudes into the lumen of the bowel and acts as a 'foreign body', which is then propelled by peristalsis distally along the gut, dragging the bowel behind.

In adults and in some children, a polyp, carcinoma, intestinal lymphoma or an inverted Meckel's diverticulum may form the apex of the intussusception.

The intussusceptum has its blood supply cut off by direct pressure of the outer layer and by

*John Peyer (1653–1712), Swiss Anatomist.

stretching of its supplying mesentery, so that, untreated, gangrene will occur.

Clinical features in infants
Intussusception usually occurs in previously healthy children commonly aged between 3 and 12 months. Boys are affected twice as often as girls.

The history is of paroxysms of abdominal colic typified by screaming and pallor. There is vomiting and usually the passage of blood and/or slime per rectum, giving the appearance of redcurrant jelly. On examination, the child is pale and anxious, and a typical attack of screaming may be observed. Palpation of the abdomen, after sedation if necessary, reveals a sausage-shaped tumour anywhere except in the right iliac fossa (RIF). Occasionally, the tumour cannot be felt because it is hidden under the costal margin. Rectal examination nearly always reveals 'redcurrant jelly' on the examining finger and, rarely, the tip of the intussusception can be felt.

If neglected, after 24 hours the abdomen becomes distended, faeculent vomiting occurs and the child becomes intensely toxic, due to gangrene of the intussusception and associated peritonitis.

Treatment in the infant
Non-operative
Barium is run in per rectum, and X-ray confirmation of the diagnosis is established. If the intussusception is recent, it may be completely reduced hydrostatically by the pressure of the column of barium and this is confirmed radiologically.

Operative
The intussusception is reduced at laparotomy by squeezing its apex backwards out of the containing bowel. In late cases, reduction may be impossible or the bowel may be gangrenous so that resection may be necessary.

Mortality is very low in the first 24 hours but is naturally very high in the irreducible or gangrenous cases. An intussusception may recur in a small percentage of children.

Volvulus

Definition

A twisting of a loop of bowel around its mesenteric axis, which results in a combination of obstruction together with occlusion of the main vessels at the base of the involved mesentery.

Most commonly it affects the sigmoid colon, caecum and small intestine, but volvulus of the gall bladder and stomach may also occur.

Aetiology

Precipitating factors include:
- an abnormally mobile loop of intestine, e.g. congenital failure of rotation of the small intestine, or a particularly long sigmoid loop;
- an abnormally loaded loop — as in the pelvic colon of chronic constipation;
- a loop fixed at its apex by adhesions, around which it rotates;
- a loop of bowel with a narrow mesenteric attachment.

Sigmoid volvulus

This occurs usually in elderly, constipated patients. It is four times more common in men than in women. It is relatively rare in the UK (about 2% of intestinal obstructions) but is much more common in Russia, Scandinavia and Central Africa. The loop of sigmoid colon usually twists anti-clockwise, from one-half to three turns.

Clinical features

There is a sudden onset of colicky pain with characteristic gross and rapid dilatation of the sigmoid loop.

A plain X-ray of the abdomen shows an enormously dilated oval gas shadow on the left side, which may be looped on itself to give the typical 'bent inner-tube' sign. If left untreated, the strangulated bowel undergoes gangrene, resulting in death from peritonitis. The caecum is usually visible and dilated in the right lower quadrant, distinguishing it radiologically from caecal volvulus.

Treatment

A long, soft rectal tube is passed through a sigmoidoscope and advanced into the sigmoid colon. This often untwists an early volvulus and is accompanied by the passage of vast amounts of flatus and liquid faeces. If this method fails, the volvulus is untwisted at laparotomy and the bowel is decompressed via a rectal tube threaded upwards from the anus. If gangrene has occurred, the affected segment is excised and the two open ends are brought out as a double-barrelled colostomy, which is later closed (Paul–Mikulicz procedure*).

Recurrent sigmoid volvulus is an indication for elective resection of the redundant sigmoid loop.

Caecal volvulus

Caecal volvulus is usually associated with a congenital malrotation where, in contrast to the incomplete rotation which causes volvulus neonatorum (p. 182), the caecum rotates beyond the RIF so that, instead of being fixed in the RIF, it has a persistent mesentery.

Clinically, there is an acute onset of pain in the RIF with rapid abdominal distension. X-ray of the abdomen shows a grossly dilated caecum, which is often ectopically placed and is frequently located in the left upper quadrant of the abdomen.

Treatment

At laparotomy, the volvulus is untwisted. If the caecum is infarcted, a right hemicolectomy is performed. Otherwise there are three procedures to prevent recurrence.

1 A temporary caecostomy may be fashioned to decompress the caecum and initiate adhesions between the caecum and the abdominal wall.

2 The caecum may be excised as part of a right hemicolectomy.

---

*Frank Thomas Paul (1851–1941), Surgeon, Liverpool Royal Infirmary, UK. Johann von Mikulicz-Radecki (1850–1905), Professor of Surgery successively at Cracow, Konigsberg and Breslau, Poland.

3 The mesenteric pedicle attaching the caecum can be broadened to prevent further twisting. Merely fixing the caecum to the lateral wall of the abdomen is usually unsuccessful.

Small intestine volvulus in adults

This may occur where a loop of small intestine is fixed at its apex by adhesions or by a fibrous remnant of the vitello-intestinal duct (often associated with a Meckel's diverticulum). Occasionally, the apex of the volvulus bears a tumour. In Africa, primary volvulus of the small bowel is relatively common, and may be due to the loading of a loop of gut with large quantities of vegetable foodstuffs. The clinical picture is one of acute intestinal obstruction.

Treatment

Early operation with simple untwisting and treatment of the underlying cause. If gangrene is present resection must be carried out.

Volvulus neonatorum

This is considered on page 182.

Mesenteric vascular occlusions

Embolism or thrombosis of the mesenteric vessels constitutes a special variety of intestinal obstruction without occlusion of the bowel.

Aetiology
Mesenteric embolus

This may arise from the left atrium in atrial fibrillation, a mural thrombus secondary to myocardial infarction, a vegetation on a heart valve, or from an atheromatous plaque on the aorta. Occasionally, it may be a paradoxical embolus originating in the deep leg veins and crossing the septum of the heart through a patent foramen ovale (p. 82).

Mesenteric arterial thrombosis

This is usually thrombosis secondary to atheroma. Arterial occlusion may also be secondary to an aortic dissection (p. 66).

Mesenteric venous thrombosis

This is associated with portal hypertension, or may follow splenectomy for thrombocytopenic purpura, pressure of a tumour on the superior mesenteric vessels or septic thrombophlebitis secondary to Crohn's disease, for example. Both mesenteric arterial and venous thrombosis are well documented in previously healthy young women on oral contraceptives, and are also associated with thrombophilias such as antithrombin III deficiency.

Non-occlusive infarction of the intestine

This may occur in patients with grossly diminished cardiac output and mesenteric blood flow consequent upon myocardial infarction or congestive cardiac failure.

Pathology

Mesenteric vascular occlusion results in infarction of the affected bowel with bleeding into the gut wall, lumen and peritoneal cavity; gangrene and subsequent perforation of the ischaemic bowel occurs. Impaired arterial blood flow to the gut without infarction may produce the symptoms of 'intestinal angina' in which severe abdominal pain follows meals; indeed, fear of eating and thus inducing pain produces rapid loss of weight. There may be an associated steatorrhoea. Minor degrees of occlusion may be overcome by development of a collateral circulation, particularly if the block develops slowly. One or even two of the main arteries (coeliac, superior and inferior mesenteric) may be occluded without symptoms.

Clinical features

There may be some pre-existing factor such as a heart lesion or liver disease. The classical triad is acute colicky abdominal pain, rectal bleeding and shock (due to associated blood loss) in an elderly patient who has atrial fibrillation.

The abdomen is generally tender, and a vague, tender mass may be felt, which is the infarcted bowel. However, the condition is impossible to diagnose unless the clinician has a high index of suspicion.

Treatment

The shock is treated by blood transfusion. Occasionally, successes have been reported from embolectomy in very early cases before frank gangrene has occurred. Resection of the gangrenous bowel is carried out, but this is obviously impossible where the whole mesenteric supply (small intestine and right side of the colon) is affected, usually a fatal situation.

Revascularization using a saphenous vein conduit to take blood from the iliac artery to the superior mesenteric artery may be possible. Resection of definitely infarcted bowel is performed, and the bowel of dubious viability is left and inspected at subsequent laparotomy the following day.

In young patients, extensive resection of the small bowel can be managed by total parenteral nutrition on a permanent basis. Intestinal transplantation may be available for these cases in the future.

CHAPTER 23

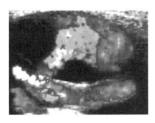

The Small Intestine

Meckel's diverticulum

Meckel's diverticulum* is the remnant of the vitello-intestinal duct of the embryo. It lies on the anti-mesenteric border of the ileum and, as an approximation, occurs in 2% of the population, 2 feet (60 cm) from the caecum and averages 2 inches (5 cm) in length.

Clinical features
It may present in numerous ways.
• *A symptomless finding* at operation or autopsy.
• *Acute inflammation*, clinically identical to acute appendicitis.
• *Perforation by a foreign body*, presenting as peritonitis.
• *Intussusception* (ileo-ileal), often gangrenous by the time the patient comes to operation.
• *Peptic ulceration* due to contained hetero-topic gastric epithelium, which bears HCl-secreting parietal cells. This particularly occurs in children and characteristically is the cause of melaena about the age of 10 years. Rarely, the peptic ulcer perforates or gives rise to post-cibal pain. The diverticulum may also contain ectopic pancreatic tissue.

• *Patent vitello-intestinal duct*, presenting as an umbilical fistula that discharges intestinal contents.
• *Raspberry tumour at the umbilicus* due to a persistent umbilical extremity of the duct.
• *Vitello-intestinal band* stretching from the tip of the diverticulum to the umbilicus, which may snare a loop of intestine to produce obstruc-tion or act as the apex of an ileal volvulus.

Special investigations
Most diverticula are incidental findings. However, the following investigations may be indicated.
• *Technetium scan*. Radio-labelled technetium (^{99m}Tc) is taken up by gastric mucosa, and scintigraphy will outline the stomach and, in addition, the Meckel's diverticulum, usually near the right iliac fossa (RIF).
• *Barium meal and follow-through* may show the diverticulum arising from the anti-mesenteric border.
Treatment involves resecting the diverticulum.

Crohn's disease

Crohn's disease† is a non-specific inflamma-tory disease of the alimentary canal, with dis-

---

*Johann Frederick Meckel (1781–1833), Professor of Anatomy and Surgery, Halle, Germany. His grand-father and father were both Professors of Anatomy.

†Burrill Bernard Crohn (1884–1983), Physician, Mount Sinai Hospital, New York, USA.

eased segments sandwiched between normal segments (i.e. it is discontinuous). It was first described in the ileum and termed 'regional ileitis'. However, this description is inaccurate, as the disease may affect any part of the alimentary tract from the mouth to the anus. Indeed, in recent years a growing number of examples of Crohn's disease affecting the large bowel alone, or with small-intestine involvement, are being encountered (see p. 206).

Aetiology

The aetiology is unknown. The presence of granulomas suggested an atypical *Mycobacterium* infection or sarcoidosis. Other possibilities include a viral or non-specific bacterial infection. Response to dietary manipulation, such as the elemental diet (see below) suggest intraluminal contents are important, and the aetiology may involve an abnormal immune response to intraluminal contents.

Acute ileitis can also be caused by the bacterium *Yersinia enterocolitica*.

Pathology

Distribution

The small bowel is affected in two-thirds of cases, with the lower ileum being the commonest site, although the disease may affect any part of the alimentary canal from the buccal mucosa to the anal verge. One-third of patients with ileal disease also have rectal or colonic manifestations.

Macroscopic appearance

In the acute stage, the bowel is bright red and swollen; mucosal ulceration and intervening oedema result in a 'cobblestone' appearance of the mucous membrane. The wall of the intestine is greatly thickened, as is the adjacent mesentery, and the regional lymph nodes are enlarged. Mesenteric fat advances over the serosal surface in affected segments. There may be skip areas of normal intestine between involved segments. Fistulae may occur into adjacent viscera.

Microscopic appearance

There is fibrosis, lymphoedema and a chronic inflammatory infiltrate through the whole thickness of the bowel with non-caseating foci of epithelioid and giant cells. Ulceration is present, with characteristic fissuring ulcers extending deep through the mucosa. These may extend through the bowel wall to form abscesses, or fistulae into adjacent viscera.

Clinical features

Crohn's disease occurs at any age, but is particularly common in young adults with a peak age of onset between 20 and 40 years of age. There is no sex difference. The typical clinical picture is a young adult with abdominal pain and diarrhoea, often with a palpable mass in the RIF. However, Crohn's disease may manifest clinically in several ways.

Acute Crohn's disease

Crohn's disease may present like appendicitis with acute abdominal pain, usually in the RIF, and vomiting. Rarely there is perforation of the bowel or acute haemorrhage. However, the history is usually of several days or weeks, and investigation may reveal anaemia, or other features may be present.

Intestinal obstruction

Following inflammatory exacerbations, fibrosis of the intestinal wall occurs leaving stenotic segments which result in intestinal obstruction. Obstruction may also follow an intraperitoneal abscess.

Fistula formation

Fistulae may develop. They may penetrate adjacent loops of gut or the bladder, or may be perianal. External faecal fistulae usually follow operative intervention.

Malabsorption

Extensive involvement of the bowel produces malabsorption with steatorrhoea and multiple vitamin deficiencies. It is exacerbated where bowel resections have already occurred.

Diarrhoea

Diarrhoea may be due to inflammation and mucosal ulceration, colonic or rectal involvement, bacterial overgrowth in obstructed segments, and malabsorption secondary either to disease or short bowel following previous surgery. Mucosal ulceration causes diarrhoea, with positive occult blood and anaemia.

Perianal disease

Ten per cent of patients with small bowel Crohn's disease also have perianal disease, ranging from fissures to fistulae (see p. 216).

Special investigations

Crohn's disease is associated with anaemia, positive occult blood and occasionally steatorrhoea. Serum albumin is low, and inflammatory markers such as C-reactive protein and the acute phase proteins are helpful markers of disease activity. Additional investigations include the following:

• *Small-bowel enema* demonstrates any fistulae or strictures (the string sign of Kantor*) in the affected segment, usually the terminal ileum, and ulcerated small bowel may show a 'cobblestone' appearance.

• *Technetium-labelled leucocyte scan* is a sensitive way to show the extent of disease activity. Leucocytes are taken up in the inflamed segments, and also localize to abscesses.

Complications

In addition to those already mentioned, the following are associated with the disease.

• *Renal calculi*: usually oxalate stones secondary to hyperoxaluria, which occurs as a consequence of steatorrhoea.

• *Biliary calculi* are more common in patients with ileal Crohn's disease, and where the ileum has been resected. They may be due to interruption of the enterohepatic bile-salt circulation.

• *Primary sclerosing cholangitis*, sacroiliitis, pyoderma gangrenosum and uveitis also occur, but are more common when the colon is also involved.

Treatment

Treatment is primarily medical, although

*John Leonard Kantor (1890–1947), Gastroenterologist, Presbyterian Hospital, New York, USA.

surgery is appropriate in the management of complications and chronic disease. Surgery is avoided where possible because of the malabsorption that may follow extensive resections of the bowel or the production of blind loops of intestine.

Medical management

Initial management is conservative. Nutritional support may be required, and an elemental diet may be useful. Acute episodes are treated with steroids and immunosuppressants such as azathioprine; parenteral nutrition may be required.

Mild symptoms are treated with anti inflammatory drugs such as mesalazine. Metronidazole may also help, and steroids may be required.

Surgical management

If found at laparotomy in the acute stage the condition should be left undisturbed since in a high proportion the acute phase may subside completely without further episodes. Where the diagnosis was mistaken for appendicitis the appendix is removed.

In the chronic stage of the disease surgery is indicated for severe or recurrent obstructive symptoms, and for the treatment of fistulae into the bladder or skin. Recognizing that the disease is recurrent and that further resections may be required, surgery should be as conservative as possible. The affected segment is either resected, or a strictureplasty is performed.

Prognosis

Recurrence of the disease after resection occurs in some 50% of cases within 10 years and repeated operations may be required over the years.

Tumours of the small intestine

One of the many mysteries of tumour formation is the rarity of growths from beyond the pylorus to the ileo-caecal valve.

Classification
Benign
• Adenoma.
• Leiomyoma.
• Lipoma.
• Hamartoma (e.g. Peutz–Jeghers syndrome,* associated with circumoral pigmentation and multiple intestinal polyps.)

Malignant
1 *Primary*:
  (a) adenocarcinoma;
  (b) lymphoma;
  (c) carcinoid;
  (d) leiomyosarcoma.
2 *Secondary invasion* (e.g. from stomach, colon or bladder or from a lymphoma).

Clinical features
Tumours of the small intestine may present with the following:
• intestinal bleeding;
• obstruction;
• intussusception;
• volvulus.

Carcinoid syndrome

Carcinoid tumours are derived from cells of neural crest origin and are APUD (**a**mine **p**recursor **u**ptake and **d**ecarboxylation) tumours. As such they may be associated with one of the multiple endocrine neoplasia (MEN) syndromes. They occur most commonly in the appendix, but may be found anywhere in the alimentary canal and occasionally in lung. They commonly secrete 5-hydroxytryptamine (5-HT, also called serotonin), in addition to other hormones, but are rarely symptomatic until they have metastasized to the liver, as the liver normally inactivates these hormones.

Pathology
Macroscopic appearance
The tumour appears as a yellowish submucosal nodule. The overlying mucous membrane is at first intact but later ulcerates. Extension to the serosa leads to fibrosis and obstruction. Usually the tumour encircles the bowel at the time of diagnosis.

Microscopic appearance
The tumour is made up of Kultschitzky cells,† which take up silver stains and arise in the crypts of the intestinal mucosa.

The tumour is very slow growing, and usually presents after the fourth decade. Up to a quarter are multiple. Carcinoids of the appendix are relatively benign but 4% eventually metastasize. They may present early as appendicitis by obstructing the appendix lumen. Those arising in the ileum and large bowel spread to the regional lymph nodes and the liver.

Clinical features
The carcinoid syndrome comprises one or more of the following features:
• enlarged liver or abdominal mass produced by the tumour and its secondaries;
• flushing with attacks of cyanosis and a chronic red-faced appearance, often precipitated by stress, or ingestion of food or alcohol;
• diarrhoea, often profuse, with noisy borborygmi;
• bronchospasm;
• pulmonary and tricuspid stenosis; lung carcinoids also cause stenosis of the left heart valves (mitral and aortic).

Special investigations
• *5-Hydroxyindole acetic acid (5-HIAA) urinary concentration.* 5-HT is broken down to 5-HIAA, which is excreted in the urine and can be estimated. The level is raised in this syndrome.

*John Law Augustine Peutz (1886–1957), Physician, The Hague, Holland. Harold Jos Jeghers (Contemporary), Professor of Medicine, New Jersey College of Medicine, Jersey City, USA.

†Nicolai Kultschitzky (1865–1925), Professor of Histology, Kharkov, Russia. After the Russian Revolution he became Lecturer in Anatomy at University College, London.

• *Computed tomography (CT) or ultrasound of the liver* to seek metastases.

Treatment

Resection of the tumour in early cases. Local deposits in the liver are also occasionally resectable. Palliation of more extensive deposits can be achieved by embolizing the hepatic arterial supply via a catheter passed through the femoral artery. Cytotoxic therapy may induce worthwhile remission.

Symptoms may be controlled by using 5-HT antagonists, e.g. methysergide and cyproheptadine, and octreotide may also be useful. Even if widespread deposits are present, the tumour is slow growing and the patient may survive for many years.

CHAPTER 24

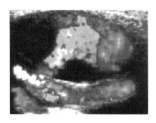

Acute Appendicitis

This is the commonest abdominal emergency and is estimated to affect one-sixth of the British population. It is, however, prevalent only in peoples on a Western diet.

Pathology

Acute appendicitis usually occurs when the appendix is obstructed by a faecolith or foreign body in the lumen, by a fibrous stricture in its wall from previous inflammation, by enlargement of lymphoid follicles in its wall secondary to a catarrhal inflammation of its mucosa, or occasionally by a carcinoid tumour near its base. Occasionally, acute appendicitis occurs proximal to an obstructing lesion (usually carcinoma) in the caecum or ascending colon. As the appendix of the infant is wide mouthed and well drained, and as the lumen of the appendix is almost obliterated in old age, appendicitis at the two extremes of life is relatively rare. However, when it does occur in these age groups it is poorly tolerated, and often diagnosed late.

The obstructed appendix acts as a closed loop; bacteria proliferate in the lumen and invade the appendix wall, which is damaged by pressure necrosis. The vascular supply to the appendix is made up of end-arteries, which are branches of the appendicular branch of the ileo-colic artery. Once these are thrombosed, gangrene is inevitable and is followed by perforation.

There is no strict time relationship for this chain of events. An appendix may occasionally perforate in under 12 hours, but conversely it is not rare to see an acutely inflamed but not perforated appendix after 3 or 4 days.

The effects of appendicular obstruction depend on the content of the appendix lumen. If bacteria are present, acute inflammation occurs; if, as sometimes happens, the appendix is empty, then a *mucocele* of the appendix results, due to continued secretion of mucus from the goblet cells in the mucosal wall.

Occasionally, appendicitis occurs in the non-obstructed appendix. Here there may be a direct infection of the lymphoid follicles from the appendix lumen, or in some cases the infection may be haematogenous (e.g. the rare streptococcal appendicitis). The non-obstructed acutely inflamed appendix is more likely to resolve than the obstructed form.

Pathological course

The acutely inflamed appendix may resolve, but if so a further attack is likely. It is not uncommon for a patient with acute appendicitis to confess to one or more previous milder episodes of pain, the grumbling appendix. More often the inflamed appendix undergoes gangrene and then perforates, either with general peritonitis or, more fortunately, with a localized appendix abscess. These possibilities can be summarized thus:

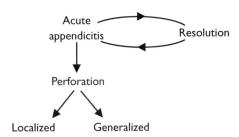

Clinical features
History
The vast majority of patients with acute appendicitis present with marked localized pain and tenderness in the right iliac fossa (RIF).

Pain. Typically the pain commences as a central peri-umbilical colic, which shifts after approximately 6 hours to the RIF, or, more accurately, to the site of the inflamed appendix as the adjacent peritoneum becomes inflamed. The appendix is a long tube (7–10 cm long), tethered proximally to the caecum near the ileo-caecal junction; distally the tip may lie anywhere from behind the caecum (retrocaecal), adjacent to the ileum, or down in the pelvis lying against the rectum or bladder. Thus, if the appendix is in the pelvic position, the pain may become suprapubic, with urinary frequency as the bladder is irritated; if it is in the high retrocaecal position, the symptoms may become localized in the right loin with less tenderness on palpation. Occasionally, the tip of the inflamed appendix extends over to the left iliac fossa and pain may localize there. The colicky central abdominal pain is visceral in origin; the shift of pain is due to later involvement of the sensitive parietal peritoneum by the inflammatory process. Typically, the pain is aggravated by movement and the patient prefers to lie still with the hips and knees flexed.

Nausea and vomiting usually occur following the onset of pain. Murphy* described the diagnostic sequence as Colicky central abdominal pain, followed by vomiting, followed by movement of the pain to the RIF.

Anorexia is almost invariable.

Constipation is usual, but occasionally diarrhoea may occur (particularly where the ileum is irritated by the inflamed appendix in the retro-ileal position).

There may be a history of previous milder attacks of similar pain.

With perforation of the appendix there may be temporary remission or even cessation of pain as tension in the distended organ is relieved; this is followed by more severe and more generalized pain with profuse vomiting as general peritonitis develops.

Examination
- Pyrexia and tachycardia are usual.
- The patient is flushed, may appear toxic and is obviously in pain.
- Movement exacerbates the pain.
- The tongue is usually coated, and a fetor oris is present.
- The abdomen shows localized tenderness in the region of the inflamed appendix. There is usually guarding of the abdominal muscles over this site with release tenderness. Coughing mimics the release test for rebound tenderness.
- Rectal examination reveals tenderness when the appendix is in the pelvic position or when there is pus in the recto-vesical or Douglas pouch.†
- In late cases with generalized peritonitis, the abdomen becomes diffusely tender and rigid, bowel sounds are absent and the patient is obviously very ill. Later still the abdomen is distended and tympanitic, and the patient exhibits the Hippocratic facies of advanced peritonitis.
- There is usually a polymorph leucocytosis.

*J. B. Murphy (1857–1916), Professor of Surgery, North Western University, Chicago, USA.

†James Douglas (1675–1742), Obstetrician and Anatomist, London.

Differential diagnosis and special investigations

The differential diagnosis of appendicitis includes most of the causes of acute abdominal pain. The special investigations performed are directed at excluding these possibilities, as well as confirming appendicitis.

The differential diagnoses should be considered systematically under the following headings.

• Other intra-abdominal causes of acute pain.
• The urinary tract.
• The chest.
• Gynaecological emergencies in female patients.
• The central nervous system (CNS).

Intra-abdominal disease

The following commonly simulate appendicitis.
• *Non-specific mesenteric adenitis*, particularly in young children, following upper respiratory tract infection. This may coexist with appendicitis, so the diagnosis is best confirmed at the time of appendicectomy.
• *Meckel's diverticulitis*, often indistinguishable from appendicitis, should always be sought if the appendix is normal at exploration.
• *Acute Crohn's ileitis*, affects young adults, usually with a long history of recurrent pain.

• *Acute intestinal obstruction*, with colicky pain and vomiting, but noisy bowel sounds and distended bowel on X-ray.
• *Gastroenteritis*, with diarrhoea and vomiting but more diffuse and less severe tenderness. Vomiting usually precedes any colic.
• *Perforated peptic ulcer*, normally a sudden onset; RIF pain may occur as fluid tracks down the paracolic gutter.
• *Acute cholecystitis*, where the initially colicky pain is fore-gut pain, so in the epigastrium. A distended, inflamed gall bladder may descend to the RIF.
• *Pancreatitis*, a central pain with central and sometimes RIF tenderness, diagnosed by a raised serum amylase concentration.
• *Acute colonic diverticulitis*, usually affecting the left colon but may give RIF pain if the sigmoid colon is sufficiently mobile, or if there is inflammation of a solitary caecal diverticulum. The age group differs from the usually younger patient with appendicitis.

The urinary tract

• *Testicular torsion* may occasionally present with peri-umbilical pain and vomiting. It is mandatory to examine the testes of all boys with abdominal pain, to exclude both torsion and maldescent (see p. 360).
• *Renal colic and acute pyelonephritis*. The urine

A MASS IN THE RIGHT ILIAC FOSSA

The causes of a mass in the right iliac fossa are best thought of by considering the possible anatomical structures in this region.
• Appendix abscess or appendix mass.
• Carcinoma of caecum (differentiated from the above by usually an older age group, a longer history, often the presence of diarrhoea, positive occult blood with anaemia and finally the barium enema examination).
• Crohn's disease (always to be thought of when there is a local mass in a young patient with diarrhoea).

• A distended gall bladder (which may quite often extend down as far as the right iliac fossa).
• Pelvic kidney (or renal transplant).
• Ovarian or tubal mass.
• Aneurysm of the common or external iliac artery.
• Retroperitoneal tumour arising in the soft tissues or lymph nodes of the posterior abdominal wall or from the pelvis.
• Ileo-caecal tuberculosis (rare in the UK, common in India).
• Psoas abscess—now rare.

must be tested for blood and pus cells in every case of acute abdominal pain. The patient with ureteric colic is usually restless and moving about, with pain radiating from loin to groin. Remember, however, that an inflamed appendix adherent to the ureter or bladder may produce dysuria and microscopic haematuria or pyuria; if reasonable doubt exists, it is safer to remove the appendix.

The chest

Basal pneumonia and pleurisy may give referred abdominal pain, which may be surprisingly difficult to differentiate, especially in children. Auscultation may reveal a rub, and chest X-ray may demonstrate a pneumonia.

Gynaecological emergencies

The commonest pitfalls are acute salpingitis, ectopic pregnancy ('every woman is pregnant until proved otherwise') and ruptured cyst of the corpus luteum. A ruptured or torted ovarian cyst presents with sudden severe RIF pain radiating to the loin, and the patient with salpingitis has a more diffuse bilateral lower abdominal pain and a vaginal discharge. Ultrasound helps to visualize the distended uterine tube in salpingitis and ectopic pregnancy. A pregnancy test may help confirm the presence of an ectopic pregnancy. In all women of childbearing age, laparoscopy may be helpful in the differential diagnosis.

The CNS

The pain preceding the eruption of herpes zoster affecting the 11th and 12th dorsal segments, the irritation of these posterior nerve roots in spinal disease (invasive tumour or tuberculosis) and the lightning pains of tabes dorsalis, all occasionally mimic appendicitis.

Nothing can be so easy, nor anything so difficult, as the diagnosis of acute appendicitis. The tyro may smile indulgently at the long list of differential diagnoses given in the text books but, as year follows year, he or she will experience the chagrin of making most, if not all, of these errors.

Treatment

The treatment of acute appendicitis is appendicectomy, except under the following circumstances:

• The patient is moribund with advanced peritonitis. Here the only hope is to improve the condition by intravenous drip and naso-gastric aspiration, antibiotics and other resuscitative measures.

• The attack has already resolved; in such a case, appendicectomy can be advised as an elective procedure, but there is no immediate emergency.

• An appendix mass has formed without evidence of general peritonitis (see below).

• Where circumstances make operation difficult or impossible, e.g. at sea. Here reliance must be placed on a conservative regimen and the hope that resolution or local abscess will form, rather than on one's surgical skill with a razor blade and a bent spoon.

Antibiotic prophylaxis is given preoperatively. When at operation peritonitis is discovered, antibiotic therapy is continued; metronidazole and gentamicin, or a cephalosporin, are effective for both the anaerobic and aerobic bowel organisms, but this regimen may need to be supplemented or changed when the bacteriological sensitivities of the cultured pus become available after 24–48 hours. After appendicectomy, a drain is inserted when there is severe inflammation of the appendix bed, when a local abscess is present or where closure of the appendix stump is not perfectly sound. Very occasionally, the inflamed and adherent appendix cannot be safely removed, and in such circumstances the area of the appendix requires adequate drainage and subsequent 'interval appendicectomy' in about 3 months.

The appendix mass

Not uncommonly the patient will present with a history of 4 or 5 days of abdominal pain and with a localized mass in the RIF. The rest of the abdomen is soft, bowel sounds are present and the patient obviously has no evidence of general peritonitis. In these circumstances, the inflamed appendix is walled off by adhesions to the omentum and adjacent viscera, with or without the presence of a local abscess. Immediate surgery in such circumstances is difficult.

Treatment

Initial treatment is conservative. The outlines of the mass are marked on the skin, the patient is put to bed on a fluid diet and a careful watch kept on the general condition, temperature and pulse. Metronidazole is commenced, but prolonged antibiotics are *not* given, as these may merely produce a chronic inflammatory mass honeycombed with abscesses (the so-called 'antibioticoma').

On this regimen, 80% of appendix masses resolve. In the remaining cases the abscess obviously enlarges over the next day or two and the temperature fails to subside. In these circumstances, drainage of the abscess is instituted. In neglected cases an appendix abscess may burst spontaneously through the abdominal wall, into the rectum, or into the general peritoneal cavity.

If resolution occurs, appendicectomy is carried out after an interval of 3 months to allow the inflammatory condition to settle completely. Unless interval appendicectomy is

performed there is considerable risk of a further attack of acute appendicitis.

Appendicitis in pregnancy

Appendicitis in pregnancy is no rarer or commoner than appendicitis in the general community, but it has a higher mortality and morbidity because it is confused with other complications of pregnancy. Differentiation must be made from pyelitis, vomiting of pregnancy, red degeneration of a fibroid or torsion of an ovarian cyst.

Because the appendix is displaced by the enlarging uterus, pain and tenderness are higher and more lateral than in the usual circumstances. There is considerable danger of abortion, particularly in the first trimester.

Acute abdominal pain

Appendicitis may be confused with many other causes of abdominal pain. When evaluating someone with abdominal pain, it is important to get as much information as possible about the pain, such as where it started and where it went; what made it worse and what made it better; whether it recurred or was this the first episode; was it colicky or was it constant? The question 'What happened next?' is particularly useful.

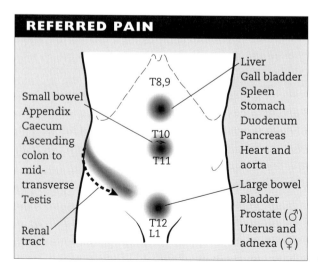

REFERRED PAIN

Small bowel
Appendix
Caecum
Ascending
colon to
mid-
transverse
Testis

Renal
tract

T8,9
T10
T11
T12
L1

Liver
Gall bladder
Spleen
Stomach
Duodenum
Pancreas
Heart and
aorta

Large bowel
Bladder
Prostate (♂)
Uterus and
adnexa (♀)

Fig. 24.1 Location of referred pain for the abdominal organs.

Location of referred pain for the abdominal organs (Fig. 24.1)

The location of referred pain from abdominal viscera can help locate the source. It is useful to consider the viscera in terms of their embryology. Thus, epigastric pain is generally from foregut structures, such as stomach, duodenum, liver, gall bladder, spleen, and pancreas; peri-umbilical pain is midgut pain from small bowel and ascending colon; suprapubic pain is hindgut pain, originating in the colon, rectum and other structures of the cloaca such as the bladder, uterus and fallopian tubes. Testicular pain may also be peri-umbilical, reflecting the intra-abdominal origin of this organ before its descent into the scrotum.

CHAPTER 25

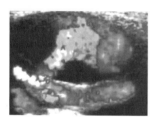

The Colon

Constipation and diarrhoea

Constipation and diarrhoea are two symptoms frequently attributable to diseases of the large bowel. There are, of course, many causes of these common complaints, due not only to lesions of the large intestine but also to other parts of the alimentary canal being affected or to general diseases. It is useful here to consider the commoner causes of these two symptoms.

Constipation

1 *Organic obstruction*:
(a) carcinoma of the colon;
(b) diverticular disease.

2 *Painful anal conditions*:
(a) fissure-*in-ano*;
(b) prolapsed piles.

3 *Adynamic bowel*:
(a) Hirschsprung's disease;
(b) senility;
(c) spinal cord injuries and disease;
(d) myxoedema;
(e) Parkinson's disease.

4 *Drugs*:
(a) aspirin;
(b) opiate analgesics;
(c) anticholinergics;
(d) ganglion blockers.

5 *Habit and diet*:
(a) dyschezia (rectal stasis due to faulty bowel habit);
(b) dehydration;
(c) starvation;
(d) lack of bulk in diet.

Diarrhoea

1 *Specific infections*:
(a) food poisoning (e.g. *Salmonella*);
(b) dysentery (amoebic and bacillary);
(c) cholera;
(d) viral enterocolitis.

2 *Inflammation or irritation of the intestine*:
(a) ulcerative colitis;
(b) tumours of the large bowel;
(c) diverticular disease;
(d) Crohn's disease.

3 *Drugs*:
(a) antibiotics and antibiotic-induced colitis;
(b) erythromycin (stimulates the motilin receptor);
(c) purgatives;
(d) digitalis.

4 *Loss of absorptive surface*:
(a) bowel resections and short circuits;
(b) sprue and coeliac disease;
(c) idiopathic steatorrhoea.

5 *Pancreatic dysfunction*: steatorrhoea due to lipase deficiency.

6 *Post-gastrectomy and vagotomy*: cause unknown.

7 General diseases:
(a) anxiety states;
(b) thyrotoxicosis;

(c) uraemia;

(d) carcinoid syndrome (p. 192);

(e) Zollinger–Ellison syndrome (p. 271).

Diverticulosis and diverticulitis

Background

Diverticula of the colon consist of out-pouchings of mucous membrane through the muscle wall of the bowel. Because they lack the normal muscle coats, they are examples of 'false' diverticula, in contrast to a Meckel's diverticulum of the small bowel, which is a true diverticulum. They lie alongside the taenia coli, often overlapped by the appendices epiploicae. In the colon, diverticula are found most commonly in the sigmoid and descending colon, and become increasingly rare in passing from the left to right side of the colon. They are unusual before the age of 40 years, but they are found in about 30% of all post-mortems of elderly people. The sex distribution is roughly equal. Although colonic diverticula are so common in Western communities, they are extremely rare amongst people of the developing countries.

Pathogenesis

Hypertrophy of the muscle of the sigmoid colon produces high intraluminal pressures, which cause herniation of the mucosa at the sites of potential weakness in the bowel wall, which correspond to the points of entry of the supplying vessels to the bowel (Fig. 25.1). The aetiology of the muscular hypertrophy is unclear, but may relate to the nature of the intraluminal contents. Diets that are low in bulk tend not to distend the sigmoid colon, permitting high intramural pressures to develop, while high-fibre diets or bulking agents distend the colon and reduce intraluminal pressure. It may be that the modern, refined, low-roughage diet may be responsible for the Western nature of the disease.

Diverticulitis

This results from infection of one or more diverticula. An inflamed diverticulum may do one of three things.

1 *Perforate*:

(a) into the general peritoneal cavity to cause peritonitis;

(b) into the pericolic tissues with formation of a pericolic abscess;

Fig. 25.1 The relationship of diverticula of the colon to the taenia coli and to the penetrating blood vessels. (a) normal colon, (b) colon with diverticula; both shown in transverse section.

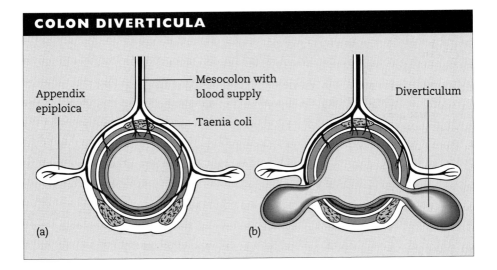

COLON DIVERTICULA

Appendix epiploica

Mesocolon with blood supply

Taenia coli

Diverticulum

(a)   (b)

(c) into adjacent structures (e.g. bladder, small bowel, vagina) forming a fistula.

2 *Produce chronic infection* with inflammatory fibrosis, resulting in obstructive symptoms — acute, chronic, or acute on chronic.

3 *Haemorrhage*, as a result of erosion of a vessel in the bowel wall. The bleeding varies from acute and profuse to a chronic occult loss.

Clinical features

Acute diverticulitis

This is well nicknamed 'left-sided appendicitis': an acute onset of central abdominal pain, which shifts to the left iliac fossa (LIF) accompanied by fever, vomiting and local tenderness and guarding. A vague mass may be felt in the LIF and also on rectal examination. Perforation into the general peritoneal cavity produces the signs of general peritonitis. A pericolic abscess is comparable to an appendix abscess but on the left side; a tender mass accompanied by a swinging fever and leucocytosis.

Chronic diverticular disease

This exactly mimics the local clinical features of carcinoma of the colon (p. 207); there may be diarrhoea alternating with constipation which progresses to a large-bowel obstruction with vomiting, distension, colicky abdominal pain and constipation. (Note: small-bowel obstruction from adhesion of a loop of small intestine to the inflammatory mass is not uncommon.) There may be episodes of pain in the LIF, passage of mucus or bright red blood per rectum or of melaena, or there may be anaemia due to chronic occult bleeding. Examination reveals tenderness in the LIF and there is often a thickened mass in the region of the sigmoid colon, which may also be felt per rectum.

More unusual presentations are the following.

• *Sudden severe rectal haemorrhage*: bleeding from a diverticulum is the most likely cause of a sudden, profuse, bright red bleed in an elderly, often hypertensive, patient.

• *Colo-vesical fistula*: fistula into the bladder with the passage of faeces and gas bubbles (*pneumaturia*) in the urine. Diverticulitis is the commonest cause of colo-vesical fistula, others being carcinoma of the colon, carcinoma of the bladder, Crohn's disease and trauma.

Special investigations

• *Sigmoidoscopy*: if the affected segment is low in the colon, there may be an oedematous block to the passage of the instrument beyond about 15 cm. Rigid sigmoidoscopes only view the rectum, so do not visualize colonic diverticula. Fibre-optic sigmoidoscopes are longer, as well as flexible, and do allow 'sigmoidoscopy'.

• *Barium enema* demonstrates diverticula as globular out-pouchings, which often show a signet-ring appearance because of the filling defect produced by contained pellets of faeces (faecoliths). Diverticular disease is characterized by stricture formation, which may closely simulate an annular carcinoma. More often the oedema and thickening produce a 'saw-tooth' narrowed segment in the sigmoid. This examination should not be performed in the acute phase to prevent iatrogenic perforation of friable and inflamed bowel.

• *Colonoscopy* may allow the affected segment to be inspected, but often the rigid and narrow sigmoid in this condition makes onward passage of the instrument impossible.

• *Computed tomography (CT) scanning* is preferable to barium enema in the acute phase and can help exclude other causes of lower abdominal pain in difficult cases.

Differential diagnosis

The important differential diagnosis is from neoplasm of the colon. It is impossible to be certain of this differentiation clinically or even on special investigations unless a positive biopsy is obtained by flexible sigmoidoscopy or colonoscopy to establish definitively the diagnosis of carcinoma. Even at laparotomy it is difficult to be sure whether one is dealing with carcinoma or diverticular disease; indeed, these two common conditions may coexist.

Treatment

Acute diverticulitis

This is managed conservatively; the patient is placed on a fluid diet and antibiotics (metronidazole with penicillin and gentamicin, or a cephalosporin, are the combinations of choice). The great majority settle on this regimen.

A *pericolic abscess* is treated initially conservatively in a similar way to an appendix abscess (p. 198), but if the abscess is enlarging, drainage is indicated. This is often followed by the formation of a faecal fistula and is therefore best combined with a defunctioning transverse colostomy.

General peritonitis from rupture of an acute diverticulitis is a dangerous condition. Laparotomy is performed, the affected segment of colon resected and a defunctioning colostomy fashioned. Full antibiotic therapy is given.

Acute obstruction due to diverticulitis requires laparotomy to establish the diagnosis and a transverse colostomy to relieve the obstruction. It is important to determine whether or not the obstruction is caused by an adherent loop of small intestine, which is by no means uncommon. Following this emergency procedure, elective resection of the affected segment of colon can be be carried out and the colostomy subsequently closed. In experienced hands, an intra-operative antegrade colonic lavage is performed followed by a primary anastomosis, with or without covering loop colostomy.

Chronic diverticular disease

If the diagnosis is made with considerable certainty and symptoms are mild, this can be treated conservatively. The bowels are regulated by means of a lubricant laxative (e.g. Milpar). A high-roughage diet (fruit, vegetables, wholemeal bread and bran) is prescribed. If, however, symptoms are severe or if carcinoma cannot be excluded, laparotomy and resection of the sigmoid colon is performed.

Colo-vesical fistula is treated by preliminary defunctioning colostomy. The affected segment of the colon is then resected and the fistula into the bladder is sutured; the colostomy is subsequently closed.

Angiodysplasia

This term is applied to one or multiple, small (less than 5 mm) mucosal or submucosal vascular malformations, usually a dilated vein or sheaf of veins. Because they occur most commonly in the elderly, they are considered to be degenerative vascular anomalies. The caecum and ascending colon are the sites most usually involved, although they may be found anywhere in the small or large bowel.

Clinical features

They are usually asymptomatic, and were unknown before the advent of mesenteric angiography and colonoscopy. Their only clinical manifestation is bleeding, which may take the form of continuous chronic intestinal blood loss, presenting with anaemia, or recurrent acute dark or bright red rectal haemorrhage, which may be occasionally severe and life threatening. Recurrent bleeding is common. They account for some 5% of such emergency cases.

Special investigations

• *Colonoscopy* is the investigation of choice, although it is often difficult to visualize the caecum in these elderly patients. The lesions appear as bright red 0.5–1-cm diameter submucosal lesions with small, dilated vessels visible on close inspection. They are invisible on barium enema.
• *Mesenteric angiogram*. Actively bleeding angiodysplasias may be detected on angiography as contrast medium leaks into the bowel lumen.

Treatment

Blood transfusion is necessary if heamorrhage is severe. Colonoscopic electrocoagulation is often curative. Resection, usually a right hemicolectomy, is sometimes required.

Colitis

Colitis, inflammation of the colon, presents with diarrhoea and often lower abdominal pain, and blood and mucus per rectum. The five main causes of colitis are:

1 *ulcerative colitis*;

2 *Crohn's colitis*;

3 *antibiotic-associated colitis*, e.g. pseudo-membranous colitis due to *Clostridium difficile*, (see p. 14);

4 *infective colitis*, e.g. *Campylobacter* and amoebic colitis;

5 *ischaemic colitis*, due to mesenteric ischaemia, occurring spontaneously or following ligation of the inferior mesenteric artery in aortic surgery.

Ulcerative colitis

Ulcerative colitis is an inflammatory disease of the rectum extending for a variable distance proximally in the colon. Females are more often affected than males, and it is found in any age from infancy to the elderly, but the maximum incidence is between the ages of 20 and 40 years.

Aetiology

The aetiology of ulcerative colitis is unknown, although it appears to combine environmental stimuli, autoimmune responses and genetic factors (association with human leucocyte antigen (HLA) B27).

Pathology

The rectum and sigmoid colon are principally affected, but the whole colon may be involved. (Note that the sigmoid is the site of election for all the major diseases of the colon: colitis, volvulus, carcinoma, polyposis and diverticulitis. Why it deserves this notoriety is unknown.)

Initially, there is oedema of the mucosa, with contact bleeding and petechial haemorrhage, proceeding to ulceration; the ulcers are shallow and irregular. Oedematous tags of mucosa between the ulcers form pseudo-polyps. The wall of the colon is oedematous and fibrotic and therefore is rigid with loss of its normal haustrations. The changes are confluent, with no unaffected 'skip lesions' as found in Crohn's disease. Surprisingly, the inflamed colon does not become adherent to its neighbouring intra-abdominal viscera.

Microscopically, the principal locus of the disease is mucosal; small abscesses form within the mucosal crypts ('crypt abscesses'). These abscesses break down into ulcers whose base is lined with granulation tissue. The walls of the colon are infiltrated with polymorphs and round cells; there is oedema and submucosal fibrosis. In the chronic, burnt-out disease the mucosa is smooth and atrophic; the bowel wall is thinned.

Clinical features

Manifestations of ulcerative colitis may be fulminant, intermittent or chronic. The commonest scenario is of diarrhoea, with blood and mucus. There may be accompanying cramplike abdominal pains. Examination reveals nothing except some tenderness in the LIF, and blood on the glove of the examining finger after rectal examination. The rectal mucosa may feel oedematous.

In severe attacks there is fever, toxaemia, severe bleeding and risk of perforation. Anorexia and loss of weight occur in the acute episodes.

Special investigations

Investigations aim to make the diagnosis, differentiate it from Crohn's colitis, exclude complications and assess the proximal extent.

• *Sigmoidoscopy* reveals oedema of the mucosa with contact bleeding in the early mild cases, proceeding to granularity of the mucosa and then frank ulceration with pus and blood in the bowel lumen. Biopsy will give confirming histological evidence of the diagnosis.

• *Colonoscopy* enables the whole of the large bowel to be inspected, the proximal extent to be noted, and biopsy material to be obtained.

• *Barium enema* shows a ragged surface,

indicating ulceration. Oedema and fibrosis produce loss of haustration and in the chronic case the typical smooth, narrow 'drainpipe' colon.

• *Examination of the stools* reveals pus and blood either to the naked eye or under the microscope, but no specific organism has ever been grown.

Differential diagnosis

Ulcerative colitis may be difficult to differentiate from other causes of diarrhoea (p. 200), especially the dysenteries and carcinoma, or Crohn's disease of the large bowel (Table 25.1). Differentiation from colonic Crohn's disease may be particularly difficult, even when the resected colon is examined by an expert pathologist. Indeed, about 10% of cases have to be labelled 'non-specific colitis'.

Table 25.1 Differentiating Crohn's colitis from ulcerative colitis.

Complications
Local

• Toxic dilatation, where the colon dilates in a fulminant colitis, leading to perforation.
• Haemorrhage (acute, or chronic with progressive anaemia).
• Stricture.
• Malignant change (see below).
• Perianal disease: fistula-*in-ano*, fistula into the vagina, fissures and perianal abscesses.

General

General complications include toxaemia, loss of weight, anaemia, arthritis, pyoderma gangrenosum, uveitis, skin rashes and ulceration of the legs. Primary sclerosing cholangitis is also associated with ulcerative colitis, as it is with Crohn's disease.

Malignant change

Patients with ulcerative colitis who have had chronic total colitis (affecting the whole large bowel), particularly if the first attack was in childhood, have a high risk of developing carcinoma of the colon. Statistics indicate a risk

CROHN'S AND ULCERATIVE COLITIS

	Crohn's colitis	Ulcerative colitis
Clinical features	Perianal disease, e.g. fissure-*in-ano* and fistula common	Perianal disease rare
	Gross bleeding uncommon	Often profuse haemorrhage
	Small bowel may also be affected	Small bowel not affected
Pathology		
Macroscopic differences	Any part of colon may be involved (skip lesions)	Disease extends proximally from rectum
	Transmural involvement	Mucosal involvement only
	Fistulae in adjacent viscera	No fistulae
	No polyps	Pseudo-polyps of regenerating mucosa
	Thickened bowel wall	No thickening of bowel wall
Microscopic differences	Granulomas present	No granulomas

of 5–12% of patients with colitis of 20 years' duration develop malignant change. Patients should therefore be offered annual or biannual colonoscopy with multiple biopsies to seek the dysplasia that heralds malignant change.

Even in the absence of a total, or pan-colitis, patients with ulcerative colitis are at far greater risk of developing carcinoma of the large bowel than a normal individual. More-over, the tumours occurring in the colitics are more likely to affect a younger age group, be anaplastic and be multiple compared with those arising in previously healthy bowel. Often the condition is only diagnosed late, as both the patient and doctor attribute the symptoms (bleeding, diarrhoea and pus) to the colitis.

Treatment

Initially this is medical in the uncomplicated case, but surgery is required when medical treatment fails or when complications supervene.

Medical treatment

A high-protein diet is prescribed with vitamin supplements, iron and potassium (the last to replace electrolyte loss in the stools). Blood transfusion is given if the patient is severely anaemic. Diarrhoea may be controlled with codeine phosphate or loperamide. Corticos-teroids given systemically, by rectal infusion or in combination will often produce remission in an acute attack. Salicylates such as mesalazine, or sulphasalazine (salazopyrine, sulphonamide/ salicylate combination) are used to maintain a remission.

Patients with ulcerative colitis are often highly intelligent, tense and anxious, and treat-ment should be supplemented with simple psychotherapy in the form of sympathy and reassurance.

Surgery

The indications for surgery are:
• fulminating disease not responding to medical treatment (defined as the passage of

more than six bloody motions per day, with fever, tachycardia and hypoalbuminaemia);
• chronic disease not responding to medical treatment;
• long-standing disease (as prophylaxis against malignant change);
• the complications of colitis already listed.

The procedure usually comprises total removal of the colon and rectum with either a permanent ileostomy or an ileo-anal anasto-mosis with an interposed pouch of ileum (Parks' pouch*). Occasionally, the disease of the rectum is relatively mild and the anal sphincter can be preserved with anastomosis between the ileum and rectum (colectomy with ileo-rectal anastomosis).

Most patients requiring surgery for ulcera-tive colitis are either on corticosteroids or have recently received them. Surgical proce-dures must therefore be covered by increased dosage of corticosteroids, which can then be tailed off gradually in the post-operative period.

Crohn's colitis

Crohn's disease,† although most commonly found in the terminal ileum (see p. 189), may occur anywhere in the alimentary tract from the mouth to the anus. It may be confined to the large bowel, or there may be involvement of both the small and large intestine.

Clinical features

Colonic Crohn's disease closely mimics ulcera-tive colitis in its clinical manifestations. However, unlike ulcerative colitis, the affected segment of colon commonly becomes adher-ent to adjacent structures with abscess forma-tion and fistulation. Perianal inflammation with abscesses and multiple fistulae-in-ano is also common and indeed may be the first manifestation of the disease.

---

*Sir Alan Parks (1920–82), Surgeon, St Marks Hospi-tal, London.
†Burrill Bernard Crohn (1884–1983), Physician, Mount Sinai Hospital, New York, USA.

Treatment

This is similar to that of Crohn's disease of the small intestine (see p. 189). Resection of extensively involved large bowel may require total excision with a permanent ileostomy. Restorative proctocolectomy and Park's pouch formation is not performed for Crohn's disease because of the immediate risks of sepsis and fistulation, and the chance of recurrence.

Tumours

Classification

Benign

- Adenomatous polyp.
- Papilloma.
- Lipoma.
- Neurofibroma.
- Haemangioma.

Malignant

1 *Primary*:
   (a) carcinoma;
   (b) lymphoma;
   (c) carcinoid tumour (see p. 192).
2 *Secondary*: invasion from adjacent tumours, e.g. stomach, bladder, uterus and ovary.

Carcinoma

Carcinomas affecting the large bowel are common; they are next in frequency to cancers of the lung in males, and cancer of the breast in females. They are the second commonest cause of death from malignant disease in this country.

Tumours may occur at any age. Females are affected more often than males (although interestingly the incidence of rectal cancer is roughly equal in the two sexes). The sigmoid is the commonest site in the colon, although the rectum accounts for one-third of all the large-bowel cancers. Five per cent of tumours of the large bowel are multiple (synchronous).

Predisposing factors

Pre-existing polyps, ulcerative colitis (see above) and a number of inherited colo-rectal cancer syndromes are risk factors for the development of carcinoma of the large bowel. Inherited syndromes such as familial adenomatous polyposis and hereditary non-polyposis colon cancer account for a significant proportion of colo-rectal cancers, and potential carriers should be offered screening (see below). Family history alone is sufficient to increase the risk, and it has been estimated that one first-degree relative contracting colon cancer aged over 45 years increases one's lifetime risk from 1 in 50 to 1 in 17; if the relative was diagnosed before 45 the lifetime risk increases to 1 in 10.

Familial adenomatous polyposis

This is a rare disease, but it is important because it invariably proceeds to carcinoma of the colon unless treated and accounts for 0.5% of all colon cancers. It has an autosomal dominant inheritance, the affected familial adenomatous polyposis (FAP) gene being located on chromosome 5q21. New mutations are relatively common. The polyps first appear in adolescence; symptoms of bleeding and diarrhoea commence about the age of 21 years and malignant change occurs between 20 and 40 years of age. Affected individuals also have hypertrophy of the retinal pigment layer which is a useful, non-invasive screening test. Variants such as *Gardner's syndrome** exist where colonic polyps are associated with desmoid tumours and osteomas of mandible and skull.

Treatment comprises a total colectomy with excision of the rectum, and formation of an ileo-anal pouch. If the polyps are not profuse in the lower rectum, it is possible to resect the colon while leaving a stump of rectum to which an ileo-rectal anastomosis is performed, and then carry out regular diathermy of the polyps in the rectal stump through a sigmoidoscope.

Hereditary non–polyposis colon cancer

This accounts for around 5% of colo-rectal

*E. J. Gardner (1909–?), Geneticist, later Professor of Zoology, Utah State University, USA.

cancers, and is also dominantly inherited. It results from one of at least four different gene mutations all affecting DNA mismatch repair, which leads to genomic instability. Tumours tend to occur in the right colon, and arise before the age of 50 years. Occurrence of colon cancer in at least three family members spanning two generations, with one before the age of 50 years strongly suggests this syndrome.

Pathology

Macroscopically, the tumours can be classified into the following groups:
- papilliferous;
- malignant ulcer;
- annular;
- diffuse infiltrating growth;
- colloid tumour.

Microscopically, these are all adeno-carcinomas.

Spread

- *Local*: encircling the wall of the bowel and invading the coats of the colon, eventually involving adjacent viscera (small intestine, stomach, duodenum, ureter, bladder, uterus, abdominal wall, etc.).
- *Lymphatic*: to the regional lymph nodes, eventually spreading via the thoracic duct, and may involve supraclavicular nodes in late cases.
- *Blood stream*: to the liver via the portal vein, thence to the lung.
- *Trans-coelomic*: producing deposits of malignant nodules throughout the peritoneal cavity.

Staging

Carcinoma of the colon is traditionally staged according to the classification of Dukes,* and depends upon the extent of transmural extension and lymph-node spread (see p. 221).

Clinical features

The manifestations of carcinoma of the colon can be divided, as with any tumour, into those

*Cuthbert Esquire Dukes (1890–1977), Pathologist, St Marks Hospital, London.

produced by the tumour itself, by the presence of secondaries and by the general effects of the tumour.

Local effects

The most common symptom is a change in bowel habit, either constipation, diarrhoea or the two alternating with each other. The diarrhoea may be accompanied by mucus (produced by the excessive secretion of mucus from the tumour), or bleeding, which may be bright, melaena or occult.

A constricting neoplasm, commonly found in the left (descending) colon, may present with the features of intestinal obstruction, either acute, chronic or acute on chronic (see p. 177). Rarely the tumour may present with perforation, either into the general peritoneal cavity or locally with the formation of a pericolic abscess, or by fistulae into adjacent viscera, e.g. a gastro-colic fistula or colo-vesical fistula.

The effects of secondary deposits

The patient may present with jaundice, or abdominal distension due to ascites, or with hepatomegaly.

The general effects of malignant disease

Presenting features may be anaemia, anorexia or loss of weight.

Tumours of the left side of the colon, where the contained stool is solid, are typically constricting growths, so obstructive features predominate. In contrast, tumours of the right side tend to be proliferative and here the stools are semi-liquid, therefore obstructive symptoms are relatively uncommon and the patient with a carcinoma of the caecum or ascending colon often presents with anaemia and loss of weight.

Examination

This should be directed to four main headings.
1 The presence of a mass palpable either per abdomen or per rectum (a sigmoid tumour may prolapse into the pouch of Douglas).

2 Clinical evidence of intestinal obstruction.

3 Evidence of spread (hepatomegaly, ascites, jaundice or supraclavicular nodes).

4 Clinical evidence of anaemia or loss of weight suggesting malignant disease.

Special investigations

• *Occult blood in the stool* is frequently present.

• *Sigmoidoscopy* will reveal tumours in the recto-sigmoid region and allow positive evidence by biopsy to be obtained. Even if the tumour is not reached directly, the presence of blood or slime coming down from above is strongly suspicious of malignant disease.

• *Colonoscopy*, using the fibre-optic colonoscope, enables the higher reaches of the colon to be inspected and a biopsy to be obtained.

• *Barium enema* will usually reveal the growth, either as a stricture or filling defect ('apple-core' deformity). It is important to remember that a negative barium enema does not definitely exclude the presence of a small tumour, particularly in the presence of extensive diverticulosis. False-positive X-rays may result from the presence of faecal material in the bowel lumen. It is by no means easy to differentiate radiologically between a carcinomatous stricture and one produced by diverticular disease.

• *CT scan*. In elderly patients who tolerate bowel preparation poorly, a CT scan may give sufficient information for the diagnosis of colonic cancer, and identify any liver involvement.

Rarely, if there is reasonable doubt as to the diagnosis, laparotomy is indicated.

Differential diagnosis

Diseases producing local symptoms

• Diverticular disease.

• Ulcerative colitis.

• The dysenteries and other causes of diarrhoea and constipation (see p. 200).

Diseases producing similar general manifestations

A useful quintet characterized by anaemia, a rather lemon-yellow tinge of the skin, loss of weight and general malaise are:

1 carcinoma of the large bowel;

2 carcinoma of the stomach;

3 carcinoma of the pancreas;

4 uraemia;

5 pernicious anaemia.

These five common conditions are often misdiagnosed for one another.

Treatment

Pre-operative treatment: the bowel is cleared by enemas and oral stimulant laxatives (e.g. Picolax). Metronidazole and gentamicin (or a cephalosporin) are given at the time of surgery. The haemoglobin level is checked and blood transfusion given if necessary.

The principle of operative treatment is wide resection of the growth together with its regional lymphatics. In the unobstructed case, the bowel can be prepared beforehand and primary resection with restoration of continuity can be achieved. In the obstructed case, where bowel preparation is contra-indicated, the primary goal is to relieve obstruction. It may be possible to achieve primary resection with restoration of continuity at the same time, but the poor vascularity and high incidence of colonic anastomotic breakdown means that this is undertaken only after serious consideration. The options would be to use an extended right colonic resection round to the splenic flexure, or bring out a defunctioning colostomy.

The incurable case

Even if liver secondaries are present, the best palliation is achieved by resection of the primary tumour. If this is impossible, palliative short-circuit or colostomy is performed to relieve the obstruction. Irradiation and cytotoxic therapy may give temporary alleviation.

Prognosis

Dukes' A tumours are usually curable with over 90% 5-year survival. Survival with Dukes' B tumours, where the disease is still confined to the bowel wall, is around 65%, and the presence of lymph-node metastases gives a 30% survival. If the apical lymph node, i.e. the node at the highest point of lymphatic drainage, is free from disease (C1) prognosis is better than C2 disease where the apical node is involved.

Colonic surgery

The different colonic resections are based on the blood supply to the colon coming from the superior mesenteric artery (midgut components, i.e. caecum, ascending colon and two-thirds of the transverse colon) and the inferior mesenteric artery (distal transverse colon, descending colon, sigmoid and rectum) together with a free anastomosis between the principal arteries via the marginal artery (of Drummond). Because survival of colonic cancer is, in the case of Dukes' C disease, dependent upon the adequacy of resection (clearing all affected lymph nodes), surgery for cancer involves taking as much of the lymphatic drainage as possible. In practice this means resecting as far down the principal artery as possible, as the lymphatic drainage runs along side the arterial inflow. In non-cancer operations, more conservative surgical techniques may be employed.

Colostomy

When bowel is brought to the surface and opened it is termed a stoma (meaning mouth); in the case of the colon such an opening is termed a colostomy. Stomas may be permanent (e.g. when the distal bowel has been removed) or temporary when there is a possibility of restoring continuity at a future date.

Indications for colostomy formation

The common indications for colostomy formation are:
• to divert faeces to allow healing of an anastomosis or fistula;
• to decompress a dilated colon, as a prelude to resection of the obstructing lesion;
• removal of the distal colon and rectum.

Types of colostomy

Loop colostomy

The colon is brought to the surface and the anti-mesenteric border opened. A rod or similar device is often used to stop the opened bowel loop from falling back inside. A loop colostomy is used to temporarily divert faeces and is simple to reverse.

End colostomy

An end (or terminal) colostomy is fashioned by dividing the colon and bringing the proximal end to the surface. It may be used as a definitive procedure in someone undergoing total rectal excision, or following perforated diverticula disease where the diseased bowel is removed and gross faecal contamination makes performing a primary anastomosis to restore continuity undesirable. In the latter, the distal bowel may be closed off and left within the abdomen (a Hartmann's procedure) or brought to the surface at a separate place as a mucus fistula.

Double-barrelled colostomy (Paul–Mikulicz*)

A double-barrelled colostomy comprises proximal and distal colon brought out adjacent to each other, rather like a loop colostomy, but with the intervening colon removed. This type of colostomy is not commonly used because the distal bowel is usually too short, but is useful in the treatment of sigmoid volvulus, where there is usually sufficient distal colon.

Complications of colostomy formation

• Retraction, where the colon disappears down the hole out of which it was brought. Retraction is either real and due to tension, or apparent and due to necrosis of the terminal bowel.
• Stenosis, where the opening becomes smaller. This may be due to ischaemia, or poor

*Frank Thomas Paul (1851–1941), Surgeon, Liverpool Royal Infirmary, UK. Johann von Mikulicz-Radecki (1850–1905), Professor of Surgery successively at Cracow, Konigsberg and Breslau, Poland.

apposition of colonic mucosa with the skin edge.

• *Paracolostomy hernia*, where peritoneal contents herniate through the abdominal wall defect made to accommodate the stoma.

• *Prolapse*, where the colon intussuscepts out of the stoma.

• *Lateral space small-bowel obstruction*, due to failure to obliterate the space between the terminal colon and the lateral abdominal wall.

In addition there are psychological problems, excess gas production with certain foods, leakage and skin excoriation due to ill-fitting stoma appliances or poorly constructed stomas.

Stoma appliances: principles

Modern-day stoma appliances have made the management of stomas straightforward. The principal components are the collecting pouch, or bag, into which the faeces are collected, and the adhesive flange, which adheres to the skin and keeps the pouch in position. The flange is cut to fit the stoma closely, and any exposed skin is covered with a barrier paste.

Colostomies contrast with ileostomies by the nature of the effluent. Ileostomy effluent is very irritant and causes severe skin excoriation. For this reason an ileostomy is constructed with a spout to keep the effluent off the skin, in contrast to a colostomy which is flush.

Management of a colostomy

In the first few weeks after performing a colostomy, the faecal discharge is semi-liquid, but this gradually reverts to normal, solid stools. The colostomy appliances, which are both waterproof and windproof, allow the patient to lead a normal life with little risk of leakage or unpleasant odour.

Although there is obviously no sphincteric control of the colostomy opening, most patients find that they pass a single stool a day, usually after breakfast. This can be helped by preparations such as Fybogel or Celevac, which produce a bulky, formed stool. Patients are best advised to avoid large amounts of vegetables or fruit, which may produce diarrhoea.

CHAPTER 26

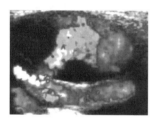

The Rectum and Anal Canal

The distribution around the anal canal of various conditions is shown in Fig. 26.1.

Bright red rectal bleeding (Table 26.1)

The passage of bright red blood per rectum is a common symptom, which the patient usually attributes to 'piles'; indeed haemorrhoids are by far the commonest cause of rectal bleeding. It is important, however, to bear in mind a list of possible causes of this symptom.

General causes

Bleeding diatheses (rare).

Local causes

1 Haemorrhoids.
2 Fissure-*in-ano*.
3 Tumours of the colon and rectum:
 (a) benign;
 (b) malignant.
4 Diverticular disease.
5 Ulcerative colitis.
6 Trauma.
7 Angiodysplasia of the colon.
8 Rarely, massive haemorrhage from higher up the alimentary canal — even a bleeding duodenal ulcer may produce bright red blood per rectum instead of the usual melaena, although such cases are commonly accompanied by haematemesis.

Haemorrhoids

Functional anatomy

Continence is partly a function of the anal sphincters, and partly a consequence of the anal cushions. The anal cushions comprise highly vascular tissue lining the anal canal, with a rich blood supply from the rectal arteries, which anastomose with the draining veins both through capillaries and through direct arterio-venous shunts. The draining veins form saccules, commonly just below the dentate line, which then drain via the superior rectal vein. The venous saccules are supported by smooth muscle to form the cushions, which are arranged such that they lie in the 3, 7 and 11 o'clock positions. Apposition of these subepithelial vascular cushions is important for continence of gas and fluid.

Classification

Haemorrhoids (or piles, the words are synonymous) may be classified according to their relationship to the anal orifice into internal, external and intero-external. Internal haemorrhoids are congested vascular cushions with dilated venous components draining into the superior rectal veins. External haemorrhoids is a term that should be abandoned, as it is applied to a conglomeration of quite different entities including perianal haematoma ('thrombosed external pile') the 'sentinel pile' of

DISTRIBUTION OF ANAL PATHOLOGY

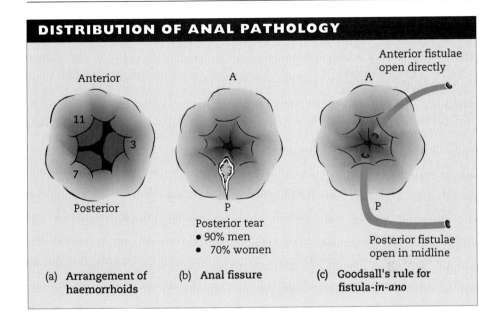

(a) Arrangement of haemorrhoids

(b) Anal fissure

(c) Goodsall's rule for fissula-in-*ano*

Fig. 26.1 Distribution of different conditions around the anal canal.

Table 26.1 Differentiating the common causes of rectal bleeding.

fissure-*in-ano* and perianal skin tags. Strictly speaking, internal piles that prolapse should be termed intero-external haemorrhoids, but this term is seldom employed except by literary perfectionists. In this chapter, which aims at being neither archaic nor pedantic, the terms 'external' and intero-external' haemorrhoids will not be further employed.

RECTAL BLEEDING

	Blood	Pain
Piles	Bright red, blood on paper and in pan. May prolapse	Painless, unless prolapsed and thrombosed
Fissure	Bright red, blood on paper and outside of stool	Painful, pain lasting long after passing stool
Colon and rectal cancer	Blood often mixed in with stool, especially if proximal tumour	Usually painless, unless locally infiltrating when causes tenesmus
Diverticular disease	Large volume of blood in the pan	Painless
Ulcerative colitis	Blood and mucus mixed with loose stool	Painless, unless coexistent fissure

Pathology

Internal haemorrhoids, or piles, are abnormal anal cushions, usually congested as a result of straining at stool, and traumatized by the passage of hard stool. The anal cushions are particularly prominent in pregnancy due to the venous congestion caused by the large gravid uterus, and the laxity of the supporting tissues due to the influence of progesterone. With the patient in the lithotomy position the usual arrangement is that three major piles occur at 3, 7 and 11 o'clock, exactly corresponding to the arrangement of the anal cushions.

Grading haemorrhoids

• *First-degree haemorrhoids* are confined to the anal canal—they bleed but do not prolapse.
• *Second-degree haemorrhoids* prolapse on defaecation, then reduce spontaneously.
• *Third-degree haemorrhoids* prolapse on defaecation but may be replaced manually by the patient.

To this grading a fourth degree has been added by some authors comprising haemorrhoids which remain persistently prolapsed outside the anal margin.

Predisposing factors

Most haemorrhoids are idiopathic, but they may be precipitated or aggravated by factors that produce congestion of the superior rectal veins. These include compression by any pelvic tumour (of which the commonest is the pregnant uterus), cardiac failure, excessive use of purgatives, chronic constipation and a rectal carcinoma. Rarely, they may complicate portal hypertension, as the pile-bearing area is at the site of portal–systemic anastomosis between the superior and inferior rectal veins. In such cases, the piles are the dilated, thin-walled superior rectal veins, akin to the varices in the oesophagus (p. 251).

Clinical features

Rectal bleeding is almost invariable; this is bright red and usually occurs at defaecation. In the case of first-degree piles this is the only symptom. More extensive piles prolapse

and may produce a mucus discharge and pruritus ani. The prolapsed piles may result in soiling.

Note that pain is not a feature of internal haemorrhoids except when these undergo thrombosis (see below). When a patient complains of 'an attack of piles', it often means that some acute painful condition has developed at the anal margin. Apart from thrombosed internal piles, the common causes of such anal pain to be considered are:
• fissure-*in-ano*;
• perianal haematoma;
• perianal or ischio-rectal abscess;
• tumour of the anal margin;
• proctalgia fugax: benign episodic pain relieved by digital dilatation of the anal sphincter.
Every patient presenting with the story suggestive of internal haemorrhoids is submitted to the following procedure.

1 *Examination of the abdomen* to exclude palpable lesions of the colon or aggravating factors for haemorrhoids, e.g. an enlarged liver or a pelvic mass.

2 *Rectal examination.* Internal haemorrhoids are not palpable but prolapsing piles are immediately obvious. The presence of prolapsing piles does not exclude a lesion higher in the bowel.

3 *Proctoscopy*, which will visualize the internal haemorrhoids.

4 *Sigmoidoscopy* is performed routinely, again to eliminate a lesion higher in the rectum — proctitis, polyp or carcinoma.

5 *A barium enema* is carried out in any case where symptoms such as alteration in bowel habit point to some more sinister condition than internal haemorrhoids.

6 *Colonoscopy* may be indicated to visualize and biopsy any lesion thus revealed.

Complications

• *Anaemia*: following severe or continued bleeding.
• *Thrombosis*: this occurs when prolapsing piles are gripped by the anal sphincter ('strangulated piles'). The venous return is occluded and thrombosis of the pile occurs. The prolapsed

haemorrhoids are swollen often to the size of large plums, purplish black and tense, and are accompanied by considerable pain and distress. Suppuration or ulceration may occur. After 2 or 3 weeks the thrombosed piles become fibrosed, often with spontaneous cure.

Treatment

Before commencing treatment, it is essential to exclude either any predisposing cause or an associated and more important lesion, e.g. carcinoma of the rectum.

Conservative management

Ideally the patient should avoid straining at stool, and aim to pass a firm, soft motion daily. A bulk laxative, together with advice on an adequate fluid intake, are often required.

Sclerotherapy

This is suitable for first- and second-degree piles. Two to three millilitres of 5% phenol in almond oil (or arachis oil) is injected above each pile as a sclerosing submucous perivenous injection. (The phenol sterilizes the oil, which is the main sclerosant). Because the injection is placed high in the anal canal it is painless. One or more repeat injections may be required at monthly intervals.

Banding

Application of a small O-ring rubber band to areas of protruding mucosa results in strangulation of the mucosa, which falls away after a few days. It can be successfully applied to first- and second-degree piles, but care must be taken to position the bands above the dentate line, lest the patient should feel the application.

Surgery

Haemorrhoidectomy is performed for third-degree piles.

Thrombosed strangulated piles

Conservative management is instituted for these. The patient is placed in bed with the foot of the bed elevated. Opiate analgesia is given for the severe pain which is also eased by local cold compresses. Often the thrombosed piles fibrose completely with spontaneous cure. Many surgeons now carry out haemorrhoidectomy at once in these patients.

Specific complications of haemorrhoidectomy

Acute retention of urine

Due to acute anal discomfort post-operatively.

Stricture

This only occurs when excessive amounts of mucosa and skin are excised. It is important to leave a bridge of epithelium between each excised haemorrhoid.

Post-operative haemorrhage

This may be reactionary, usually on the night of the operation, or secondary, about the seventh or eighth day. The bleeding may not be apparent externally, as the source of haemorrhage may be above the anal sphincter, with the blood filling the large bowel with only a little escaping to the exterior.

General treatment comprises blood transfusion if haemorrhage is severe as evidenced by the general appearance of the patient, a pulse raised above 100 and a systolic blood pressure below 100.

Local treatment is carried out under general anaesthetic in the operating theatre. The blood is washed out of the rectum with warm saline. Occasionally in reactionary haemorrhage a bleeding point is seen and can be diathermied or ligated. More often there is a general oozing from the operation field and the anal canal requires packing with gauze round a wide-bored rubber tube, which allows evacuation of flatus and escape of any blood from the bowel. The tube and gauze are removed after 48 hours.

Perianal haematoma

This lesion, which is also termed a thrombosed external pile, is produced by thrombosis within the inferior rectal venous plexus. Unlike internal haemorrhoids, it is covered by squamous epithelium supplied by somatic nerves and is therefore painful. The onset is acute, often after straining at stool, with sudden pain and the appearance of a lump at the anal verge. Local examination shows a tense, smooth, dark-blue, cherry-sized lump at the anal margin.

Untreated, this perianal haematoma either subsides over a few days, eventually leaving a fibrous tag, or ruptures, discharging some clotted blood.

Treatment

In the acute phase, immediate relief is produced by evacuating the haematoma through a small incision, conveniently performed under local anaesthetic. If seen when the haematoma is already discharging or becoming absorbed, hot baths are prescribed and the patient reassured that all will soon be well.

Anal fissure

A fissure is a tear at the anal margin, which usually follows the passage of a constipated stool. The site is usually posterior in the midline (90% of males, 70% of females), occasionally anteriorly in the midline, and rarely multiple. The posterior position of the majority of fissures is explained by the anatomical arrangement of the external anal sphincter; its superficial fibres pass forward to the anal canal from the coccyx, leaving a relatively unsupported V posteriorly. The anterior fissures of females may be associated with weakening of the perineal floor following tears at childbirth. Multiple fissures may complicate Crohn's disease of the colon.

Clinical features

Acute anal pain is characteristic. It is stinging in nature and lasts for a while after the passage of stool, sometimes 2 or more hours later. Fissure is the commonest cause of pain at the anal verge (see list, p. 214). There is often slight bleeding, and, because of the pain, the patient is usually constipated. On examination the anal sphincter is in spasm, and there may be a 'sentinel pile' protruding from the anus, which represents the torn tag of anal epithelium. The fissure can usually be seen by gently pulling open the anal verge. It may be impossible to do a rectal examination without anaesthetic; the fissure may then be palpable as a crack in the anal canal.

Treatment

Early small fissures may heal spontaneously. A local anaesthetic ointment together with a lubricant laxative may give relief. More recently, application of glyceryl trinitrate (GTN) cream has been shown to aid healing, by relaxing the anal sphincter and allowing the torn epithelium to heal.

More intractable cases usually respond to stretching the anal sphincter by insertion of a well-lubricated plastic dilator twice daily, or dividing the internal sphincter submucosally under general anaesthetic. It is important to assess the anal tone prior to performing an anal stretch or sphincterotomy, as incontinence may result, particularly in patients who have suffered previous obstetric injury.

A chronic recurring fissure-in-ano requires excision.

Ano-rectal abscesses

Classification (Fig. 26.2)

• *Perianal*: resulting from infection of a hair follicle, a sebaceous gland or perianal haematoma.

• *Ischio-rectal*: from infection of an anal gland leading from the anal canal into the submucosa, spread of infection from a perianal abscess, or penetration of the ischio-rectal fossa by a foreign body. The abscess may track as a horseshoe behind the rectum to the opposite ischio-rectal fossa.

• *Submucous*: infected fissure or laceration of the anal canal.

• *Pelvi-rectal*: spread from pelvic abscess (rare).

PERIANAL ABSCESSES

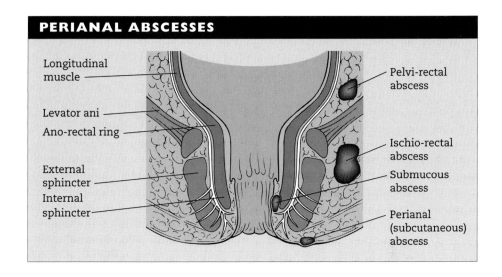

Longitudinal muscle

Levator ani

Ano-rectal ring

External sphincter

Internal sphincter

Pelvi-rectal abscess

Ischio-rectal abscess

Submucous abscess

Perianal (subcutaneous) abscess

Fig. 26.2 The anatomy of perianal abscesses.

Treatment

Early surgical drainage to prevent rupture and the possible formation of a fistula-*in-ano*.

Fistula-*in-ano*

Definitions

• A *fistula* is an abnormal communication between two epithelial surfaces, e.g. between a hollow viscus and the surface of the body or between two hollow viscera.
• A *sinus* is a granulating track leading from a source of infection to a surface.

Aetiology

The term fistula-*in-ano* is loosely applied to both fistulae and sinuses in relation to the anal canal. The great majority result from an initial abscess forming in one of the anal glands that pass from the submucosa of the anal canal to open within its lumen. Growth of bowel organisms, as opposed to skin flora, from an ano-rectal abscess is suggestive of the presence of a fistula. Rarely, fistulae are associated with Crohn's disease, ulcerative colitis and carcinoma of the rectum (occasionally, also, tuberculosis).

Anatomical classification (Fig. 26.3)

Anal fistulae are classified according to their position and relation to the internal and external anal sphincters.

• Submucous ⎫
• Subcutaneous ⎬ Superficial
• Intersphincteric ⎫
• Trans-sphincteric ⎬ Low anal
• Suprasphincteric—high anal
• Ano-rectal.

Superficial fistulae may be either subcutaneous or submucous, and are superficial tracks resulting from rupture respectively of subcutaneous and submucous abscesses. Intersphincteric and trans-sphincteric fistulae are examples of *low anal fistulae*, in which the track is below the ano-rectal ring. They differ in their penetration through the external sphincter, and most are at a low level with the track passing through the subcutaneous part of the sphincter. Suprasphincteric fistulae, with tracks close to the ano-rectal ring, are examples of *high anal fistulae*. Ano-rectal fistulae, fortunately rare, extend above the ano-rectal junction.

Fistulae with external openings posterior to the meridian in the lithotomy position usually

PERIANAL FISTULAE

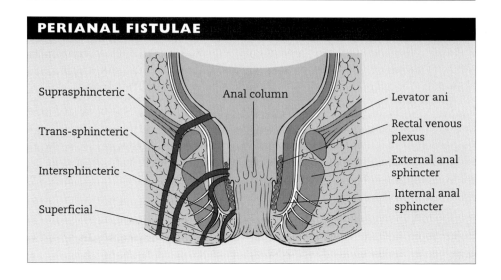

Suprasphincteric

Trans-sphincteric

Intersphincteric

Superficial

Anal column

Levator ani

Rectal venous plexus

External anal sphincter

Internal anal sphincter

Fig. 26.3 The anatomy of perianal fistulae.

open in the midline of the anus, whilst those with anterior external openings usually open directly into the anus — Goodsall's law* (Fig. 26.1).

Clinical features

There is usually a story of an initial ano-rectal abscess, which discharges. Following this there are recurrent episodes of perianal infection with persistent discharge of pus. Examination reveals the external opening of a fistula. The internal opening may be felt per rectum, but probing of the track is painful and should be deferred until the patient is anaesthetized. Accurate assessment of the extent of the fistula track, in particular its relation to the anal sphincter, is crucial. Where doubt exists, magnetic resonance imaging (MRI) can demonstrate the anatomy of a fistula very clearly.

Treatment

Superficial and low-level anal fistulae are laid open and allowed to heal by granulation. Because no sphincter, or only the subcutaneous part of the external and internal sphinc-

*David Goodsall (1843–1906), Surgeon, St Mark's Hospital, London.

ters, is divided in this procedure there is no loss of anal continence. Fistulae can only be treated in this manner when they quite definitely lie below the level of the ano-rectal ring, therefore careful assessment is important.

In high fistulae (suprasphincteric, and transsphincteric close to the ano-rectal ring) only the lower part of the fistula is laid open. A nonabsorbable strong ligature (e.g. nylon), termed a seton, is passed through the upper part of the track and left in place for 2 or 3 weeks so that the sphincter is fixed by scar tissue by the time of subsequent division of the upper part of the tract at a second operation, or by repeated tightening of the ligature. Laying open of the whole track of a suprasphincteric fistula in error will completely divide the sphincters and result in incontinence.

Stricture of the anal canal

Classification

- *Congenital.*
- *Traumatic*, particularly post-operative, after too radical excision of the skin and mucosa in haemorrhoidectomy.
- *Inflammatory*: lymphogranuloma inguinale (mostly female), Crohn's disease, ulcerative colitis.

- *Post-irradiation.*
- *Infiltrating neoplasm.*

Treatment
Depends on the underlying pathology and may call for repeated dilatation, plastic reconstruction, defunctioning colostomy or, in the case of malignant disease, excision of the rectum.

Prolapse of the rectum

This may be partial or complete.

Partial prolapse is confined to the mucosa, which prolapses an inch or two from the anal verge. Palpation of the prolapse between the finger and thumb reveals that there is no muscular wall within it. It may occur in infants who, unlike the usual textbook description, are not wasted but often perfectly healthy. Treatment of these babies requires nothing more than reassurance of the parents that the condition is self-curing. In adults it usually accompanies prolapsing piles or sphincter incompetence, and may present with pruritus ani.

Complete prolapse involves all layers of the rectal wall. It usually occurs in elderly females. Apart from the discomfort of the prolapse there is associated incontinence due to the stretching of the sphincter and mucus discharge from the prolapsed mucosal surface.

Treatment
Treatment of partial prolapse in adults comprises excision of the redundant mucosa, or a submucosal phenol-in-oil injection in order to produce sclerosis. In children, as already mentioned, self-cure without active treatment is the fortunate rule.

Many methods have been described for dealing with complete prolapse, including the Thiersch wire* operation where a wire or nylon suture is passed around the anal orifice to narrow it and keep the prolapse reduced.

---

*Karl Thiersch (1822–95), Professor of Surgery, Erlangen then Leipzig. Devised the split skin graft.

Today two procedures are commonly performed. The first is fixation of the rectum in the pelvis by an abdominal operation such as wrapping the mobilized rectum in polyvinyl sponge, which produces a brisk fibrous reaction welding the rectum to the pelvic tissues. The alternative procedure (Delorme's procedure) involves a less traumatic perineal approach, with excision of the mucosa and bunching of the bowel muscle to form a doughnut-like ring, which holds the rectum in the pelvis rather as a ring pessary may control vaginal prolapse.

Pruritus ani

There are four principal causes of pruritus ani.

1 *Local causes within the anus or rectum.* Any factor that causes moisture and sogginess of the anal skin, e.g. lack of cleanliness, excessive sweating, leakage of mucus from haemorrhoids, proctitis, colitis, fistula-*in-ano*, rectal neoplasm or threadworms.

2 *Skin diseases*: scabies, pediculosis, fungal infections, *Candida albicans*.

3 *General diseases associated with pruritus*: diabetes mellitus, Hodgkin's disease, obstructive jaundice.

4 *Idiopathic*: here very often the original cause has disappeared but the pruritus persists because of continued scratching of the anal region by the patient.

Treatment
Directed to the underlying cause. The idiopathic group often responds dramatically to hydrocortisone ointment and attention to local hygiene.

Tumours

Pathology
Benign
- Adenoma.
- Papilloma.
- Lipoma.
- Endometrioma.

Malignant

1 *Primary*:
   (a) adenocarcinoma;
   (b) squamous carcinoma of lower anal canal;
   (c) melanoma;
   (d) carcinoid tumour;
   (e) rodent ulcer of anal verge;
   (f) lymphoma;

2 *Secondary*: invasion from prostate, uterus or pelvic peritoneal deposits.

Rectal polyps

There are five common types of benign polyp found in the rectum.

1 *Juvenile polyp*, occurs in children and young adolescents, and looks like a cherry on a stalk. It is always benign, and presents with bleeding and may prolapse during defaecation.

2 *Metaplastic polyp*, a small, 2–3-mm, sessile, wart-like lesion. Often multiple, always benign, and not truly metaplastic, it is an incidental finding on sigmoidoscopy.

3 *Villous adenoma*, appears like an anemone with many fronds growing from its base on the rectal wall. Often grows very large, and produces large amounts of mucus. Liable to malignant change, so best completely removed.

4 *Adenomatous polyp*, is a benign polyp, which may undergo malignant change. Multiple polyps present in familial adenomatous polyposis (p. 207).

5 *Pseudo-polyp*, associated with colitis is not a true polyp but is oedematous mucosa against a background of ulcerated, mucosa-denuded bowel wall.

Diagnosis is by biopsy. Because of the propensity for malignant change of villous adenomas and adenomatous polyps, these should always be excised in full to ensure that no area of malignant change is missed. Small polyps may be excised in the clinic; larger polyps will require an operating sigmoidoscope with diathermy coagulation.

Carcinoma of the rectum
Pathology

The sexes are equally affected. It occurs in any age group from the twenties onwards, but is particularly common in the age range 50–70 years. Carcinoma of the rectum accounts for approximately one-third of all tumours of the large intestine. Predisposing factors (as with carcinoma of the colon) are pre-existing adenomas, familial adenomatous polyposis and ulcerative colitis.

Macroscopic appearance

The tumours may be:
• papilliferous;
• ulcerating (commonest);
• stenosing (usually at recto-sigmoid);
• colloid.

Microscopic appearance

About 90% are adenocarcinomas. Another 9% are colloid (adenocarcinoma with profuse production of mucus) and the remainder are the highly anaplastic carcinoma simplex. At the anal verge squamous carcinoma may occur, but a malignant tumour protruding through the anal canal is more likely to be an adenocarcinoma of the rectum invading the anal skin.

Spread

1 *Local*:
   (a) circumferentially around the lumen of the bowel;
   (b) invasion through the muscular coat;
   (c) penetration into adjacent organs, e.g. prostate, bladder, vagina, uterus, sacrum, sacral plexus, ureters and lateral pelvic wall.

2 *Lymphatic*: to regional lymph nodes along the inferior mesenteric vessels. At a late stage there is invasion of the iliac lymph nodes and of the groin lymph nodes (by retrograde spread) and involvement of the supraclavicular nodes via the thoracic duct.

3 *Blood*: via the superior rectal venous plexus, thence the portal vein to the liver and then lungs.

4 *Trans-coelomic*: seeding of the peritoneal cavity.

Staging

The extent of spread of rectal tumours is

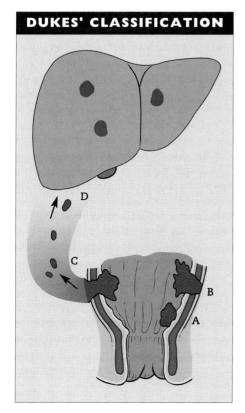

DUKES' CLASSIFICATION

Fig. 26.4 Dukes' classification of tumours of the large bowel: A, confined to the bowel wall; B, penetrating wall; C, involving regional lymph nodes; D, distant spread.

conveniently classified by Dukes' method* (Fig. 28.4).

A The tumour is confined to the rectal wall, with no spread beyond its muscle layers.

B The growth has completely breached the rectal wall.

C The regional lymph nodes are involved.

D Distant spread has occurred, e.g. to the liver or invasion into the bladder.

Prognosis

Depends largely on the stage of progression of the tumour and its histological degree of

*Cuthbert Esquire Dukes (1890–1977), Pathologist, St Marks Hospital, London

differentiation. The more advanced its spread and the more anaplastic its cells, the worse the prognosis.

Clinical features

The patient may present with:
- local disturbances due to the presence of the tumour in the rectum;
- manifestations of secondary deposits;
- the general effects of malignant disease.

Effects of secondary deposits and malignant disease are similar to those of carcinoma of the colon (p. 208) with the addition that rarely carcinoma of the rectum may spread to the groin nodes as a late phenomenon. With carcinoma at the anal verge this commonly occurs.

Local symptoms

Bowel disturbance (constipation and/or diarrhoea occur in 80% of cases), and bleeding, which is almost invariable and is the presenting complaint in about 60% of patients. There may also be mucus discharge, rectal pain and tenesmus.

Examination

Abdominal palpation is negative in early cases, but careful attention must be paid to the detection of hepatomegaly, ascites or abdominal distension. Other general features that may be detected in late cases are enlarged supraclavicular nodes, nodes in the groin or jaundice. Rectal examination reveals the tumour in 90% of cases.

Special investigations

- *Sigmoidoscopy* enables the great majority of tumours to be inspected and a biopsy to be taken.
- *Barium enema* is indicated if the growth is not visualized sigmoidoscopically, if a second tumour is suspected (5% of tumours in the large bowel are multiple) or if there is ulcerative colitis of familial polyposis.

Differential diagnosis of a rectal tumour

Differential diagnosis of a palpable tumour in the rectum must be made from:

- benign tumours;
- carcinoma of the sigmoid colon prolapsing into the pouch of Douglas and felt through the mucosal wall;
- secondary deposits in the pelvis;
- ovarian or uterine tumours;
- extension from carcinoma of the prostate or cervix;
- endometriosis;
- lymphogranuloma inguinale;
- amoebic granuloma;
- diverticular disease;
- the rare malignant tumours of the rectum (see p. 220);
- faeces (these give the classical physical sign of indentation).

The beginner may mistake the normal cervix for a palpable tumour, and should not be caught out by the presence of a ring pessary or tampon in the vagina, which are readily felt per rectum.

Treatment
Curative
Surgery depends upon the distance of the tumour from the anal verge.

Upper-third tumours can be resected with restorative anastomosis between the sigmoid colon and the lower rectum (anterior resection).

Lower-third tumours, less than 5 cm from the anal verge, are usually treated by abdomino-perineal excision of the rectum, with a terminal colostomy. Adjunctive radiotherapy may reduce the incidence of local recurrence after abdomino-perineal resection.

Mid-third rectal tumours can usually be treated by anterior resection, provided that satisfactory distal clearance can be obtained. The operation is easier in the female, where the wider pelvis facilitates dissection.

Palliative procedures
Even if secondaries are present, palliation is best achieved when possible by excision of the primary tumour. A colostomy may be necessary for intestinal obstruction, but this does not relieve the bleeding, mucus discharge and sacral pain.

In completely inoperable cases, deep X-ray therapy, diathermy or laser of the tumour may give temporary relief, as may cytotoxic drugs.

CHAPTER 27

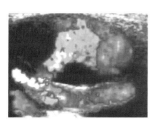

Peritonitis

Aetiology

Bacteria may enter the peritoneal cavity via four portals.

1 *From the exterior*: penetrating wound or infection at laparotomy; peritoneal dialysis.

2 *From intra-abdominal viscera*:

    (a) gangrene of a viscus, e.g. acute appendicitis, acute cholecystitis, diverticulitis or infarction of the intestine;

    (b) perforation of a viscus, e.g. perforated duodenal ulcer, perforated appendicitis, rupture of intestine from trauma;

    (c) post-operative leakage of an intestinal suture line.

3 *Via the blood stream*: as part of a septicaemia (pneumococcal, streptococcal or staphylococcal). This has been wrongly termed primary peritonitis; in fact, it is secondary to some initial source of infection.

4 *Via the female genital tract*: acute salpingitis or puerperal infection.

Approximately 30% of all cases of peritonitis in adults result from post-operative complications, 20% from acute appendicitis and 20% from a perforated peptic ulcer.

Pathology

Peritonitis of bowel origin usually shows a mixed flora (*Escherichia coli*, *Streptococcus fae-*
calis, *Pseudomonas*, *Klebsiella* and *Proteus*, together with the anaerobic *Clostridium* and *Bacteroides*). Gynaecological infections may be chlamydial, gonococcal or streptococcal. Blood-borne peritonitis may be streptococcal, pneumococcal, staphylococcal or tuberculous. In young children, a rare gynaecological infection is due to *Pneumococcus*.

The pathological effects of peritonitis are as follows.

1 Widespread absorption of toxins from the large, inflamed surface.

2 The associated paralytic ileus (p. 229) with:

    (a) loss of fluid;

    (b) loss of electrolytes;

    (c) loss of protein.

3 Gross abdominal distension with elevation of the diaphragm, which produces a liability to lung collapse and pneumonia.

Clinical features

Peritonitis is inevitably secondary to some precipitating lesion, which may itself have definite clinical features, e.g. the onset may be an attack of acute appendicitis, or a perforated duodenal ulcer, with appropriate symptoms and signs.

Early peritonitis is characterized by severe pain; the patient wishes to lie still because any movement aggravates the agony. Irritation of the diaphragm may be accompanied by pain referred to the shoulder tip. Vomiting is frequent. The temperature is usually elevated and the pulse rises progressively. Examination at this time shows localized or generalized tenderness, depending on the extent of the peritonitis. The abdominal wall is held rigidly and rebound tenderness is present. The abdomen is silent or the transmitted sounds of the heart beat and respiration may be detected. Rectal examination may show tenderness in the pouch of Douglas.

In advanced peritonitis the abdomen becomes distended and tympanitic, signs of free fluid are present, the patient becomes increasingly toxic with a rapid, feeble pulse, vomiting is faeculent and the skin is moist, cold and cyanosed (the Hippocratic facies).

Special investigations

These are of only limited value; diagnosis depends on the clinical features.

• *Chest X-ray* (performed with the patient erect) may reveal free gas under the diaphragm in cases of a perforated abdominal viscus (seen in 70% of perforated peptic ulcers). A chest X-ray may also exclude pulmonary infection as a differential diagnosis.

• *Abdominal X-ray* may also demonstrate free gas, or may demonstrate another cause of peritonitis.

• *Serum amylase* helps differentiate acute pancreatitis.

• *Full blood count* usually reveals a marked leucocytosis.

Differential diagnosis

This is from intestinal obstruction and from ureteric or biliary colic, in all of which the patient tends to be restless. Basal pneumonia, myocardial infarction, intraperitoneal haemorrhage or leakage of an aortic aneurysm are other fairly common misdiagnoses.

Principles of treatment

In this section only an outline of treatment is given, as specific causes of peritonitis may require specific therapy; these are dealt with in their appropriate chapters.

1 *Relieve pain* with opiates, e.g. intravenous morphine.

2 *Gastric aspiration* by means of naso-gastric tube reduces the risk of inhalation of vomit under anaesthesia and prevents further abdominal distension by removing swallowed air.

3 *Fluid and electrolyte replacement* by intravenous therapy. Blood or blood substitutes may be required in the presence of shock.

4 *Antibiotic therapy*, usually to deal with the broad spectrum of bowel organisms, e.g. gentamicin and metronidazole, but therapy is guided, where possible, by checking the sensitivity of the responsible organisms.

5 *Surgery* is indicated if the source of infection can be removed or closed, e.g. the repair of a perforated ulcer or removal of the gangrenous, perforated appendix.

Any localized collection of pus requires drainage and later surgery may be required for the evacuation of residual abscesses, e.g. subphrenic or pelvic collections.

Conservative treatment is indicated, at least initially, where the infection has been localized, e.g. an appendix mass, or where the primary focus is irremovable, as in pancreatitis or postpartum infection. Where the patient is moribund or where there is a lack of surgical facilities, as on board ship, reliance is placed on intravenous therapy, gastric aspiration and antibiotics.

Particular causes of peritonitis

Peritoneal dialysis peritonitis

Patients with chronic renal failure on peritoneal dialysis are prone to peritonitis either from organisms entering via the indwelling dialysis catheter (usually skin flora such as *Staphylococcus*), or from perforation of a viscus, in which case the flora is generally a mixture of colonic organisms. Diagnosis is made by the presence of abdominal pain, and turbid dialysate. Single organisms are treated by intravenous and intraperitoneal antibiotics. Multiple organisms suggest perforation and require laparotomy as well as antibiotics.

Non-specific bacterial peritonitis

Patients with hepatic cirrhosis and ascites have a protein-rich medium for the culture of organisms, as well as being immunosuppressed by their disease. Infection is by blood-borne organisms, is confirmed by peritoneal tap and is treated with intravenous antibiotics.

Pneumococcal peritonitis

This may be secondary to the septicaemia accompanying a pneumococcal lung infection, or, uncommonly these days, may result from an ascending infection from the vagina in girls between the age of 4 and 10 years.

Clinically, there is peritonitis of sudden onset accompanied by severe toxaemia and fever. The white-cell count is elevated above 20×10^9/L.

Treatment

Usually laparotomy is performed because a perforated appendicitis is suspected. Clear or turbid fluid containing fibrin flakes is discovered without an obvious primary cause. A slide made of the pus shows the characteristic Gram-positive pneumococci lying in pairs. The condition responds to penicillin therapy.

Haemolytic streptococcal peritonitis

This may occur in children, secondary or streptococcal infection of the tonsil, otitis media, scarlet fever or erysipelas.

Staphylococcal peritonitis

This very rarely complicates staphylococcal septicaemia, which more often produces intra-abdominal or perinephric abscesses.

Tuberculous peritonitis

Tuberculous peritonitis is always secondary to tuberculosis elsewhere although the primary focus may no longer be active. It usually occurs as a result of local spread from the mesenteric lymph nodes or via the female genital tract, although it may complicate generalized miliary tuberculosis.

With the diminution of tuberculosis elsewhere, tuberculous peritonitis is becoming increasingly rare in this country. It is seen most often in immigrants from developing countries and patients who are immunosuppressed, either therapeutically or by disease (e.g. acquired immune deficiency syndrome (AIDS)).

Pathology

The peritoneum is studded with tubercles in the initial phase, with an accompanying serous effusion. Later the tubercles coalesce, local abscesses may develop and the intra-abdominal viscera become matted together with dense fibrous adhesions.

Clinical features

It may present either as acute peritonitis, ascites or intestinal obstruction secondary to gross adhesions. Diagnosis is usually made only at operation.

Treatment

Treatment comprises anti-tuberculous chemotherapy. Operation may be required for the relief of intestinal obstruction from adhesions.

Bile peritonitis

This may occur as a result of:
• traumatic rupture of the gall bladder or its ducts (open or closed injury, iatrogenic damage from liver biopsy or percutaneous cholangiography);
• leakage from the liver, gall bladder or its ducts after a biliary tract operation;
• perforation of an acutely inflamed gall bladder;
• transudation of the bile through a gangrenous but non-perforated gall bladder;
• spontaneous perforation of the gall bladder;
• idiopathic — a rare but well-recognized condition in which bile peritonitis occurs without obvious cause, possibly a small perforation due to a calculus, which then becomes sealed.

Bile peritonitis is only a rare accompaniment of acute cholecystitis, because unlike the appendix, which when inflamed rapidly undergoes gangrene, the inflamed gall bladder is usually thickened and walled off by adhesions. In addition, again unlike the appendix, which only receives an end-artery supply from the ileo-colic artery, the gall bladder has an additional blood supply from the liver bed, therefore frank gangrene of the inflamed gall bladder is unusual.

The patient presents with all the features of general peritonitis. Laparotomy is required to deal with the underlying cause, but the mortality is approximately 50%. As with all other causes of peritonitis, not surprisingly it is the elderly patient with late disease who does badly.

Localized intraperitoneal collections of pus

Following peritonitis, pus may collect in the subphrenic spaces or in the pelvis. These are the most dependent parts of the peritoneal cavity when the patient lies supine.

Subphrenic abscess
Anatomy (Fig. 27.1)
The subphrenic region lies between the diaphragm above and the transverse colon with mesocolon below and is divided further by the liver and its ligaments. The right and left *subphrenic spaces* lie between the diaphragm and the liver and are separated from each other by the falciform ligament. The right and left *subhepatic spaces* are below the liver, the right forming Morison's pouch* and the left being the lesser sac, which communicates with the former through the foramen of Winslow.†
The right *extraperitoneal space* lies between the bare area of the liver and the diaphragm. About

*James Rutherford Morison (1853–1939), Professor of Surgery, University of Durham.
†Jacob Winslow (1669–1760), Danish, became Professor of Anatomy and Surgery in Paris.

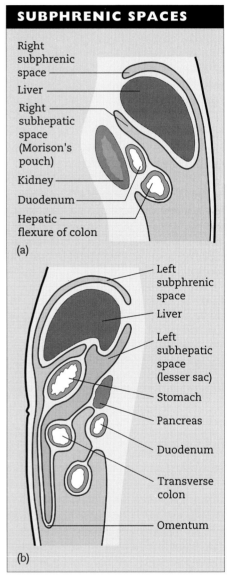

SUBPHRENIC SPACES

Right subphrenic space
Liver
Right subhepatic space (Morison's pouch)
Kidney
Duodenum
Hepatic flexure of colon
(a)

Left subphrenic space
Liver
Left subhepatic space (lesser sac)
Stomach
Pancreas
Duodenum
Transverse colon
Omentum
(b)

Fig. 27.1 The anatomy of the subphrenic spaces. (a) right; (b) left.

two-thirds of subphrenic abscesses occur on the right side. Rarely, they are bilateral.

Aetiology
A localized collection of pus may occur in the subphrenic region following general peritonitis.

Usually, the underlying cause is a peritonitis involving the upper abdomen — leakage following biliary or gastric surgery or a perforated peptic ulcer. Rarely, infection occurs from haematogenous spread or from direct spread from a primary chest lesion, e.g. empyema.

Clinical features

Subphrenic infection usually follows general peritonitis after 10–21 days, although if antibiotics have been given an abscess may be disguised and may only become manifest weeks or even months after the original episode. There may be no localizing symptoms, the patient presenting with malaise, nausea, loss of weight, anaemia and pyrexia; hence, the aphorism 'pus somewhere, pus nowhere, pus under the diaphragm'. At least half the cases have a fever that continues from the original peritonitis, although the standard description is of a swinging temperature, which commences some 10 days after the initial illness.

Localizing features are pain in the upper abdomen, lower chest or referred to the shoulder tip with localized upper abdominal or chest-wall tenderness. There may be signs of fluid, or collapse at the lung base. In late cases, a swelling may be detected over the lower chest wall or upper abdomen.

Special investigations

1 *Full blood count*: the white-cell count is raised in the region of 15–20 × 10⁹/L, with a polymorph leucocytosis.

2 *Chest X-ray* may show the following (Fig. 27.2):
    (a) elevation of the diaphragm on the affected side;
    (b) pleural effusion and/or collapse of the lung base;
    (c) gas and a fluid level below the diaphragm.

3 *Ultrasound* may show diminished or absent mobility of the diaphragm, and may demonstrate the subphrenic abscess.

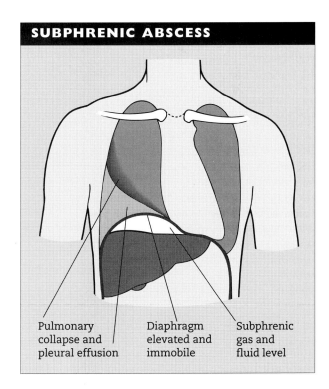

SUBPHRENIC ABSCESS

| Pulmonary collapse and pleural effusion | Diaphragm elevated and immobile | Subphrenic gas and fluid level |

Fig. 27.2 Diagram of the radiological appearance of a right subphrenic abscess. The diaphragm is raised (and fixed on screening), a fluid level is present beneath it and there is a sympathetic pleural effusion with compression and/or collapse of the lung base.

4 *Computed tomography (CT)* will demonstrate an abscess, and also locate any other peritoneal collections of pus.

Treatment

In early cases, where there is absence of gas and free fluid on X-ray, the patient is placed on broad-spectrum antibiotic therapy. If there is rapid response, the diagnosis is one of a spreading cellulitis of the subphrenic space.

If there is clinical or radiological evidence of a localized abscess, or if resolution fails to occur on chemotherapy, percutaneous drainage may be carried out under ultrasound or CT control. If this fails, or if the abscess is loculated, surgical drainage is performed. Depending on the location of the abscess, this is carried out either by a posterior extraperitoneal approach through the bed of, or just below, the 12th rib, or an anterior approach via a subcostal incision.

Pelvic abscess

A pelvic abscess may follow any general peritonitis, but it is particularly common after acute appendicitis (75%), or after gynaecological infections. In the male the abscess lies between the bladder and the rectum, in the female between the uterus and posterior fornix of the vagina anteriorly, and the rectum posteriorly (pouch of Douglas*).

*James Douglas (1675–1742), Anatomist and Obstetrician, London.

Left untreated the abscess may burst into the rectum or vagina, or may discharge onto the abdominal wall, particularly if there has been a previous abdominal laparotomy incision at the time of the original episode of peritonitis. Occasionally, the abscess may rupture into the peritoneal cavity.

Clinical features

• *General*: swinging pyrexia, toxaemia, weight loss with leucocytosis.
• *Local*: diarrhoea, mucus discharge per rectum, the presence of a mass felt on rectal or vaginal examination, which is occasionally large enough to be palpated abdominally.

Treatment

An early pelvic cellulitis may respond rapidly to a short course of chemotherapy, but there is the risk that the prolonged antibiotic treatment of an unresolved infection may produce a chronic inflammatory mass studded with small abscess cavities in the pelvis. It is safer therefore, where there is an established pelvic abscess, to withhold chemotherapy and await pointing into the vagina or rectum through which surgical drainage can be carried out. Very often even this is not required, as firm pressure by the finger in the rectum may be followed by rupture of the abscess through the rectal wall.

CHAPTER 28

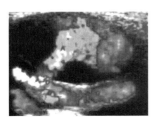

Paralytic Ileus

The word ileus comes from the Greek verb 'to roll', from which it became applied to colic and hence to obstruction. Obstructions are subdivided into mechanical and paralytic, which is produced by lack of intestinal motility. It is therefore a bad habit to say that a patient has 'an ileus' when one really means a 'paralytic ileus', as the word ileus alone implies merely intestinal obstruction.

Paralytic (or adynamic or neurogenic) ileus can be defined as a state of atony of the intestine. Its principal clinical features are:

- abdominal distension;
- absolute constipation;
- vomiting;
- absence of intestinal movements, and hence, of colicky pain.

Aetiology

The state of paralytic ileus may be produced by a large number of factors, sometimes coexisting.

Reflex paralytic ileus

This probably results from interference with the autonomic nerve supply of the gut; it may complicate fractures of the spine or pelvis, application of a plaster cast, retroperitoneal haemorrhage and retroperitoneal surgery, intestinal ischaemia, ureteric colic and occasionally parturition. Where the colon alone is affected it has been termed colonic pseudo-obstruction (Ogilvie's syndrome*).

Peritonitis

Perhaps as a result of toxic paralysis of intrinsic nerve plexuses, the bowel in peritonitis becomes atonic. There may be an associated mechanical obstruction produced by kinking of loops of bowel by fibrinous adhesions, so that frequently the paralytic ileus is complicated by mechanical obstruction.

Metabolic factors

Severe potassium depletion, uraemia and diabetic coma may result in paralytic ileus.

Drugs

Paralytic ileus is produced by heavy dosage of anticholinergic agents and anti-parkinsonian drugs.

Post-operative

Some degree of paralytic ileus occurs after every laparotomy. Its aetiology is complex, including sympathetic over-action, the effects of manipulation of the bowel, potassium depletion (where there has been excessive pre-operative vomiting), peritoneal irritation from

*Sir Heneage Ogilvie (1887–1971), Surgeon, Guy's Hospital, London.

blood or associated peritonitis and the atony of stomach and the large bowel, which occurs after every abdominal operation for a period of some 24–48 hours.

The distension that occurs on the first and second post-operative day is probably produced by swallowed air. This air passes through the small intestine (where peristalsis usually returns quickly) to the colon, which is atonic and produces a functional hold up.

Paralytic ileus that persists for more than 48 hours post-operatively probably has some other aetiological factor present.

Pathology
The deleterious effects of paralytic ileus are similar to those of a simple mechanical obstruction.
• There is severe loss of fluid, electrolytes and protein into the gut lumen and in the vomitus or gastric aspirate.
• Gross gaseous distension of the gut, produced mainly from swallowed air that cannot pass through the bowel, impairs the blood supply of the bowel wall and allows toxic absorption to occur.

Clinical features
Paralytic ileus is most commonly seen in the post-operative stage of peritonitis or of major abdominal surgery. There is abdominal distension, absolute constipation and effortless vomiting. Pain is not present, apart from the discomfort of the laparotomy wound and the abdominal distension. On examination the patient is anxious and uncomfortable. The abdomen is distended, silent and tender. A plain X-ray of the abdomen will show gas distributed throughout the small and large gut and some fluid levels may be present on an erect abdominal X-ray.

The paralytic ileus may merge insidiously into a mechanical obstruction produced by adhesions or bands following abdominal surgery, and an important, often extremely difficult, differential diagnosis lies between these two conditions. The diagnosis is important, as paralytic ileus is treated conservatively whereas mechanical obstruction usually calls for urgent operation.

Differential diagnosis
Differentiating paralytic ileus from mechanical obstruction can be achieved with the following criteria.
• *Duration*: paralytic ileus rarely lasts more than 3 or 4 days; persistence of symptoms after this time is suspicious of mechanical obstruction.
• *Bowel sounds*: the presence of bowel sounds is important. An absolutely silent abdomen is diagnostic of paralytic ileus, whereas noisy bowel sounds indicate mechanical obstruction.
• *Pain*: paralytic ileus is relatively painless, whereas colicky abdominal pain is present in mechanical obstruction.
• *Timing*: if symptoms commence after the patient has already passed flatus or had a bowel action it is very likely that a mechanical obstruction has supervened. The other possibility to consider is that there has been a leakage from an anastomosis and that peritonitis is now present.
• *X-ray appearances*: a plain X-ray of the abdomen showing a localized loop of distended small intestine without gas shadows in the colon or rectum is strongly suggestive of mechanical obstruction, in contrast to the diffuse appearance of gas throughout the small and large bowel in paralytic ileus.

Treatment
Prophylaxis
Biochemical imbalance is corrected pre-operatively. The bowel is handled gently at operation. Post-operatively, gastric distension due to air swallowing may require naso-gastric suction.

In the established case
Naso-gastric suction is employed to remove swallowed air and prevent gaseous distension. The aspiration of fluid also helps to relieve the associated gastric dilatation. Intravenous fluid and electrolyte therapy is instituted with careful biochemical control. Pethidine, which

has relatively little effect on intestinal motility compared with the other opiates, may be used to allay discomfort, and combined with a phenothiazine such as prochlorperazine for nausea. Eventually, patience is rewarded and recovery from the ileus will occur unless it is secondary to some underlying cause, such as infection.

In the absence of any evidence of mechanical obstruction or infection, prolonged stubborn ileus is occasionally treated pharmacologically. Motility stimulants such as metoclopramide and cisapride, together with erythromycin (which stimulates the motilin receptor) may be tried. Metoclopramide is a dopamine antagonist that stimulates gastric emptying and small intestinal transit. Cisapride stimulates motility by promoting acetyl choline release in the gut wall.

CHAPTER 29

Hernia

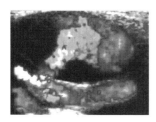

General considerations

A hernia is a protrusion of any viscus or part of a viscus through its coverings into an abnormal situation. Most hernias occur as diverticula of the peritoneal cavity and therefore have a sac of parietal peritoneum. The common varieties of hernias through the abdominal wall, in order of frequency, are:
- inguinal (indirect or direct);
- femoral;
- umbilical and para-umbilical;
- incisional;
- ventral and epigastric.

Aetiology
Hernias occur at sites of weakness in the abdominal wall. This weakness may be congeni-
tal, e.g. persistence of the processus vaginalis of testicular descent giving rise to a congenital inguinal hernia, or failure of complete closure of the umbilical scar. It may occur at the site of penetration of structures through the abdominal wall, e.g. the femoral canal, or the layers of the abdominal wall may be weakened following a surgical incision (incisional hernia), either by poor healing as a result of infection, haematoma formation or poor technique, or by damage to nerves that results in paralysis of the abdominal muscles.

Hernias should also be thought of as portents of other diseases, as they are often associated with pathological increases in intra-abdominal pressure by conditions such as:
- chronic cough, secondary to chronic bronchitis;

A LUMP IN THE GROIN

A patient presenting with a lump in the groin is a common clinical problem. Whenever one considers the differential diagnosis of a mass situated in a particular area, a two-stage mental process is required: first, what are the anatomical structures in that particular region, and second, what pathological entities may arise therefrom?

In considering the groin, let these possibilities pass through your mind.
1 *The hernial orifices:*
  (a) inguinal hernia;
  (b) femoral hernia.
2 *The testicular apparatus:*
  (a) hydrocele of the cord;
  (b) ectopic testis.
3 *The vein:* saphena varix.
4 *The artery:* femoral aneurysm.
5 *The lymph nodes:* lymphadenopathy due to infection, neoplasm or lymphoma.
6 *The psoas sheath:* psoas abscess.
7 *The skin and subcutaneous tissues:* lipoma.

- constipation, perhaps due to colonic carcinoma;
- urinary obstruction, due to prostatic disease;
- pregnancy;
- abdominal distension with ascites;
- weak abdominal muscles, e.g. in gross obesity or muscle wasting in cachexia.

Fig. 29.1 The differences between (a) a reducible, (b) an irreducible and (c) a strangulated hernia.

Varieties

A hernia at any site may be (Fig. 29.1):

- reducible;
- irreducible;
- strangulated.

Reducible hernia

The contents of a reducible hernia can be replaced completely into the peritoneal cavity.

Irreducible hernia

A hernia becomes irreducible, or incarcerated, usually because of adhesions of its contents

TYPES OF HERNIA

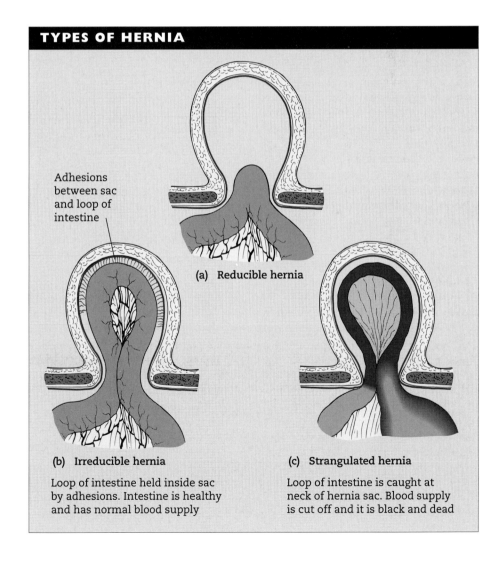

Adhesions between sac and loop of intestine

(a) Reducible hernia

(b) Irreducible hernia

Loop of intestine held inside sac by adhesions. Intestine is healthy and has normal blood supply

(c) Strangulated hernia

Loop of intestine is caught at neck of hernia sac. Blood supply is cut off and it is black and dead to the inner wall of the sac, or sometimes as a result of adhesions of its contents to each other to form a mass greater in size than the neck of the sac. Occasionally, inspissated faeces within the loops of bowel in the hernia prevent reduction.

Strangulated hernia

When strangulation occurs, the contents of the hernia are constricted by the neck of the sac to such a degree that their circulation is cut off. Unless relieved, gangrene is inevitable and, if gut is involved, perforation of the gangrenous loop will eventually occur.

Clinical features
Reducible hernia

A reducible hernia simply presents as a lump that may disappear on lying down and that is usually not painful, although it may be accompanied by some discomfort. Examination reveals a reducible lump with a cough impulse.

Irreducible hernia

If the hernia will not reduce but is painless and there are no other symptoms, irreducibility is diagnosed. The absence of a cough impulse alone does not indicate strangulation, because in an irreducible femoral hernia, for example, the neck is often plugged by omentum, which prevents the cough impulse from being felt.

Strangulated hernia

If strangulation supervenes, the patient complains of severe pain in the hernia of sudden onset and also of central abdominal colicky pain. The other symptoms of intestinal obstruction — vomiting, distension and absolute constipation — soon appear. Examination reveals a tender, tense hernia that cannot be reduced and has no cough impulse. The overlying skin becomes inflamed and oedematous and there are the signs of intestinal obstruction with distension, abdominal tenderness and noisy bowel sounds. These features are much less marked when omentum rather than intestine is contained within the sac.

The three common types of hernia to strangulate are, in order of frequency, femoral, indirect inguinal and umbilical.

Inguinal hernia

May be classified into:
• *indirect* — entering the internal inguinal ring and traversing the inguinal canal;
• *direct* — pushing through the posterior wall of the inguinal canal medial to the internal ring.
See Table 29.1 (p. 236) for a summary of the differences between indirect and direct inguinal hernias.

The anatomy of the inguinal canal is the key to the understanding of these hernias.

Anatomy (Fig. 29.2)

The inguinal canal represents the oblique passage taken through the lower abdominal wall by the testis and cord (the round ligament in the female). It is 4 cm long and passes downwards and medially, and from deep to superficial, from the internal to the external inguinal rings, lying parallel to, and immediately above, the inguinal ligament.
• *Anteriorly*: skin, superficial fascia and external oblique aponeurosis cover the full length of the canal; the internal oblique covers its lateral third.
• *Posteriorly*: the conjoint tendon (representing the fused common insertion of the internal oblique and transversus abdominis muscles into the pubic crest) forms the posterior wall of the canal medially, the transversalis fascia lies laterally.
• *Above*: the lowest fibres of the internal oblique and transversus abdominis.
• *Below*: lies the inguinal ligament.

The internal ring represents the point at which the spermatic cord pushes through the transversalis fascia; it is demarcated medially by the inferior epigastric vessels as they pass upwards from the external iliac artery and vein.

The external ring is an inverted V-shaped defect in the external oblique aponeurosis and

INGUINAL CANAL

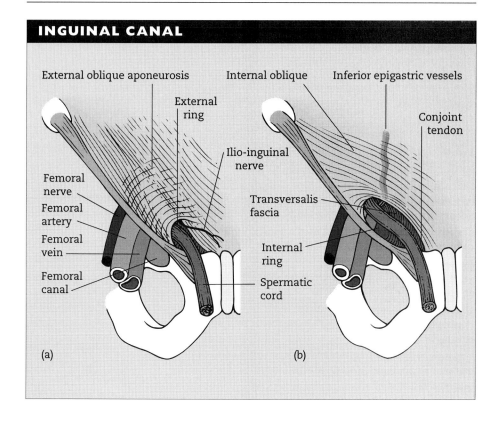

External oblique aponeurosis   Internal oblique   Inferior epigastric vessels

External ring

Conjoint tendon

Ilio-inguinal nerve

Femoral nerve

Femoral artery

Transversalis fascia

Femoral vein

Internal ring

Femoral canal

Spermatic cord

(a)   (b)

Fig. 29.2 The anatomy of the inguinal canal: (a) with the external oblique aponeurosis intact; (b) aponeurosis laid open.

lies immediately above and medial to the pubic tubercle.

The inguinal canal transmits the spermatic cord (round ligament in the female) and the ilio-inguinal nerve.

Indirect inguinal hernia

This passes through the internal ring, along the canal in front of the spermatic cord, and, if large enough, emerges through the external ring and descends into the scrotum. If reducible, such a hernia can be completely controlled by pressure with one fingertip over the internal inguinal ring, which lies 1–2 cm

above the point where the femoral artery passes under the inguinal ligament, i.e. 1–2 cm above the femoral pulse. This can be felt at the mid-inguinal point, halfway between the anterior superior iliac spine and the symphysis pubis.

If the hernia protrudes through the external ring, it can be felt to lie above and medial to the pubic tubercle and is thus differentiated from a femoral hernia, which emerges through the femoral canal below and lateral to this landmark (see Fig. 29.3, p. 237).

Indirect hernias may be congenital, due to persistence of the processus vaginalis; these present at or soon after birth or may arise in adolescence. The acquired variety may occur at any age in adult life and here the sac is formed as an out-pushing of the abdominal peritoneum.

The narrow internal opening through the internal inguinal ring accounts for two impor-

INDIRECT AND DIRECT INGUINAL HERNIAS

	Indirect	Direct
Origin	Pass through internal ring, lateral to inferior epigastric vessels	Pass through posterior wall of inguinal canal, medial to inferior epigastric vessels
Congenital or acquired	May be congenital	Always acquired, rare in childhood and adolescence
Control by pressure over internal ring	Yes	No
Strangulates	Commonly, because of narrow neck (internal ring)	Occasionally, because usually wide necked
Extends down into scrotum	Often	Rarely
Reduces on lying	Not readily	Spontaneously
Recurrence after surgery	Uncommon	More common

Table 29.1 Characteristic differences that help differentiate indirect and direct inguinal hernias.

tant features of the indirect hernia. First, the hernia often does not reach its full size until the patient has been up and around for a little time, and then does not reduce immediately when the subject lies down, because it takes a little time for the hernial contents to pass in or out of the sac through its narrow neck. Secondly, the indirect hernia has a distinct tendency to strangulate at the site of this narrow orifice.

Direct inguinal hernia

This pushes its way directly forward through the posterior wall of the inguinal canal. Because it lies medial to the internal ring, it is not controlled by digital pressure applied over the ring immediately above the femoral pulse. On inspection the hernia is seen to protrude directly forwards (hence its name) compared with the oblique route downwards towards the scrotum of an indirect inguinal hernia.

Other points that differentiate a direct from an indirect hernia are that the direct is always acquired and is therefore extremely rare in infancy or adolescence; it has a large orifice and therefore appears immediately on standing, disappearing again at once when the patient lies down. Moreover, because of this large opening, strangulation is extremely rare.

Although clinically it is usually quite easy to tell the difference between the two types of inguinal hernia, the ultimate differentiation can only be made at operation; the inferior epigastric vessels demarcate the medial edge of the internal ring; therefore an indirect sac will pass lateral, and a direct hernia medial to these vessels. Quite often a direct and indirect hernia coexist; they bulge on either side of the inferior epigastric vessels like the legs of a pair of pantaloons.

Sixty per cent of inguinal herniae occur on the right side, 20% on the left and 20% are bilateral.

Treatment

Congenital inguinal herniae in infants do not obliterate spontaneously; the patent processus vaginalis is ligated and the hernial sac excised at the age of about 1 year (herniotomy). In

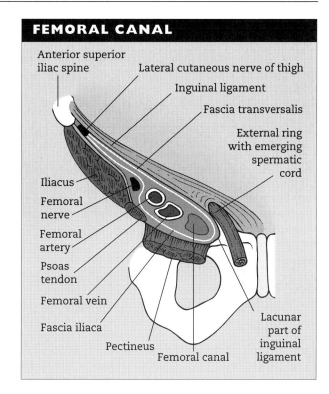

FEMORAL CANAL

Anterior superior iliac spine

Lateral cutaneous nerve of thigh

Inguinal ligament

Fascia transversalis

External ring with emerging spermatic cord

Iliacus

Femoral nerve

Femoral artery

Psoas tendon

Femoral vein

Fascia iliaca

Pectineus

Femoral canal

Lacunar part of inguinal ligament

Fig. 29.3 The anatomy of the femoral canal and its surrounds to show the relationships of a femoral hernia.

adults, operation is usually advised. This comprises excision of the sac and repair of the weakened inguinal canal, commonly performed either by plicating the posterior wall with a nylon suture, or reinforcing the posterior wall with a nylon or polypropylene mesh (Liechtenstein repair).

A truss is only prescribed in patients who are of very poor general condition and are unable to stand operation, although they often have difficulty keeping a truss correctly in place. But even in such cases, a painful hernia that threatens strangulation is much better repaired as an elective procedure, if necessary under local anaesthesia, rather than as an emergency should strangulation supervene.

Recurrent inguinal hernias may be due to causes such as infection, haematoma or poor technique, but are most likely to be a failure to appreciate the underlying cause of the increased intra-abdominal pressure that initi-

ated the hernia in the first place (e.g. continuing constipation, or bladder neck obstruction by a large prostate).

Femoral hernia

Anatomy

A femoral hernia passes through the femoral canal. This is a gap normally about 1.5 cm in length, which just admits the tip of the little finger and which lies at the medial extremity of the femoral sheath containing the femoral artery and vein. The boundaries of the femoral canal (Fig. 29.3) are as follows.

- *Anteriorly*: the inguinal ligament.
- *Medially*: the sharp edge of the lacunar part of the inguinal ligament (Gimbernat's ligament*).

*Manuel Gimbernat (1734–1816), Anatomist and Surgeon to King Carlos III of Spain.

HERNIA POSITIONS

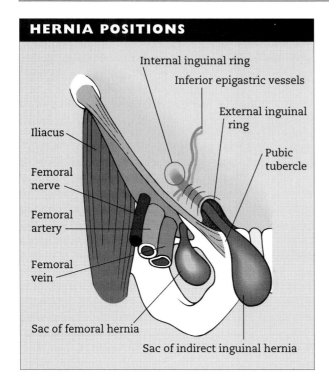

Internal inguinal ring

Inferior epigastric vessels

External inguinal ring

Iliacus

Femoral nerve

Pubic tubercle

Femoral artery

Femoral vein

Sac of femoral hernia

Sac of indirect inguinal hernia

Fig. 29.4 The relationships of an indirect inguinal and a femoral hernia compared: the inguinal hernia emerges above and medial to the pubic tubercle; the femoral hernia lies below and lateral to it.

• *Laterally*: the femoral vein.
• *Posteriorly*: the pectineal ligament (of Astley Cooper*), which is the thickened periosteum along the superior pubic ramus.

The canal contains a plug of fat and a lymph node (the node of Cloquet†).

Clinical features

Femoral hernias occur more commonly in females than males because of the wider female pelvis (but note that inguinal hernias are commoner than femoral in females also). They are never due to a congenital sac but are invariably acquired. Although cases do rarely occur in children they are usually seen in the middle-aged and elderly.

A non-strangulated hernia presents as a globular swelling below and lateral to the pubic

tubercle. It enlarges on standing and on coughing and may disappear when the patient lies down. However, in most cases even when the hernia is completely reduced, a swelling can still be palpated and this is due to extraperitoneal fat around the femoral sac.

As the hernia enlarges it passes through the saphenous opening in the deep fascia (the site of penetration of the great saphenous vein to join the femoral vein), and then turns upwards so that it may project above the inguinal ligament. There should not, however, be any difficulty in differentiating between an irreducible femoral and inguinal hernia — the neck of a femoral hernia always lies below and lateral to the pubic tubercle, whereas the sac of an indirect inguinal hernia extends above and medial to this landmark (Fig. 29.4).

The neck of the femoral canal is narrow and has a particularly sharp medial border. For this reason irreducibility and strangulation are extremely common in this type of hernia.

*Sir Astley Cooper (1768–1841), Surgeon, Guy's Hospital, London.
† Hippolyte Cloquet (1787–1840), Professor of Anatomy, Paris.

Richter's hernia

A Richter's hernia* is particularly likely to occur in the femoral sac. In this type of hernia only part of the wall of the small intestine herniates through the defect, where it is then strangulated. Because the lumen of the bowel is not completely encroached upon, symptoms of intestinal obstruction do not occur, although the knuckle of bowel may become completely necrotic and indeed perforate into the hernial sac and thence into the peritoneal cavity.

Treatment

All femoral hernias should be repaired by excision of the sac and closure of the femoral canal because of their great danger of strangulation.

Umbilical hernia

Exomphalos

This is a rare condition in which there is failure of all or part of the mid-gut to return to the abdominal cavity in fetal life. The bowel is contained within a translucent sac protruding through a defective anterior abdominal wall. Untreated, this ruptures with fatal peritonitis or rupture may occur during delivery.

Treatment

Immediate surgical repair if possible. Where the sac is massive it is protected with dressing soaked in mild antiseptic. Gradual epithelialization takes place and later repair may then be undertaken.

Congenital umbilical hernia

This results from failure of complete closure of the umbilical cicatrix. It is especially common in black children. The vast majority close spontaneously during the first year of life.

Treatment

Surgical repair should not usually be carried out unless the hernia persists after the child is 2 years old. The parents of an infant with a congenital umbilical hernia should be reassured that the majority disappear spontaneously. Strapping the hernia or providing a rubber truss are only required to allay parental anxiety.

Para-umbilical hernia

This is an acquired hernia that occurs just above or below the umbilicus. It especially occurs in obese, multiparous, middle-aged women. The neck is narrow and, like a femoral hernia, it is particularly prone to become irreducible or strangulated. The contents are nearly always the omentum, and often in addition transverse colon and small intestine.

Treatment

The sac is excised and the edges of the rectus sheath are overlapped above and below the hernia (Mayo's operation†).

Ventral hernia

A midline ventral hernia may exist as an elongated gap between the recti in elderly wasted patients (divarication of the recti). In the majority of cases no treatment is required.

Epigastric hernia

A particular variety of ventral hernia is the epigastric hernia, which consists of one or more small protrusions through defects in the linea alba above the umbilicus. These usually contain only extraperitoneal fat but are often surprisingly painful.

Treatment

Simply suturing the defect is all that is required.

---

*August Gottlieb Richter (1742–1812), Surgeon, Göttingen, Germany.

†William Mayo (1861–1939), Surgeon, Rochester, Minnesota, USA.

Incisional hernia

An incisional hernia occurs through a defect in the scar of a previous abdominal operation. The causes, which are the same as those of a burst abdomen, are given on page 18.

There is usually a wide neck, and strangulation is in consequence rare.

Treatment

If the general condition of the patient is good, the hernia is repaired by dissecting out and suturing the individual layers of the abdominal wall. Large hernias are repaired with a sheet of nylon or polypropylene plastic mesh. If operation is considered inadvisable an abdominal belt is prescribed.

Unusual hernias

Obturator hernia

These are found particularly in thin, elderly women. The hernia develops through the obturator canal where the obturator nerve and vessels traverse the membrane covering the obturator foramen. Pressure of a strangulated obturator hernia upon the nerve may cause referred pain in its area of cutaneous distribution, so that intestinal obstruction associated with pain along the medial side of the thigh in a thin, elderly woman should suggest this diagnosis. The hernia is often of the Richter type. Contrast-enhanced computed tomography (CT) will confirm the diagnosis.

Spigelian hernia

A Spigelian hernia* passes upwards through the arcuate line into the lateral border of the lower part of the posterior rectus sheath. It presents as a tender mass to one side of the lower abdominal wall. CT scanning will confirm the diagnosis where doubt exists.

Gluteal hernia

Traverses the greater sciatic foramen.

Sciatic hernia

Passes through the lesser sciatic foramen.

Lumbar hernia

A lumbar hernia is most commonly an incisional hernia following an operation on the kidney, but may rarely occur through the inferior lumbar triangle bounded by the crest of the ilium below, the latissimus dorsi medially and the external oblique on the lateral side.

*Adrian van der Spieghel (Spigelius) (1578–1625), Professor of Anatomy and Surgery, Padua.

CHAPTER 30

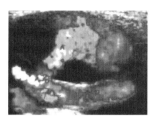

The Liver

Liver enlargement

Physical signs

The normal liver is impalpable, although it may be felt in thin adults, particularly on deep inspiration. In contrast, an infant's liver is normally palpable two fingers below the right costal margin.

The enlarged liver extends downwards below the right costal margin and may fill the subcostal angle or even extend beneath the left costal margin in gross hepatomegaly. The liver moves with respiration, is dull to percussion and the liver dullness may extend above the normal upper level of the fifth right interspace.

Causes

1 *Congenital:*
  (a) Riedel's lobe;
  (b) polycystic disease.
2 *Inflammatory:*
  (a) infective hepatitis;
  (b) portal pyaemia;
  (c) leptospirosis (Weil's disease);
  (d) actinomycosis.
3 *Parasitic:*
  (a) amoebic hepatitis and abscess;
  (b) hydatid.
4 *Neoplastic:*
  (a) primary tumour;
  (b) secondary deposits.
5 *Cirrhosis:*
  (a) portal;
  (b) biliary;
  (c) cardiac;
  (d) haemochromatosis.
6 *Haemopoietic diseases and reticuloses:*
  (a) Hodgkin's disease;
  (b) non-Hodgkin's lymphoma;
  (c) leukaemia;
  (d) polycythaemia.
7 *Metabolic diseases:*
  (a) amyloid;
  (b) Gaucher's disease.

Whenever the liver is palpable, the patient must be examined to detect any accompanying splenomegaly or lymphadenopathy. If the spleen is palpable in addition to the liver, consider cirrhosis, polycythaemia, leukaemia or amyloid as possible diagnoses. If, in addition, the lymph nodes are enlarged, the diagnosis is almost certainly a lymphoma.

Jaundice

The normal serum bilirubin is below 17 μmol/L (1 mg/dl). Excess bilirubin becomes clinically detectable when the serum level rises to over 35 mmol/L (2 mg/dl), and gives a yellow tinge to the sclera and skin, termed jaundice (or icterus).

Bilirubin metabolism (Fig. 30.1)

Knowledge of bile-pigment metabolism and excretion is essential if the pathogenesis, presentation, investigation and treatment of jaundice are to be understood.

When red cells reach the end of their life in the circulation, they are destroyed in the reticulo-endothelial system. The porphyrin ring of the haemoglobin molecule is disrupted and a bilirubin–iron–globin complex pro-

duced. The iron is released and used for further haemoglobin synthesis. The bilirubin–globin fraction reaches the liver as a lipid-soluble, water-insoluble substance. In the liver, the bilirubin is conjugated with glucuronic acid in the hepatocyte and excreted in the bile as the now water-soluble bilirubin glucuronide.

In the bowel lumen, bilirubin is reduced by bacterial action to the colourless urobilinogen. Most of the urobilinogen is excreted in the faeces, where it is broken down into urobilin, which is pigmented and which, with the other

Fig. 30.1 The metabolism of bilirubin.

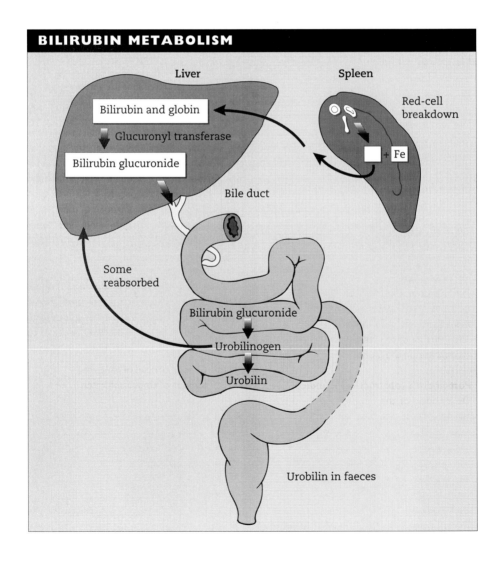

BILIRUBIN METABOLISM

Liver

Bilirubin and globin

Glucuronyl transferase

Bilirubin glucuronide

Bile duct

Spleen

Red-cell breakdown

+ Fe

Some reabsorbed

Bilirubin glucuronide

Urobilinogen

Urobilin

Urobilin in faeces

breakdown products of bilirubin, gives the stool its normal colour.

A small amount of urobilinogen is reabsorbed from the intestine into the portal venous tributaries and passes to the liver, where most of it is excreted once more in the bile back into the gut. Some, however, reaches the systemic circulation and this is excreted by the kidney into the urine. When urine is exposed to air, its contained urobilinogen is oxidized to urobilin.

Classification and pathogenesis

The causes of jaundice are classified according to which stage in the metabolism of bilirubin resulted in its accumulation.

Pre-hepatic jaundice

Increased production of (unconjugated) bilirubin by the reticulo-endothelial system, as may result from excessive destruction of red cells in haemolysis, exceeds the ability of the liver to conjugate, therefore the unconjugated bilirubin accumulates in the blood. There is no increase in conjugated bilirubin in the blood, so none is found in the urine. However, there is an increase in the amount of urobilinogen produced in the gut, so more is resorbed and overflows into the systemic circulation, where it is excreted by the kidney.

Hepatic jaundice

In the presence of hepatocellular damage, the liver is unable to conjugate bilirubin efficiently, and less is excreted into the canaliculi. Thus, both unconjugated and conjugated bilirubin accumulates in the blood.

Post-hepatic (obstructive) jaundice

Obstruction of the intrahepatic or extrahepatic bile ducts prevents excretion of conjugated bilirubin. Without pigment, the stools become pale, and the conjugated bilirubin builds up in the blood and is excreted in the urine, turning it dark brown.

Quite frequently the hepatic and post-hepatic forms coexist. For example, a stone in the common bile duct may produce jaundice partly by obstructing the outflow of bile and partly by secondary damage to the liver (biliary cirrhosis). Similarly, tumour deposits in the liver and cirrhosis may both result in jaundice partly by actual destruction of liver tissue and partly by intrahepatic duct compression.

Causes

Pre-hepatic jaundice

This is caused by increased production of bile pigments due to haemolytic disorders, e.g. spherocytosis, incompatible blood transfusion.

Hepatic jaundice

This is a result of impaired bile conjugation due to the following.

• Hepatitis — viral (hepatitis viruses A, B, C), leptospirosis, glandular fever.
• Cirrhosis.
• Cholestasis from drugs, e.g. chlorpromazine.
• Liver poisons, e.g. paracetamol overdosage; chlorinated hydrocarbons such as carbon tetrachloride, chloroform and halothane; phosphorus.
• Liver tumours.

Post-hepatic jaundice

This is caused by obstruction to biliary drainage due to the following.

1 *Obstruction within the lumen*: gall stones.
2 *Pathology in the wall*:
  (a) congenital atresia of common bile duct;
  (b) traumatic stricture;
  (c) chronic cholangitis;
  (d) tumour of bile duct.
3 *External compression*:
  (a) pancreatitis;
  (b) tumour of head of pancreas;
  (c) tumour of ampulla of Vater.

Diagnosis

This is based on history, examination and special investigations.

History

A family history of anaemia, splenectomy or gall stones suggests a congenital red-cell defect. Clay-coloured stools and dark urine accompanying the episodes of jaundice indicate hepatic or post-hepatic causes. Enquire after recent blood transfusions, drugs (chlorpromazine, paracetamol, methyldopa, repeated exposure to halothane), injections and alcohol consumption. Has there been contact with cases of viral hepatitis? What is the patient's occupation? (Farmers and sewer workers are at risk of leptospirosis.)

Usually painless jaundice of sudden onset with liver tenderness in a young person is viral in origin. Attacks of severe colic, rigors and intermittent jaundice suggest a stone. Remorselessly progressive jaundice, often accompanied by continuous pain radiating to the back, is suspicious of malignant disease. Recent onset of diabetes suggests carcinoma of the pancreas.

Examination

The colour of the jaundice is important; a lemon-yellow tinge suggests haemolytic jaundice (due to combined anaemia and mild icterus). Deep jaundice suggests the hepatic or post-hepatic types.

Other signs of cirrhosis should be sought: spider naevi, liver palms, gynaecomastia, testicular atrophy, flapping tremor, encephalopathy, splenomegaly and occasionally finger clubbing. There may also be ascites and leg oedema, but these may be associated with intra-abdominal malignant disease as well as cirrhosis.

Examination of the liver itself is helpful; in viral hepatitis the liver is slightly enlarged and tender, in cirrhosis the liver edge is firm, although the liver may be shrunken and impalpable. A grossly enlarged, knobbly liver suggests malignant disease.

If the gall bladder is palpable and distended, it is probable that the cause of the jaundice is not a stone (Courvoisier's law,* see p. 260). The liver is usually smoothly enlarged in post-hepatic obstructive jaundice.

A pancreatic tumour may be palpable or a

*Ludwig Courvoisier (1843–1918), Professor of Surgery, Basle, Switzerland.

separate primary focus of malignant disease may be obvious, e.g. a melanoma.

Splenomegaly suggests cirrhosis of the liver, blood disease or a lymphoma. In the latter there may also be obvious lymphadenopathy.

Special investigations (Table 30.1)

The pre-hepatic causes of jaundice are relatively easy to distinguish from hepatic and post-hepatic, but the latter two are often very difficult to differentiate one from the other and, as already stated, are often associated with each other. Laboratory tests are of some help but are by no means diagnostic. Imaging techniques are valuable in visualizing the liver, gall bladder and pancreas, while endoscopic cannulation of the bile ducts, or trans-hepatic duct puncture enable the bile-duct system to be outlined. However, it is not unusual for the diagnosis to be established finally only at laparotomy.

Bilirubin is not excreted by the kidney except in its water-soluble (conjugated) form. It is therefore absent from the urine in pre-hepatic jaundice (hence the old term 'acholuric jaundice'), although present when there is post-hepatic obstruction.

In pre-hepatic jaundice, large amounts of bilirubin are excreted into the gut, therefore the urobilinogen in the faeces is raised, the amount absorbed from the bowel increases and there is therefore greater spillover into the urine.

In hepatic damage the urinary urobilinogen may also be raised because of the inability of the liver to re-excrete the urobilinogen reabsorbed from the bowel.

In post-hepatic obstruction, very little bile can enter the gut, therefore the urobilinogen must be low in both the faeces and the urine.

The important laboratory findings in the various types of jaundice can now be summarized.

• *Urine*: the presence of bilirubin indicates obstructive jaundice, either intra- or post-hepatic. Excess of urobilinogen indicates pre-hepatic jaundice or sometimes liver damage,

DIAGNOSIS OF JAUNDICE

Test	Pre-hepatic	Hepatic	Obstructive
Urine	Urobilinogen	Urobilinogen	No urobilinogen. Bilirubin present
Serum bilirubin	Unconjugated bilirubin	Conjugated and unconjugated	Conjugated bilirubin
ALT (SGPT) AST (SGOT)	Normal	Raised	Normal or moderately raised
ALP	Normal	Normal or moderately raised	Raised
Blood glucose	Normal	Low if liver failure	Sometimes raised if pancreatic tumour
Reticulocyte count	Raised in haemolysis	Normal	Normal
Haptoglobins	Low due to haemolysis	Normal	Normal
Prothrombin time	Normal	Prolonged due to poor synthetic function	Prolonged due to vitamin K malabsorption; corrects with vitamin K
Ultrasound	Normal	May be abnormal liver texture, e.g. cirrhosis	Dilated bile ducts

Table 30.1 Differentiating pre-hepatic, hepatic and obstructive jaundice. (For abbreviation definitions, see text.)

whereas an absence of urobilinogen suggests obstructive causes.

• *Faeces*: absence of bile pigment indicates intra- or post-hepatic causes. The faecal urobilinogen is raised in pre-hepatic jaundice. The occult blood test may be positive, either on account of oozing oesophageal varices secondary to portal hypertension (indicating cirrhosis), or due to an ampullary carcinoma that is occluding the orifice of the common bile duct and also bleeding into the duodenum.

• *Haematological investigations*: red blood cell fragility, Coombs' test and reticulocyte count confirm haemolytic causes.

• *Serum bilirubin* is rarely higher than 100 mmol/L (5 mg/dl) in pre-hepatic jaundice, but may be considerably higher in obstructive cases. In late malignant disease it may exceed 1000 mmol/L.

• *Conjugated bilirubin*: in pre-hepatic jaundice bilirubin is present in the unconjugated form. In the pure post-hepatic obstructive jaundice the bilirubin is mainly in the conjugated form, whereas in hepatic jaundice it is present in the mixed conjugated and unconjugated forms due to a combination of liver destruction and intra-hepatic duct blockage.

• *Alkaline phosphatase (ALP)* is produced by cells lining the bile canaliculi. It is normal in pre-hepatic jaundice, raised in hepatic jaundice, and considerably raised in post-hepatic jaundice and in primary biliary cirrhosis. A raised ALP and normal bilirubin are features of obstruction of some, but not all of the intrahepatic bile ducts (NB: a different isoenzyme of ALP is produced by bone, and isolated elevated levels should be typed to determine origin).

• *Serum proteins* are normal in pre-hepatic jaundice, have a reversed albumin/globulin ratio with depressed albumin synthesis in hepatic jaundice and are usually normal in post-hepatic jaundice, unless associated with liver damage.

• *Haptoglobin* levels are low in pre-hepatic jaundice. Haptoglobin binds free haemoglobin released after haemolysis, and once bound the complex is catabolized faster than haptoglobin alone.

• *Serum transaminases*, such as alanine transaminase (ALT) and aspartate transaminase (AST) are raised in acute viral hepatitis and in the active phase of cirrhosis. Gamma glutamyl transferase (GGT) is a more sensitive indicator of liver disease, and is often raised before the transaminases.

• *Prothrombin time* is normal in pre-hepatic jaundice, prolonged but correctable with vitamin K in post-hepatic jaundice (where functioning liver tissue is still present) and prolonged but not correctable in advanced hepatic jaundice, where not only is absorption of fat-soluble vitamin K impaired but also the damaged liver is unable to synthesize prothrombin.

• *Ultrasound scanning* is extremely useful as well as non-invasive. Gall stones within the gall bladder can be demonstrated with a high degree of accuracy. Unfortunately, stones within the bile ducts are often missed because of duodenal gas overlying the distal ducts. Dilatation of the duct system within the liver is a good indication of duct obstruction; thus, if the ducts are not dilated, an obstructive cause for the jaundice is unlikely.

• *Computed tomography (CT) and magnetic resonance imaging (MRI)* are useful in addition to ultrasound in the demonstration of intrahepatic lesions (e.g. tumour deposits, abscess, cyst), which may then be accurately needled for biopsy material under imaging control. A mass in the pancreas can usually be demonstrated, but differentiation between carcinoma and chronic pancreatitis is difficult.

• *Abdominal X-ray* may show gall stones (10% are radio-opaque).

• *Endoscopic retrograde cholangio-pancreatography (ERCP)*, where the ampulla of Vater* is cannulated using an endoscope passed via the mouth, may demonstrate the location and indicate the nature of an obstructing lesion within the bile ducts. A peri-ampullary tumour is also directly visualized at this examination, and can be biopsied.

• *Percutaneous trans-hepatic cholangiography (PTC)*, where a needle is passed percutaneously into the liver substance and a dilated bile duct is cannulated, may be necessary where ERCP is not possible.

Both ERCP and PTC may be used to introduce stents across obstructing bile duct lesions to decompress the bile ducts and resolve the jaundice. More recently, magnetic resonance cholangiopancreatography (MRCP) has become available, and offers non-invasive high-resolution imaging of the biliary tree. However, it does not permit therapeutic decompression.

Needle biopsy. If the ultrasound scan reveals no dilatation of the duct system, an obstructive lesion is unlikely and needle biopsy of the liver will give valuable information regarding hepatic pathology (e.g. hepatitis or cirrhosis). If the ultrasound demonstrates focal lesions in the liver, a biopsy can be obtained under scanning control. Needle biopsy is potentially dangerous in the presence of jaundice. The prothrombin time, if prolonged, should first be corrected by administration of vitamin K. Should bleeding occur following biopsy, an immediate laparotomy may be necessary.

Laparotomy. As most causes of post-hepatic obstructive jaundice can be relieved surgically, it is occasionally necessary to submit a doubtful case to laparotomy even though it is suspected that the aetiology is entirely hepatic, lest an easily remediable condition (e.g. stones in the common bile duct) is overlooked.

*Abraham Vater (1648–1751), Professor of Anatomy, Wittenberg, Germany.

Summary of investigations of jaundice.
The investigations of jaundice may be grouped as follows, to be more manageable.

- *Exclusion of pre-hepatic causes*: haptoglobin level, reticulocyte count, Coomb's test.
- *Liver synthetic function* (hepatocellular dysfunction): prothrombin time, albumin.
- *Liver cell damage*: transaminases, γ-glutamyl transferase.
- *Bile duct obstruction*: alkaline phosphatase, ultrasound of bile ducts, PTC, ERCP, MRCP and CT for pancreatic lesion.
- *Intrahepatic mass*: cross-sectional imaging, such as ultrasound and CT, with needle biopsy.

Congenital abnormalities

Riedel's lobe*

This is a projection downwards from the right lobe of the liver of normally functioning liver tissue. It may present as a puzzling and symptomless abdominal mass.

Polycystic liver

This is often associated with polycystic disease of the kidneys (and occasionally pancreas), and comprises multiple cysts. The liver may reach a very large size but functions normally. Haemorrhage into the cysts and cholangitis are occasional complications.

Liver trauma

This may be due to penetrating wounds (gunshot or stab), or closed crush injuries, often associated with fractures of the ribs and injuries to other intra-abdominal viscera, especially the spleen. Severe abdominal trauma is becoming increasingly common, and accurate pre-operative diagnosis of the source of the haemorrhage may be impossible.

---

*Bernhard Riedel (1846–1916), Professor of Surgery, Jena, Germany. Also described Riedel's thyroiditis.

Clinical features

Following injury, the patient complains of abdominal pain. Examination reveals generalized abdominal tenderness together with the signs of progressive bleeding. CT scanning, if available, can be very helpful in showing the lesion and differentiation from a ruptured spleen. Occasionally, there is delayed rupture of a subcapsular haematoma, so that abdominal pain and shock may not be in evidence until some hours after the initial injury.

Treatment

If the patient's vital observations are stable, and a definite diagnosis made by CT scanning, the patient can initially be managed conservatively with blood transfusion and careful observation. Repeat scanning is undertaken to monitor progress.

If bleeding continues, and there is the risk of overlooking damage to other viscera, a laparotomy is performed. Minor liver tears can be sutured. Packing of the injury with a gauze pack, removed after 48 hours, may be life saving in severe trauma when the patient's condition is deteriorating. If bleeding continues, the relevant main hepatic arterial branch should be tied, and if the bleeding continues in spite of this, major hepatic lobar resection may be necessary.

Antibiotic cover must be given because of the danger of infection of areas of devitalized liver, and is particularly important where packing is employed. Occasionally, liver transplantation may be needed to manage gross trauma to both lobes.

Acute infections of the liver

Possible sources of infection are:

- arterial, as part of a general septicaemia — this is unusual;
- portal, from an area of suppuration drained by the portal vein;
- biliary, resulting from an ascending cholangitis;
- spread from adjacent infection, e.g. subphrenic abscess or acute cholecystitis.

Pyogenic liver abscess

Pyogenic liver abscess is a consequence of infection either in the portal territory, leading to a portal pyaemia (pyelophlebitis), or in the biliary tree. Multiple abscesses are common. Common infecting organisms include *Escherichia coli*, *Streptococcus faecalis* and *Streptococcus milleri*.

Clinical features

The condition should be suspected in patients who develop rigors, high swinging temperature, a tender palpable liver and jaundice. A previous history of abdominal sepsis, such as Crohn's disease, appendicitis or diverticulitis may be obtained. The clinical course is often insidious, with a non-specific malaise for over a month before presentation and diagnosis.

Special investigations

• *Blood culture*, carried out before treatment is commenced, is often positive.
• *Ultrasound or CT scanning* of the liver may identify and localize hepatic abscesses, as well as identifying the source of the pyaemia.

Treatment

A large abscess can be drained percutaneously under ultrasound guidance; smaller abscesses are treated by parenteral antibiotic therapy alone.

Portal pyaemia (pyelophlebitis)

Infection may reach the liver via the portal tributaries from a focus of intra-abdominal sepsis, particularly acute appendicitis or diverticulitis. Multiple abscesses may permeate the liver; in addition, there may be septic thrombi in the intrahepatic radicles of the portal vein, and infected clot in the portal vein itself. The condition has become very rare since the advent of antibiotics.

Biliary infection

Multiple abscesses in the liver may occur in association with severe suppurative cholangitis

secondary to impaction of gall stones in the common bile duct. Clinically the features are those of *Charcot's intermittent hepatic fever** — pyrexia, rigors and jaundice. (Rigors represent a bacteraemia and are commonly due to infection in either the renal or biliary tract.)

Urgent drainage of the bile ducts is performed, either by endoscopic sphincterotomy or, if necessary, by open operation. Adequate intravenous fluid replacement is important to prevent renal failure (hepato-renal syndrome, see p. 254); mannitol may be indicated particularly perioperatively.

Amoebic liver abscess

This particular type of portal infection is secondary to an *Entamoeba histolytica* infection of the large intestine. From there, amoebae travel via the portal circulation to the liver where they proliferate. The amoeba produces a cytolytic enzyme that destroys the liver tissue producing an amoebic abscess, which is sterile, although amoebae may be found in the abscess wall.

A liver CT scan and ultrasound are the most valuable special investigations.

Treatment

The majority respond to medical treatment with metronidazole. Ultrasonographically directed percutaneous drainage is required infrequently in non-responding cases.

Hydatid disease of the liver

The liver is the site of 75% of hydatid cysts in humans.

Pathology

Dogs are infected with the ova of *Echinococcus granulosus* (*Taenia echinococcus*) as a result of eating sheep offal. The tapeworms develop in the dog's small intestine from whence ova are

*Jean Charcot (1825–1893), First Professor of Neurology at Saltpêtrière Hospital, Paris.

discharged in the faeces. Humans (as well as sheep) ingest the ova from contaminated vegetables, etc.; the ova penetrate the stomach wall to invade the portal tributaries and thence pass to the liver. Occasionally, the hydatids may pass on to the lungs. Hydatid disease is therefore common in sheep-rearing communities, e.g. Australia, Iceland, Cyprus, southern Europe, Africa and Wales. Public health measures, e.g. destruction of stray dogs, has resulted in a marked drop in incidence.

Clinical features

A cyst may present as a symptomless mass. The contents may die and the walls become calcified so that this inactive structure may be a harmless post-mortem finding.

The active cyst may, however:

- *rupture* into the peritoneal cavity, pleural cavity, alimentary canal or biliary tree;
- *become infected*;
- *produce obstructive jaundice* by pressure on intrahepatic bile ducts, although jaundice is much more often due to intrabiliary rupture and release of cysts into the bile ducts.

Special investigations

- *Plain X-ray* of the liver may show a clear zone produced by the cyst, or may show flecks of calcification in the cyst wall.
- *Ultrasound and CT scan* localize the cyst.
- *Serological tests* depend on the sensitization of the patient to hydatid fluid, which contains a specific antigen, leakage of which induces the production of antibodies. Among the various tests now available, hydatid immunoelectrophoresis is the one of choice. This depends on the formation of a specific arc of precipitation produced by the interaction of the serum from the infected patient with the antigen as compared with a control.
- *Blood count*: there may be *eosinophilia*, which is not specific but should at least arouse clinical suspicion.

Treatment

A calcified cyst should be left alone. Other cysts should be treated to prevent complications. Treatment with albendazole may result in shrinkage or even disappearance of the cysts. Failure to respond or the presence of complications are indications for surgery. The cyst is exposed and aspirated. It is then possible to excise the cyst, taking care not to liberate daughter cysts that are present within the cyst.

Cirrhosis

Definition

Cirrhosis of the liver is a consequence of chronic hepatic injury, with healing by regeneration and fibrosis. Fibrosis leads to further cell damage and destruction of hepatic architecture, progressing to liver failure and portal hypertension.

Aetiology

A convenient classification of the cirrhoses is as follows.

1 *Parenchymal*:
   (a) alcoholic;
   (b) post-hepatic—follows hepatitis B and C.

2 *Biliary*:
   (a) primary biliary cirrhosis (Hanot's cirrhosis) — an autoimmune disease characterized by raised serum anti-mitochondrial antibodies;
   (b) secondary to prolonged biliary obstruction.

3 *Hepatic venous out-flow obstruction*:
   (a) Budd–Chiari syndrome (hepatic venous occlusion);
   (b) severe chronic congestive cardiac failure.

4 *Metabolic*:
   (a) iron overload—haemochromatosis;
   (b) copper overload — hepatolenticular degeneration (Kinnier Wilson's disease).

5 *Other causes*:
   (a) chronic active hepatitis — an autoimmune disease;
   (b) schistosomiasis;
   (c) nutritional (deficient protein diet);
   (d) idiopathic (cryptogenic).

In countries with a high consumption of alcohol (France and USA), alcohol is the commonest aetiological factor. In the tropics schistosomiasis heads the list (Egyptian splenomegaly). In the UK, 50% of cirrhosis cases are alcoholic.

Consequences of cirrhosis

1 Hepatocellular failure:
(a) impaired protein synthesis — prolonged prothrombin time and low albumin;
(b) impaired metabolism of toxins — encephalopathy;
(c) impaired bilirubin metabolism — jaundice.
2 Portal hypertension (see below).
3 Ascites: due to combination of hypoalbuminaemia and portal hypertension.
4 Malignant change: hepatoma.

Hepatic encephalopathy

Characterized by mental changes, flapping tremor and hepatic coma. This occurs in the presence of a portal–systemic shunt allowing nitrogenous breakdown products from the intestine via the portal tract into the systemic circulation without the interposition of the hepatic detoxifying filter.

Clinical features of cirrhosis

A number of clinical signs, separate from those of portal hypertension (see below), are seen in cirrhosis. These include gynaecomastia, testicular atrophy, amenorrhoea, spider naevi, finger clubbing and palmar erythema ('liver palms').

Portal hypertension

The normal portal pressure is between 8 and 15 cmH$_2$O. In portal hypertension this pressure may be raised to 50 cmH$_2$O or more.

Aetiology

Portal hypertension results from an obstruction in the portal tree. The causes are classified according to the site of the block.

1 *Pre-hepatic* (obstruction of the portal venous in-flow into the liver):
(a) congenital malformation;
(b) spreading portal vein thrombosis in the neonatal period from an umbilical infection;
(c) occlusion by tumour or pancreatitis.
2 *Hepatic* (obstruction of the portal flow within the liver): the cirrhoses.
3 *Post-hepatic* (obstruction of the hepatic veins); Budd–Chiari syndrome.*
(a) Idiopathic hepatic venous thrombosis in young adults of both sexes. A possible complication of oral contraceptives in women. In many cases there is an underlying haematological neoplasm, for example polycythaemia or monoclonal gamma-globulinopathy.
(b) Congenital obliteration.
(c) Blockage of hepatic vein by tumour invasion.

By far the commonest cause of portal hypertension is cirrhosis, yet there is no strict relationship between the severity of the liver disease and the extent of portal hypertension, which is not therefore entirely explained on the basis of mechanical obstruction.

Pathological effects

The four important effects of portal hypertension are:
1 the development of a collateral portal–systemic venous drainage;
2 splenomegaly;
3 ascites (in hepatic and post-hepatic portal hypertension only);
4 the manifestations of hepatic failure (in severe cirrhosis).

Collateral channels

Portal obstruction results in the development of collateral channels between the portal and systemic venous circulations (Fig. 30.2). The sites of these channels are as follows.
• Between the left gastric vein and the

*George Budd (1808–82), Professor of Medicine, Kings College Hospital, London. Hans Chiari (1851–1916), Professor of Pathology, Prague.

SYSTEMIC SHUNTS IN PORTAL HYPERTENSION

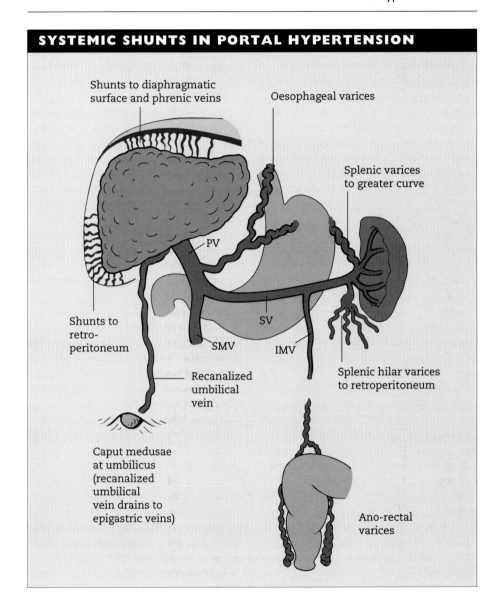

Fig. 30.2 The sites of occurrence of portal–systemic communications in patients with portal hypertension. PV, portal vein; SMV, superior mesenteric vein; IMV, inferior mesenteric vein; SV, splenic vein.

oesophageal veins, forming gastric and oesophageal varices. These are the largest and clinically the most important connections.

• Between the superior and inferior rectal veins with development of anal canal varices.

• Along the obliterated umbilical vein to the superior and inferior epigastric veins, forming a caput medusae around the umbilicus.

• Retroperitoneal and diaphragmatic anastomoses, which present technical hazards to the surgeon at the time of liver transplantation.

The oesophageal varices, and to a much lesser extent anal varices, may result in gastrointestinal haemorrhage, which is the most serious complication of portal hypertension.

Splenomegaly

Progressive splenic enlargement occurs as a result of portal congestion together with some degree of hypertrophy of the splenic substance itself. This is often associated with the haematological changes of hypersplenism — leucopenia and thrombocytopenia. Anaemia accompanying splenomegaly can be accounted for entirely by gastrointestinal bleeding and is not a result of splenic enlargement.

Ascites

This is due to a combination of factors. The raised portal pressure itself increases transudation of fluid into the peritoneal cavity but alone will not produce ascites, which is not therefore seen in the pre-hepatic obstruction. Liver damage results in a low serum albumin, therefore a low plasma osmotic pressure and consequent deficient reabsorption of ascitic fluid. Liver damage is associated with increased aldosterone level with sodium retention. Increased lymphatic pressure in the cirrhotic liver results in lymph transudation from the liver surface, and this high lymphatic pressure is also a feature in the post-hepatic block.

The effects of liver failure
- Jaundice.
- Encephalopathy.

CAUSES OF ASCITES

- Heart failure.
- Renal failure.
- Liver failure.
- Carcinomatosis.
- Chronic peritonitis, e.g. tuberculous.

Clinical features

To the surgeon, portal hypertension presents as three problems:

1 as a differential diagnosis of jaundice or hepatomegaly;
2 as a cause of gastrointestinal haemorrhage;
3 as one of the causes of ascites.

Special investigations

In addition to history and examination (which includes a careful search for the stigmata of liver disease), the following investigations are indicated.
- *Fibre-optic endoscopy* will demonstrate varices and differentiate between bleeding from this source and from a peptic ulcer or multiple gastric erosions, both of which are common in patients with cirrhosis.
- *Liver function tests and prothrombin time.*
- *Liver biopsy* if necessary.
- *Splenic venogram* or the venous phase of a selective superior mesenteric arteriogram to delineate the exact site of the portal obstruction before elective surgery is undertaken.
- *Magnetic resonance angiography* may substitute for splenic venography in the accurate demonstration of portal obstruction.

Treatment

The mere demonstration of oesophageal varices on endoscopy is not an indication for surgery. Nothing more is required than treatment of the underlying condition on medical lines, e.g. cirrhosis is managed by a high-calorie, well-balanced diet with added protein in malnourished patients (provided liver damage is not severe), and with avoidance of precipitating factors such as alcohol. Surgical intervention is only indicated if haemorrhage occurs and is not controllable endoscopically.

The management of haemorrhage from oesophageal varices

Haemorrhage from oesophageal varices is particularly dangerous, especially in patients with liver damage. In these subjects the liver is further injured by the hypotension of blood loss, and portal–systemic encephalopathy may be precipitated due to the absorption of large amounts of nitrogenous breakdown products from the 'meal of blood' within the intestine. Prognosis is better in the small group of patients with normal liver function and a pre-hepatic block.

Establishing the diagnosis

An attempt must be made to confirm the diagnosis. The presence of established liver disease, an enlarged spleen and proven varices does not necessarily mean that bleeding is from the varices. Such patients are prone to bleeding from gastric erosions and are commonly affected by peptic ulceration. Fibre-optic endoscopy should always be performed in order to visualize the bleeding point and to exclude non-variceal haemorrhage. Active bleeding may, however, prevent a satisfactory view at endoscopy.

Immediate treatment

The immediate treatment of haemorrhage is blood replacement by transfusion. Nitrogenous absorption from the bowel is reduced by emptying as much of the blood as possible from the colon by means of an enema, giving neomycin by mouth to reduce bacterial decomposition of blood in the gut, withholding protein from the diet and maintaining nourishment by means of glucose given by mouth or intravenously. If bleeding continues, more vigorous methods may be required, but here careful decision must be taken; if the patient is in advanced hepatic failure with jaundice, ascites, a low serum albumin, impaired clotting, thrombocytopenia and pre-coma or coma, then it is wise practice to refrain from further treatment, as the prognosis is hopeless and further procedures merely add to the discomfort of an already dying patient.

Stopping the haemorrhage

The bleeding may be arrested by a number of manoeuvres.

• *Endoscopic variceal injection* with a sclerosant or banding (the application of small rubber bands to ligate the varices). These procedures can stop bleeding with minimal trauma to the patient, although there are the risks of perforation of the oesophagus and repeated injections may produce ulceration or fibrosis.

• *Intravenous Pitressin* (20 units by slow intravenous injection), which produces a marked fall in portal venous pressure and temporary cessation of bleeding by mesenteric arteriolar constriction. Therapeutic doses cause intestinal colic.

• *Passing a Sengstaken tube* via the mouth into the oesophagus and cardia. The balloons on the end are inflated and produce direct pressure on the varices.

• *Trans-jugular intrahepatic portal–systemic shunt (TIPS)*: a metal stent is inserted angiographically via the jugular vein, and passed through the liver substance from hepatic vein to portal vein, so decompressing the portal system.

• *Portal–azygos disconnection*, in which the varices around the lower end of the oesophagus and the upper stomach are divided at the cardio-oesophageal junction using the circular stapling gun, in order to interrupt the communications between the two systems of veins within the wall of the lower oesophagus.

• *Portal–caval anastomosis* between the portal vein and the inferior vena cava constructed surgically, which shunts the portal blood directly into the venous systemic circulation and thus lowers the portal pressure. If the portal vein itself is occluded by a thrombus or is congenitally abnormal, portal–caval anastomosis is impossible. The portal system can be shunted to the systemic system by a variety of techniques. Unfortunately, shunt procedures (surgical or radiological), in which an anastomosis is made between the portal and systemic circulations, are likely to precipitate encephalopathy, and such patients often have to be maintained indefinitely on a low-protein diet.

Control of the bleeding allows the surgeon to assess the patient as a candidate for liver transplantation. Laparotomy should be avoided if possible if a subsequent transplant is planned, as the resulting vascular adhesions will add greatly to the dangers of the transplant operation. If the patient is not a candidate for a transplant, definitive surgery to prevent further bleeding may be contemplated.

Treatment of ascites

• *Paracentesis* gives immediate relief if discomfort is intense, but it has the disadvantage that the patient loses protein, which should therefore be replaced at the time (10 g albumin per litre of ascites removed).
• *Diet*: low sodium, high protein diet; intravenous albumin.
• *Diuretics*: spironolactone often combined with a thiazide or loop diuretic.
• *Peritoneo-venous shunt* (LeVene or Denver): a silicone rubber catheter with a pressure-activated valve, which shunts ascitic fluid from the peritoneal cavity back into the venous systems via the internal jugular vein.
• *Iatrogenic portal–systemic shunt*. A shunt either created surgically, by anastomosis of portal vein or superior mesenteric vein to the vena cava, or more recently using a TIPS (see above).

Intractable ascites due to hepatic cirrhosis is an indication for liver transplantation, which is performed after failure of medical therapy, and before the creation of shunts, which make transplantation more difficult.

Hepato-renal syndrome

Renal failure is often associated with ascites and liver failure, particularly alcoholic cirrhosis. It is a consequence of depletion of the intravascular volume, as may be caused by diuretic therapy or surgery. The mechanism of the renal failure is a reduction in intrarenal blood flow brought about by increased glomerular afferent arteriolar tone, but the cause of this is unknown. The glomerular filtration rate falls as the blood flow is diverted away from the renal cortex. Established renal failure in the presence of liver disease is difficult to treat, and is best avoided by maintaining hydration during surgery.

Liver neoplasms

Classification
Benign (rare)
• Cavernous haemangioma.
• Adenoma.

Malignant
1 *Primary* (rare in the UK):
  (a) hepatoma;
  (b) cholangiocarcinoma.
2 *Secondary* (common):
  (a) portal spread (from alimentary tract);
  (b) systemic blood spread (from lung, breast, testis, melanoma, etc.);
  (c) direct spread (from gall bladder, stomach and hepatic flexure of colon).

Hepatoma
About 50% occur in cirrhotics, especially those with nutritional deficiencies, and is common in Central Africa (50% of cancer deaths) and South-East Asia associated with hepatitis B and C infection.

The tumour forms a large, solitary mass, or there may be multiple foci throughout the liver. Spread occurs through the liver substance and metastasis outside this organ is late.

Clinically, there is massive liver swelling, which develops in a cirrhotic. Blood-stained ascites collects and there is a rapid downward course.

Serum α-fetoprotein is usually raised significantly in patients with hepatoma, and its presence confirmed on ultrasound or CT scanning.

Cholangiocarcinoma
This is much less common (20% of primary tumours). It is an adenocarcinoma arising from the intrahepatic bile duct system, which may complicate chronic sclerosing cholangitis. It usually presents with jaundice. Spread occurs directly through the liver substance and regional nodes with a fatal outcome.

Secondaries

The liver is an extremely common site for secondary deposits, which are found in about one in three post-mortems carried out on patients who have died of advanced malignant disease. Necrosis at the centre of metastases leads to the typical umbilication of these tumours.

The clinical effects of secondary deposits in the liver are as follows.

• *Hepatomegaly*: the liver is large, hard and irregular.
• *Jaundice*: due to liver destruction and intrahepatic duct compression.
• *Hepatic failure*.
• *Portal vein obstruction*: producing oesophageal varices and ascites.
• *Inferior vena cava obstruction*: producing leg oedema.

Treatment of liver tumours

A primary hepatoma, confined to one lobe, can be treated by hepatic lobectomy. It may be possible to relieve the jaundice in cholangiocarcinoma by passing a plastic tube (stent) upwards along the common bile duct through the growth into the dilated radicles above the obstruction or downwards by percutaneous intubation. This relieves the jaundice often for months and occasionally for more than a year.

In cirrhotic patients with a small (under 3-cm) primary hepatic tumour confined to the liver, transplantation has proved to be a valuable form of treatment. Lobar resection in such patients is not possible because of the lack of hepatic reserve.

Resection of secondary tumours is seldom of value but may be considered when isolate deposits are confined to one lobe. Pain may be relieved by ligation of the hepatic artery and occasionally temporary response follows the use of cytotoxic drugs.

CHAPTER 31

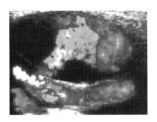

The Gall Bladder and Bile Ducts

Congenital anomalies

Developmentally, a diverticulum grows out from the ventral wall of the foregut (primitive duodenum), which differentiates into the hepatic ducts and the liver. A lateral bud from this diverticulum becomes the gall bladder and cystic duct.

Anomalies are found in 10% of subjects and these are of importance to the surgeon during cholecystectomy.

The principal developmental abnormalities include the following:

• A long cystic duct travelling alongside the common hepatic duct to open near the duodenal orifice. This occurs in 10% of cases.
• Congenital absence of the gall bladder.
• Reduplication of the gall bladder.
• Congenital obliteration of the ducts (biliary atresia, one of the causes of neonatal jaundice).
• Absence of the cystic duct, the gall bladder opening directly into the side of the common bile duct.
• A long mesentery to the gall bladder, which allows acute torsion of the gall bladder to occur with consequent gangrene and rupture.
• Anomalies of the arrangement of the blood vessels supplying the gall bladder are common; for example, the right hepatic artery crosses in front of the common hepatic duct instead of behind it in 25% of subjects.

• Cystic dilatation of the main bile ducts (choledochal cyst).

Cholelithiasis

Gall stones are rare in children, the incidence increasing with each decade. In the UK they are found in approximately 10% of women in their forties increasing to 30% after the age of 60 years. They are about half as common in men. Stones are particularly common in the Mediterranean races, and the highest incidence is found among the Indians of New Mexico.

The aphorism that gall stones occur in fair, fat, fertile females of 40 is only an approximation to the truth; people of either sex, any age, colour, shape or fecundity may have gall stones, but certainly the incidence is higher in overweight, middle-aged women. To understand gall stones it is first necessary to understand bile.

Bile composition and function

Bile is a combination of cholesterol, phospholipids (principally lecithin), bile salts (chenodeoxycholic acid and cholic acid) and water. Bile also contains conjugated bilirubin, the breakdown product of haemoglobin, which is quite distinct from bile salts. Cholesterol is not water soluble and is carried in the bile in water-soluble micelles, in which the hydrophobic cholesterol is carried within a 'shell' of phospholipid and bile salts. Once in the gut, bile salts act as a detergent, breaking up and emulsifying fats to facilitate their absorption. The bile salts themselves are resorbed in the gut, pass back via the portal venous drainage to the liver, from where they are once again secreted in the bile. This circulation of bile salts is termed the *enterohepatic circulation*, permitting a relatively small pool of bile salts to circulate up to 10 times a day. Diversion or absence of bile from the gut, as may occur in obstructive jaundice, results in a malabsorption of fat and the fat-soluble vitamins (A, D, E and K).

Gall stones

There are three common varieties of stone (Fig. 31.1).

1 *Cholesterol* (20%): these occur either as a solitary, oval stone (the cholesterol solitaire) or as two stones, one indenting the other, or as multiple mulberry stones associated with a strawberry gall bladder (see below). A cut section shows crystals radiating from the centre of the stone; the surface is yellow and greasy to the touch.

2 *Bile pigment* (5%), which are small, black, irregular, multiple, gritty and fragile.

3 *Mixed* (75%): multiple, faceted one against the other, and can often be grouped into two or more series, all of the same size, suggesting 'generations' of stones. The cut surface is laminated with alternate dark and light zones of pigment and cholesterol respectively.

This traditional classification into three groups is an over-simplification; calculi with widely different appearances simply represent different combinations of the same ingredients.

Cholesterol stones

These may be associated with a high blood

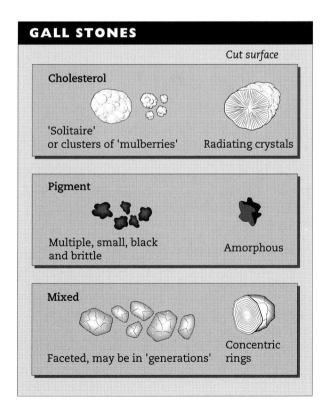

GALL STONES

Cut surface

Cholesterol

'Solitaire' or clusters of 'mulberries'   Radiating crystals

Pigment

Multiple, small, black and brittle   Amorphous

Mixed

Faceted, may be in 'generations'   Concentric rings

Fig. 31.1 The varieties of gall stones.

cholesterol, but there is little evidence to suggest this as a cause. There is a definite correlation between cholesterol stones and the contraceptive pill and pregnancy, as well as an increase with age. Family history, obesity and low dietary fibre are also risk factors. The supersaturated bile from such patients is termed 'lithogenic' (stone-forming) bile. Bile may also become supersaturated with cholesterol due to a deficiency of bile salts, which may occur as a result of interruption of the enterohepatic circulation, as may occur after resection of the terminal ileum.

Cholesterol stones form in the gall bladder when supersaturated bile is further concentrated. It may be that an excess of mucus production by the gall bladder wall is an important factor in aggregating it into calculi. In other cases, clumps of bacteria or desquamated mucosa, perhaps resulting from an episode of infection, may form the nucleus on which crystals may deposit. When the cholesterol precipitates on the gall bladder wall (cholesterosis), it forms yellow submucous aggregations of cholesterol with an appearance similar to a strawberry skin ('strawberry gall bladder').

Pigment stones

Pigment stones are composed of calcium bilirubinate, with some calcium carbonate. They occur in the haemolytic anaemias, e.g. spherocytosis and sickle-cell disease, where excess of circulating bile pigment is deposited in the biliary tract. If such stones are found in the gall bladder of children or adolescents, haemolytic anaemia should be suspected, particularly if there is a family history of calculus.

Mixed stones

It is now considered that the majority of mixed stones have the same metabolic origin as cholesterol stones, i.e. some slight alteration in the composition of bile enabling precipitation of cholesterol together with bile pigment.

The pathological effects of gall stones

• *Silent*: gall stones lying free in the lumen of

the gall bladder produce no pathological disturbance of the wall and the patient is symptom-free.

• *Impaction in gall bladder*, either at the exit of the gall bladder or in the cystic duct. Water is absorbed from the contained bile, which becomes concentrated and produces a chemical cholecystitis. This is usually at first sterile but may then become secondarily infected from organisms secreted from the liver into the bile stream (acute cholecystitis can be produced in animals with sterile bile by ligating the cystic duct). If a stone impacts in the outlet of an empty gall bladder, the walls of the organ may continue to secrete mucus and the gall bladder distends to form a *mucocele*.

• *Choledocholithiasis*: gall stones may migrate into the common bile duct. This may be silent, or produce an intermittent or complete obstruction of the common bile duct with pain and jaundice.

• *Gall-stone ileus*: this occurs when there is ulceration through the wall of the gall bladder into the duodenum or colon. The large gall stone may pass per rectum or produce a gall stone ileus—this is impaction in the distal ileum with resulting intestinal obstruction. (Note: gall-stone ileus is thus mechanical obstruction by an intraluminal stone, and not a paralytic ileus as such.)

In addition, the presence of gall stones in the biliary tree is associated with:

• *Acute and chronic pancreatitis*.
• *Carcinoma of the gall bladder*.

Clinical features

The following syndromes can be recognized:

• biliary colic;
• acute cholecystitis;
• chronic cholecystitis;
• obstruction and/or infection of the common bile duct.

Two or more of these syndromes may occur in the same patient.

Biliary colic

This is produced by impaction of the stone in

COLIC IN THE ABDOMEN

Colic pain is the result of smooth-muscle contraction against a resistance. The common causes of colic occur in the uterus and tubes, renal tract, intestinal tract and biliary tract.

Biliary tract
- Stone in Hartmann's pouch.
- Stone in cystic duct.
- Stone in Ampulla of Vater.

Renal tract
- Ureteric colic due to stone, blood clot or tumour.

Intestinal tract
- Mechanical obstruction.
- Appendicular colic as appendix lumen occludes.

Uterus
- Parturition.
- Menstruation.
- Ectopic pregnancy in fallopian tube.

the gall-bladder outlet (Hartmann's pouch*) or cystic duct for a short period, following which the calculus either falls back or is passed along the duct.

Contractions of the smooth muscle in the wall of the gall bladder and the cystic duct produce severe pain, usually rising to a plateau, which lasts for many hours. It is situated usually in the right subcostal region but may be epigastric, or spread as a band across the upper abdomen. Radiation of the pain to the lower angle of the right scapula is common and is accompanied by vomiting and sweating. Characteristically, the patient is restless and rolls about in agony, but an intermittent pain is rare.

Differential diagnosis is from the other acute colics, especially ureteric colic.

*Henri Hartmann (1860–1952), Professor of Surgery, Faculty of Medicine, Paris.

Acute cholecystitis
If the stone remains impacted in the gall-bladder outlet, the gall bladder wall becomes inflamed due to the irritation of the concentrated bile contained within it producing a chemical cholecystitis. The gall bladder fills with pus, which is frequently sterile on culture. In these instances the pain persists and progressively intensifies. There is a fever in the range of 38–39°C with marked toxaemia and leucocytosis. The upper abdomen is extremely tender, and often a palpable mass develops in the region of the gall bladder. This represents the distended, inflamed gall bladder wrapped in inflammatory adhesions to adjacent organs, especially the omentum. Occasionally, an empyema of the gall bladder develops or, rarely, gall bladder perforation takes place into the general peritoneal cavity. The swollen gall bladder may press against the adjacent common bile duct and may produce a tinge of jaundice, even though stones may be absent from the duct system.

Ninety-five per cent of cases of acute cholecystitis are associated with gall stones. Occasionally, fulminating acalculous cholecystitis may occur and this may be associated with typhoid fever or gas-gangrene infection.

Differential diagnosis is from acute appendicitis, perforated duodenal ulcer, acute pancreatitis, right-sided basal pneumonia and coronary thrombosis.

Chronic cholecystitis
This is almost invariably associated with the presence of gall stones. Repeated episodes of inflammation result in chronic fibrosis and thickening of the entire gall bladder wall, which may contain thick, sometimes infected, bile.

There are recurrent bouts of abdominal pain due to mild cholecystitis, which may or may not be accompanied by fever. Discomfort is experienced after fatty meals since they stimulate release of cholecystokinin which causes the gall bladder to contract onto the stones; there is often flatulence. The picture may be complicated by episodes of acute cholecystitis or symptoms produced by stones passing into the common bile duct.

Differential diagnosis is from other causes of chronic dyspepsia, including peptic ulceration and hiatus hernia. Occasionally, the symptoms closely mimic coronary insufficiency. It is as well to remain clinically suspicious — any or all of these common diseases may well occur in association with gall stones.

Stones in the common bile duct (choledocholithiasis)

This may be symptomless. More often there are attacks of biliary colic accompanied by obstructive jaundice with clay-coloured stools and dark urine, the attacks lasting for hours or several days. The attack ceases either when a small stone is passed through the sphincter of Oddi or when it disimpacts and falls back into the dilated common duct. Above the impacted stone other stones or biliary sludge may deposit. Occasionally, the jaundice is progressive and rarely it is painless.

If the obstruction is not relieved either spontaneously or by operation, the back-pressure in the biliary system results in secondary biliary cirrhosis and liver failure.

Ascending cholangitis. If infection of the common bile duct supervenes, the jaundice and pain are complicated by rigors, a high intermittent fever and severe toxaemia (the intermittent hepatic fever of Charcot). In these instances the duct system is severely inflamed and filled with pus, and the liver may be dotted with multiple small abscesses. Treatment is urgent biliary drainage.

Differential diagnosis of stone in the common bile duct is as follows.
1 With jaundice (75% of cases):
   (a) carcinoma of the pancreas or other malignant obstructions of common bile duct;
   (b) acute hepatitis;
   (c) other causes of jaundice (p. 241).
2 Without jaundice (25% of cases):
   (a) renal colic;
   (b) intestinal obstruction;
   (c) angina pectoris.

Courvoisier's law (Fig. 31.2)*
'If in the presence of jaundice the gall bladder is palpable, then the jaundice is unlikely to be due to stone.' This is an extremely useful rule provided it is quoted correctly. The principle on which it is based is that if the obstruction is due to stone, the gall bladder is usually thickened and fibrotic and therefore does not distend. Moreover, unlike obstruction due to malignant disease, calculus obstruction is not usually complete. This allows some escape of bile into the duodenum, with decompression of the gall bladder. Obstruction of the common bile duct due to other causes (e.g. carcinoma of the head of the pancreas) is usually associated with a normal gall bladder, which can dilate. However, in carcinoma of the bile ducts arising above the origin of the cystic duct, the gall bladder, distal to the obstruction, will be collapsed and empty.

Note that the law is not phrased the other way round — 'If the gall bladder is *not* palpable, the jaundice is due to stone' — as 50% of dilated gall bladders cannot be palpated on clinical examination, due to either the patient's obesity or because of overlap by the liver, which itself is usually enlarged as a result of bile engorgement.

Only rarely is the gall bladder dilated when the jaundice is due to stone. These circumstances occur where a stone impacts in Hartmann's pouch to produce a mucocele while at the same time jaundice is produced by a second stone in the common duct, or where a stone forms *in situ* in the common bile duct, the gall bladder itself being normal and therefore distensible.

Special investigations
• *Plain abdominal X-ray* reveals radio-opaque gall stones in only 10% of cases. These usually appear as rings due to calcium deposited on a central translucent organic core. Occasionally, the gall bladder may be seen to be calcified ('porcelain gall bladder').
• *Ultrasound*: this non-invasive technique is

*Ludwig Courvoisier (1843–1918), Professor of Surgery, Basle, Switzerland.

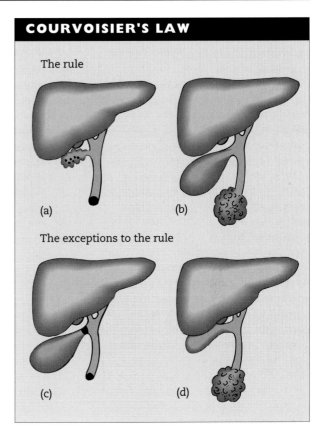

COURVOISIER'S LAW

The rule

(a)   (b)

The exceptions to the rule

(c)   (d)

Fig. 31.2 Obstructive jaundice due to stone is usually associated with a small, contracted gall bladder (a). Therefore, in the presence of jaundice, a palpable gall bladder indicates that the obstruction is probably due to some other cause—the commonest being carcinoma of the pancreas (b). Exceptions are a palpable gall bladder produced by one stone impacted in Hartmann's pouch resulting in a mucocele, another in the common duct causing obstruction (c), which is very rare or, much more commonly, the gall bladder is indeed distended but is clinically impalpable (d).

invaluable for the demonstration of stones within the gall bladder. If present, these will usually be revealed as intensely echogenic foci, which cast a clear acoustic shadow beyond them. The thickened wall of the gall bladder in chronic inflammation can also be delineated. Unfortunately, ultrasound, like computed tomography (CT), is unreliable in detecting stones in the bile ducts, especially at the lower end. However, it does demonstrate dilatation of the duct system suggesting distal duct obstruction.

• *Oral cholecystogram*: an iodine-containing preparation is given by mouth and is excreted by the liver into the bile and then concentrated in the gall bladder. The gall bladder may fill but the contained stones are outlined as defects. A diseased gall bladder, being unable to concentrate the dye, will give no shadow on X-ray. Non-filling of the gall bladder in a cholecystogram may not only represent failure of the diseased gall bladder to concentrate, but may also be accounted for by the patient having vomited the preparation, passed it through the bowel because of diarrhoea, which it sometimes induces, or because of associated liver disease, which results in failure of secretion of the compound into the bile; the gall bladder is therefore never visualized in any form of hepatic or post-hepatic jaundice.

• *Intravenous cholangiography*: contrast medium, given intravenously is excreted in high concentration in the bile, providing liver function is adequate. This investigation has a 1 in 10000 risk of anaphylaxis and is seldom used for the routine detection of gall stones, but may be useful to identify stones in the bile ducts.

• *HIDA scanning* gives similar information to a cholecystogram but, in addition, will usually outline the bile ducts. The radionuclide is excreted in the bile. Failure to opacify the gall bladder is suggestive of cholecystitis.

• *Barium meal or upper gastrointestinal endoscopy* are advisable in cases of chronic cholecystitis to exclude an associated peptic ulcer or hiatus hernia.

• *Liver function tests* are performed whenever jaundice, present or past, is a feature. Persistently raised alkaline phosphatase is suspicious of choledocholithiasis.

• *ERCP*: endoscopic intubation of the bile ducts through the ampulla of Vater enables the ducts to be visualized radiographically and contained calculi detected and removed often after first dividing the Sphincter of Oddi.

Treatment

Acute cholecystitis

At least 90% resolve on bed rest with antibiotics and pain relief. Elective cholecystectomy is usually performed about 6 weeks later because of the undoubted danger of further attacks. Cholecystectomy is routinely performed laparoscopically rather than at open operation, with the advantages of minimal scarring of the abdominal wall and rapid convalescence. The procedure requires a surgeon well trained in the technique, who can also proceed to open operation if technical difficulties are encountered at laparoscopy.

Occasionally, an empyema of the gall bladder fails to resolve. Emergency drainage (cholecystostomy) is required, either at open operation or percutaneously under ultrasound control.

Rarely, the patient presents with perforation of the acutely inflamed gall bladder and requires urgent surgery. This complication carries a high mortality.

If diagnosis is in doubt in the early stages of acute cholecystitis, laparotomy is performed. Cholecystectomy is comparatively easy in the first 24−48 hours of the illness; dissection is facilitated by the oedema of adjacent tissues, although after this time operation becomes difficult because of the inflammatory adhesions. Many surgeons advise early surgical intervention in acute cholecystitis.

Chronic cholecystitis

Cholecystectomy is performed, either by laparoscopy or laparotomy. The cystic duct is intubated and an operative cholangiogram performed by injecting radio-opaque contrast medium into the common duct. If stones are demonstrated, the common bile duct is explored, the stones removed, a T tube inserted into the common duct and a check X-ray performed. The T tube is removed 10 days post-operatively, provided a check cholangiogram taken through the tube confirms that the ducts are clear and that there is free flow into the duodenum. Alternatively, at laparoscopic cholecystectomy, the surgeon may elect to wait for a post-operative endoscopic sphincterotomy and extraction of the stones with a Dormia basket.

Obstructive jaundice due to stones

The great majority of cases resolve on conservative treatment. Subsequent cholecystectomy and exploration of the common duct is performed. Persistent or progressive jaundice, particularly in the presence of high fever, makes removal of the impacted stones and drainage of the obstructed common bile duct imperative as an emergency procedure. This can be performed by open operation or, especially in the severely ill patient, by endoscopic sphincterotomy. It is preceded by giving intravenous vitamin K, as depressed absorption of this fat-soluble vitamin lowers the serum prothrombin with consequent bleeding tendency.

Non-surgical treatment of gall stones

Gall-stone dissolution. Because cholesterol is held in solution by bile salts, dissolution of small cholesterol stones is possible by administering bile salts orally in the form of chenodeoxycholic or ursodeoxycholic acid. This therapy may be used for small, non-calcified stones in a functioning gall bladder. Treatment must be continued for many months and may be interrupted by attacks of biliary colic as small fragments of calculus pass through the bile ducts. Moreover, recurrences commonly occur after therapy is discontinued since an abnormal gall bladder remains. Obviously the indications for this treatment are limited.

Lithotripsy. Ultrasonic destruction of small stones is possible, but again there is the problem of the passage of small fragments of stone through the duct system. This may be overcome by aspirating the bile debris from the gall bladder via a catheter placed percutaneously under ultrasound control. Again, this method of treatment has disadvantages and limited indications.

The symptomless gall stone

The diagnosis of gall stones is becoming increasingly common during routine ultrasound examination of the abdomen. Cholecystectomy may be advised when the patient is young and otherwise well, as symptomless stones may eventually produce the numerous problems listed above. If the patient is elderly or unfit, symptomless stones are left untreated.

Complications of cholecystectomy

There are two special dangers after cholecystectomy, whether performed by laparotomy or laparoscopy.

1 *Leakage of bile.* This may result from:
   (a) injury to bile canaliculi in the gall-bladder bed of the liver;
   (b) injury to the common hepatic or common bile duct;
   (c) slipping of the ligature from the cystic duct;
   (d) leakage from the suture line after common bile duct exploration.

Providing the common bile duct is patent, the bile fistula will close spontaneously; if this does not occur, further exploration may be required. A percutaneous drain is usually placed to prevent generalized biliary peritonitis.

2 *Jaundice.* This may be due to:
   (a) missed stones in the common bile duct;
   (b) inadvertent ligature of the common bile duct;
   (c) cholangitis or associated pancreatitis.

Residual stones in the common duct may require operative removal. However, in the majority of cases they can be removed by endoscopic sphincterotomy or, if a T tube is still present in the common duct, by means of a Dormia basket passed along the track formed by the tube under X-ray control.

Carcinoma of the gall bladder

Pathology

This is a relatively unusual tumour, but it is associated in about 85% of cases with the presence of gall stones. It is debatable whether this is due to chronic irritation or to the carcinogenic effect of cholic acid derivatives. Fifty per cent of 'porcelain' gall bladders are associated with carcinoma. As gall stones are commoner in females, carcinoma of the gall bladder is not surprisingly four times commoner in females than males. Ninety per cent are adenocarcinoma and 10% squamous carcinoma.

There is local invasion of the liver and its ducts and lymphatic spread to the nodes in the porta hepatis; portal vein dissemination, also to the liver, may occur.

Clinical features

Carcinoma of the gall bladder usually presents with a picture closely resembling chronic cholecystitis, with right upper quadrant pain, nausea, vomiting, in addition to weight loss and, later, progressing to obstructive jaundice. At this stage a palpable mass may be present in the gall-bladder region.

Treatment

Occasionally, cholecystectomy performed for stone reveals the presence of an unexpected tumour. Under these circumstances, long-term survival may follow. If direct infiltration into the liver has already occurred, as is more common, wide local excision is only rarely possible and the prognosis is therefore usually poor, with death within months.

Cholangiocarcinoma

Pathology
The incidence of carcinoma of the bile ducts, cholangiocarcinoma, is increasing. The disease commonly occurs after 50 years of age and is more common in males. It is associated with inflammatory bowel disease, particularly in the presence of sclerosing cholangitis. Congenital hepatic fibrosis, choledochal cysts and polycystic liver are all associations.

Macroscopically, cholangiocarcinomas may occur within the liver substance, or in the larger extrahepatic bile ducts. The confluence of the left and right hepatic ducts, or the common hepatic duct with the cystic duct, are common sites.

Microscopically, they are mucin-secreting adenocarcinomas.

Clinical features
The usual presentation is with painless progressive jaundice, with dark urine and pale stools. Epigastric pain, steatorrhoea and weight loss are common. There may be hepatomegaly, usually without a palpable gall bladder because the tumour is proximal to, or at, the cystic duct confluence. Confirmation is by ERCP or percutaneous trans-hepatic cholangiography and brush cytology (poor sensitivity), and CT with needle biopsy if possible.

Treatment
The tumours are slow growing, and palliation is often achieved by endoluminal stenting at ERCP, or surgical bypass. The prognosis is poor, with no curative treatment.

CHAPTER 32

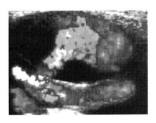

The Pancreas

Congenital anomalies

The pancreas develops as a dorsal and a ventral bud from the duodenum. The ventral bud rotates posteriorly, thus enclosing the superior mesenteric vessels; it forms the major part of the head of the pancreas and its duct becomes the main duct of Wirsung,* which in the great majority of cases has a shared opening with the common bile duct in the ampulla of Vater.† The dorsal bud becomes the body and tail and its duct becomes the accessory duct of Santorini.‡

Annular pancreas

The two developmental buds may envelop the second part of the duodenum, producing this rare form of duodenal extrinsic obstruction.

Heterotopic pancreas

This is produced by an accessory budding from the primitive foregut and occurs in some subjects. A nodule of pancreatic tissue may be found in the stomach, duodenum or jejunum. Occasionally, this produces obstructive or dyspeptic symptoms.

*Johann Georg Wirsung (1600–43), Professor of Anatomy, University of Padua, where he was murdered.
†Abraham Vater (1684–1751), Professor of Anatomy, Wittenberg, Germany.
‡Giovanni Domenico Santorini (1681–1736), Professor of Anatomy and Medicine, Venice, Italy.

Acute pancreatitis

Acute inflammation of the pancreas is a common cause of acute abdominal pain, with significant morbidity and mortality.

Aetiology

Most cases of acute pancreatitis are associated with either gall stones or alcohol, although a number of less common causes have been identified.

• *Gall stones* are present in half the cases in the UK. Often there is a common channel between common bile duct and pancreatic duct, allowing reflux of bile up the pancreatic duct, particularly when there is temporary impaction of a stone at the ampulla of Vater. Small gall stones can be recovered from the faeces of many patients with acute pancreatitis.

• *Alcohol*: the majority of non-gall-stone pancreatitis is alcohol related. This is particularly common in France and North America. Alcohol is also the commonest cause of recurrent pancreatitis. The mechanism is unclear, and it may follow either chronic alcohol abuse or binge drinking.

Other less common causes of pancreatitis include the following.

• *Post-operative*: particularly after cardiopulmonary bypass or damage to the pancreas during mobilization of the duodenum at partial gastrectomy or splenectomy.

• *Post-endoscopic retrograde cholangio-pancre-*

atography (ERCP): particularly after pancreatography and where there was difficulty cannulating the papilla with subsequent oedema and obstruction.
- *Carcinoma of the pancreas.*
- *Infection*, e.g. mumps, cytomegalovirus or Coxsackie infection.
- *Trauma*: particularly blunt trauma or crush injury.
- *Drugs*, e.g. corticosteroids, sodium valproate.
- *Hypothermia.*
- *Hypercalcaemia.*
- *Hyperlipidaemia.*
- *Vascular*: pancreatitis may occur in malignant hypertension, cholesterol emboli and polyarteritis nodosa, probably as a result of local infarction causing enzyme liberation.

Pathology

Acute pancreatitis differs from other inflammatory conditions because of the auto-digestion that may result from liberation of digestive enzymes. The pancreas is normally protected from auto-digestion by storing its enzymes in intracellular zymogen granules before secreting them as proenzymes. Trypsin, for example, is secreted as trypsinogen and converted to trypsin by the action of enterokinase in the gut. Trypsin itself then cleaves other proenzymes to produce an active form. One such enzyme is phospholipase A, which, in pancreatitis, is involved in cell wall damage and fat necrosis along with pancreatic lipase.

The mechanisms initiating auto-digestion are multiple. Duodeno-pancreatic reflux is an important factor, which may occur as a result of injury to the papilla following endoscopic cannulation, trauma or surgery in this region, or damage to the sphincter resulting from the recent passage of a stone. Duodenal fluid containing enterokinase then refluxes into the duct, activating the pancreatic proenzymes. Duodenal reflux can be shown experimentally to produce pancreatitis, and may be a common factor that underlies many of the aetiological associations mentioned above. As inflammation proceeds, local infarction may occur as arterioles thrombose, and more proenzymes leak out of the necrotic cells to be activated. Once started, pancreatitis can be rapidly progressive, with widespread auto-digestion not only confined to the pancreas.

Macroscopic pathology

At operation, the appearances are quite typical. There is a blood-stained peritoneal effusion. White spots of fat necrosis are scattered throughout the peritoneal cavity; these are produced by lipase released from the pancreas, which liberates fatty acids and glycerol from fat; these acids combine with calcium to produce insoluble calcium soaps. The pancreas is swollen, haemorrhagic or, in severe cases, actually necrotic. Occasionally, suppurative pancreatitis may occur.

Clinical features

The patient is often obese and middle-aged or elderly. Women are more often affected than men. Pain is severe, constant, usually epigastric and often radiates into the back. The patient often sits forward, and repeated retching is common. Vomiting is early and profuse. The patient is usually shocked with a rapid pulse, cyanosis (indicating circulatory collapse) and a temperature that may either be subnormal or raised up to 39.5°C (103°F). The abdomen reveals generalized tenderness and guarding. About 30% of the cases have a tinge of jaundice due to oedema of the pancreatic head obstructing the common bile duct.

A few days after a severe attack, the patient may develop a bluish discoloration in the loins from extravasation of blood-stained pancreatic juice into the retroperitoneal tissues (Grey-Turner's sign*).

Pseudo-cyst formation

As inflammation and auto-digestion progress, liquefying necrotic material and inflammatory

*George Grey-Turner (1877–1951), Professor of Surgery, University of Durham, then Foundation Professor of Surgery at the Royal Postgraduate Medical School, London.

exudate collects in the lesser sac. This fluid, walled off by the stomach in front and necrotic pancreas behind, is the pseudo-cyst, and commonly appears from day 10 onwards.

Severe cases

Severe pancreatitis is associated with haemorrhagic necrosis of the pancreas and systemic release of many vasoactive peptides and enzymes, as well as sequestration of large volumes of fluid within the abdomen. Acute lung failure occurs, characterized by increased capillary permeability and reduced oxygen transfer, and the combination of toxins and loss of circulating fluid results in acute renal failure. Several criteria predictive of the development of severe pancreatitis have been identified, and enable aggressive intensive management to be instituted at an early stage.

Differential diagnosis

The less severe episode of acute pancreatitis simulates acute cholecystitis; the more severe attack, with a marked degree of shock, is usually mistaken for a perforated peptic ulcer or coronary thrombosis. Differentiation must also be made from high intestinal obstruction and from other causes of peritonitis.

GLASGOW CRITERIA FOR SEVERE PANCREATITIS

The factors are assessed over the first 48 hours. Presence of three or more factors indicates severe pancreatitis with a high mortality.
- Age over 55 years.
- Hyperglycaemia (glucose >10 mmol/L in the absence of a history of diabetes).
- Leucocytosis (>15 × 10^9/L).
- urea >16 mmol/L (no response to intravenous fluids).
- Po$_2$ <8 kPa (60 mmHg).
- Calcium <2.0 mmol/L.
- Albumin <32 g/L.
- Lactate dehydrogenase >600 iu/L.
- Raised liver transaminases (aspartate transaminase >100 iu/L).

Special investigations

The investigation comprises tests to confirm the diagnosis and tests to assess the severity of the disease (i.e. diagnostic and prognostic).
- *Serum amylase.* Amylase is liberated into the circulation by the damaged pancreas, and exceeds the kidney's ability to excrete it, so the serum level rises. It is usually significantly raised (fivefold or more) in the acute phase, but returns to normal within 2 or 3 days. Occasionally, an overwhelming attack of pancreatitis with extensive destruction of the gland is associated with a normal amylase. Other causes of raised amylase need to be borne in mind before relying on the amylase level to diagnose pancreatitis.

RAISED SERUM AMYLASE

The causes of raised serum amylase are listed below. Only those marked with an asterisk cause a marked increase in amylase (fivefold or more).

Impaired renal excretion
- Renal failure.*
- Macroamylasaemia (amylase not cleared by kidneys due to complexing or protein binding).

Salivary gland disease
- Salivary calculi.
- Parotitis.

Metabolic causes
- Severe diabetic ketoacidosis.*
- Acute alcoholic intoxication.
- Morphine administration (causing sphincter of Oddi spasm).

Abdominal causes
- Acute pancreatitis.*
- Perforated peptic ulcer.
- Acute cholecystitis.
- Intestinal obstruction.
- Afferent loop obstruction following partial gastrectomy.
- Ruptured abdominal aortic aneurysm.
- Ruptured ectopic pregnancy.
- Mesenteric infarction.
- Trauma, open or blunt.

- *Full blood count*: there is a moderate leucocytosis, and anaemia in severe cases.
- *Blood glucose* is often raised, with glycosuria in 15% of cases.
- *Serum bilirubin* is often raised.
- *Electrocardiography* may show diminished T waves, or arrhythmia, and can cause confusion with cardiac ischaemia.
- *Abdominal X-rays* often give no direct help. The absence of free gas or of localized fluid levels assist in the differential diagnosis of perforated duodenal ulcer or high intestinal obstruction. In some cases, a solitary dilated loop of proximal jejunum may be seen (the 'sentinel loop sign'). Radio-opaque pancreatic calculi may be present in chronic cases.
- *Ultrasound* will demonstrate associated gall stones and may show enlargement of the pancreas. Ultrasonography may be obscured by gas in the upper gastrointestinal tract, resulting in poor views of the pancreas.
- *Computed tomography (CT)* produces better views of the pancreas and may confirm pancreatitis if the amylase is normal in cases that present late. At a later stage, necrotic pancreas, abscess or pseudo-cyst may be visualized.
- *Blood gases*: hypoxia occurs in severe cases.
- *Serum calcium* may be lowered, partly as a result of fat saponification; tetany may occur. The prognosis is bad in such cases.

Note that each of the three enzymes liberated by the pancreas plays a part in the overall picture of acute pancreatitis:

1 *trypsin* produces the auto-digestion of the pancreas;
2 *lipase* results in the typical fat necrosis;
3 *amylase* absorbed from the peritoneal cavity produces a rise in the serum level and is thus a helpful test in diagnosis.

Treatment

In the established case, treatment is conservative and consists of the following.
- *Analgesia*: relief of pain with pethidine (avoiding morphine, which produces sphincter spasm).
- *Fluid replacement* with colloid or blood transfusion, to treat shock and establish a diuresis. In less severe cases, electrolyte and water replacement alone may suffice.
- *Rest the pancreas* by removing stimuli for secretion: the patient is not allowed to take fluid or food by mouth, and naso-gastric aspiration is started if the patient is vomiting.
- *Antibiotics* are commenced if the pancreatitis is associated with gall stones.
- *Prophylaxis against gastric erosions* with sucralfate or an H_2-receptor antagonist (e.g. ranitidine).
- *Endoscopic sphincterotomy* performed early in the admission may be useful in gall-stone pancreatitis, especially severe cases.
- *Surgery* is indicated if the diagnosis is not certain, but should be avoided where possible. It is indicated for the drainage of an abscess or pseudo-cyst, debridement of a necrotic pancreas, or management of a complication.
- *Nutrition*: total parenteral nutrition should be instituted early in severe cases. Once on oral feeding, a low fat, high carbohydrate diet should be started, to avoid over-stimulation of the pancreas.

Attempts at treatment with drugs that reduce pancreatic enzyme activation (e.g. aprotonin) or secretion (e.g. probanthine or atropine) are of no proven benefit.

After recovery from an attack of pancreatitis, cholecystectomy is advised if gall stones are present.

Prognosis

Mortality is in the region of 10% and is directly proportional to the severity of the attack.

Complications

- *Abscess formation* with pancreatic necrosis, characterized by pyrexia and persistent leucocytosis.
- *Pseudo-cyst*, characterized by a persistently raised amylase and pain, usually in the second week, and presenting as an epigastric mass.
- *Gastrointestinal bleeding* from acute gastric erosions or peptic ulceration.
- *Renal failure* associated with shock and pancreatic necrosis.

- *Pulmonary insufficiency*: acute lung injury.
- *Further attacks* (relapsing pancreatitis).
- *Diabetes mellitus*, resulting from a severe attack with pancreatic necrosis, or chronic relapsing pancreatitis.

Chronic pancreatitis

Chronic and acute pancreatitis are clinically distinct entities, although bouts of acute pancreatitis are frequent in the course of acute pancreatitis, and the pathogenesis of chronic pancreatitis has much in common with acute pancreatitis. Chronic pancreatitis is characterized by gradual destruction of the functional pancreatic tissue.

Aetiology
In the Western world, alcoholism is the main cause of chronic pancreatitis. In parts of Asia and Africa, chronic pancreatitis is associated with malnutrition; hereditary pancreatitis and hypercalcaemia are uncommon causes.

Clinical features
The patient may present with one or more of the following:
- *Asymptomatic* (X-ray diagnosis only from pancreatic calcification).
- *Recurrent abdominal pain* radiating through to the upper lumbar region, relieved by sitting forward.
- *Steatorrhoea* due to pancreatic insufficiency, resulting in malabsorption and weight loss.
- *Diabetes* due to islet-cell damage.
- *Obstructive jaundice*, which is very difficult to differentiate, even at operation, from carcinoma of the head of the pancreas.

Special investigations
- *Serum amylase* estimations performed during attacks of pain may be elevated, but in long-standing disease are often normal, there being insufficient pancreatic tissue remaining to cause a large rise.
- *Abdominal X-ray* may show evidence of calcification or calculi.

- *CT scan* may demonstrate enlargement and irregular consistency of the gland.
- *ERCP* may show dilatation and irregularity of the pancreatic duct, and compression of the bile duct by the inflamed pancreatic head.
- *Exocrine function tests*, such as the pancreolauryl test in which fluorescein dilaurate is ingested, and is split by pancreatic esterases to release fluorescein, which is absorbed and excreted in the urine. Urinary fluorescein concentration reflects pancreatic exocrine activity. However, the differential diagnosis from a pancreatic carcinoma may only be established at laparotomy.

Treatment
The principal treatment is to remove causative factors such as alcohol consumption. Alcohol should be avoided by anyone with pancreatitis.
- *Analgesics*: the pain is often sufficient to warrant opiate analgesia, but long-term use may result in addiction. Getting the analgesia right is often one of the most difficult aspects of management.
- *Diet*: a low fat diet with pancreatic enzymes (pancreatin) by mouth.
- *Insulin* when diabetes mellitus occurs.
- *Surgery* if very frequent attacks or severe pain; partial pancreatectomy or drainage of the whole length of the pancreatic duct into a loop of intestine may be required (pancreaticojejunostomy). Occasionally, total pancreatectomy is required, with consequent diabetes and steatorrhoea.
- *Painless obstructive jaundice* may be relieved by a bypass using the gall bladder as a conduit (cholecyst-jejunostomy).

Pancreatic cysts

Classification
True (20%)
- Congenital polycystic disease of pancreas.
- Retention.
- Hydatid.
- Neoplastic: cystadenoma or cystadenocarcinoma.

False

A collection of fluid in the lesser sac (80%):

• after trauma to the pancreas;
• following acute pancreatitis;
• due to perforation of a posterior gastric ulcer (rare).

Clinical features

A pancreatic cyst presents as a firm, large, rounded, upper abdominal swelling. Initially, the cyst is apparently resonant because of loops of gas-filled bowel in front of it, but as it increases in size the intestine is pushed away and the mass becomes dull to percussion.

Treatment

True cysts require surgical excision; false cysts are drained. This may be performed internally (by anastomosis either into the stomach or into the small intestine), or percutaneously, under ultrasound control.

Pancreatic tumours

Classification

Benign

1 Adenoma.
2 Cystadenoma.
3 Islet-cell tumour:
   (a) Zollinger–Ellison tumour (non-β-cell tumour);
   (b) insulinoma (β-cell tumour — α-cells produce glucagon).

Malignant

1 *Primary*:
   (a) adenocarcinoma;
   (b) cystadenocarcinoma;
   (c) malignant islet-cell tumour.
2 *Secondary*: invasion from carcinoma of stomach or bile duct.

Islet-cell tumours

These tumours, although rare, are of great interest because of their metabolic effects even from small lesions, which may be difficult to localize even with CT and magnetic resonance imaging (MRI), or selective angiography.

Types of tumours

Islet-cell tumours are all derived from APUD cells, i.e. cells capable of amine precursor uptake and decarboxylation, and are thus sometimes termed APUDomas. They secrete a number of polypeptides according to the cell type of origin. These may be active hormones, and present relatively early, or polypeptides for which no function has been identified, and often more than one polypeptide is secreted. The islet contains at least five cell types:

1 β-cells, producing insulin;
2 α-cells, producing glucagon;
3 γ-cells, producing somatostatin;
4 F cells, producing pancreatic polypeptide;
5 enterochromaffin cell, producing serotonin.

In addition, the islet cells, which are of neuro-ectoderm origin, may produce hormones not normally found in the pancreas, such as gastrin (gastrinoma) and vasoactive polypeptide (VIPoma).

The islet-cell tumours may be associated with other neuro-ectoderm tumours elsewhere as part of a multiple endocrine neoplasia (MEN) syndrome, often involving the parathyroid and the anterior pituitary gland.

Insulinoma (β-cell islet tumour)

Ninety per cent are benign, 10% malignant and about 10% are multiple tumours. Because of the high production of insulin by the tumour, two groups of hypoglycaemic symptoms may be produced.

1 *Central nervous system phenomena*: weakness, sweating, trembling, epilepsy, confusion, hemiplegia and eventually coma, which may be fatal.
2 *Gastrointestinal phenomena*: hunger, abdominal pain and diarrhoea.

These symptoms appear particularly when the patient is hungry, or during physical exercise. They are often present early in the morning before breakfast and are relieved by eating. Often there is excessive appetite with gross weight gain.

Diagnosis: Whipple's triad*

The main diagnostic characteristics of the syndrome are:

• the attacks are induced by starvation or exercise;

• during the attack hypoglycaemia is present;

• symptoms are relieved by sugar given orally or intravenously.

Differential diagnosis of spontaneous hypoglycaemia in adults includes self-administration of insulin or alcohol, and suprarenal, pituitary or hepatic insufficiency.

Special investigations

• *Insulin levels*: raised insulin levels in the presence of hypoglycaemia. The hypoglycaemia can be prompted by a period of prolonged fasting (14–16 hours).

• *C-peptide levels* may be measured to rule out exogenous insulin administration, as these will be high in insulinoma and low when exogenous insulin is administered.

• *Localization tests* include CT, MRI and selective angiography. Ultimately, localization may not be achieved until laparotomy is performed.

Treatment

Excision of the tumour.

Gastrinoma (Zollinger–Ellison syndrome,† non-β-cell islet tumour)

This tumour of non-β-cells may be benign or malignant, multiple, and a quarter are part of an MEN syndrome. Malignant tumours are more common in sporadic forms (60%) than those related to MENs (30%), and are relatively slow growing, although eventually producing hepatic metastases. The gastrinoma secretes a gastrin-like substance into the blood stream, which produces an extremely high gastric secretion of HCl. Many patients also develop

*Allen Oldfather Whipple (1881–1963), Professor of Surgery, Columbia University, New York, USA.
†Robert Milton Zollinger (1903–92), Professor of Surgery, Ohio State University, Columbus, USA. Edward Horner Ellison (1918–70), Associate Professor at the same institution.

oesophagitis due to the high acid secretion or diarrhoea (the cause of which is not yet certain). The majority of cases develop fulminating peptic ulceration, with multiple duodenal ulcers, which relapse after cessation of medical therapy, and which rapidly recur after gastrectomy or vagotomy and drainage.

Special investigation

• *Fasting gastrin* concentration in the blood is very high.

• *Basal acid output*, measured by naso-gastric aspiration, is very high (over 15 mmol/h).

• *Localization*: as for other islet-cell tumours.

Treatment

Treatment comprises excision of the tumour or, if this is not possible, control of the high acid secretion by means of proton-pump inhibitors (e.g. omeprazole) or high doses of histamine H_2-receptor antagonists (cimetidine, ranitidine). Failure of medical treatment may require total gastrectomy.

Carcinoma
Pathology

Sixty per cent are situated in the head of the pancreas, 25% in the body and 15% in the tail.

Of the tumours of the head of the pancreas, one-third are peri-ampullary, arising from the ampulla of Vater, the duodenal mucosa or the lower end of the common bile duct.

The incidence in England and Wales is 12 per 100 000 population, with males and females now almost equally affected. It affects the middle-aged and elderly, and the incidence is rising, particularly in the USA, where deaths from this cause are now commoner than from carcinoma of the stomach. The disease is commoner in smokers.

Macroscopically, the growth is infiltrating, hard and irregular.

Microscopically, the tumours may be:

• mucus secreting (of duct origin) — adenocarcinomas;

• non-mucus secreting (of acinar origin) — acinar cell carcinoma;

- undifferentiated;
- cystadenocarcinoma (rare), papillary cystic.

Spread

1 *Direct invasion into*:
  (a) common bile duct — obstructive jaundice;
  (b) duodenum — occult or overt intestinal bleeding;
  (c) portal vein — portal vein thrombosis, portal hypertension and ascites;
  (d) inferior vena cava—bilateral leg oedema.
2 *Lymphatic*: to adjacent lymph nodes and nodes in the porta hepatis.
3 *Blood stream*: to the liver and then to the lungs.
4 *Trans-coelomic*: with peritoneal seeding and ascites.

Clinical features

Carcinoma of the pancreas may present in a variety of ways.
- *Painless progressive jaundice* is the classical presentation, but this form is rather uncommon and is most often found in the peri-ampullary type of tumour. This is because the bile duct is compressed at an early stage, before extensive painful invasion of surrounding tissues.
- *Pain*: at least 50% present with epigastric pain of a dull, continuous aching nature, which frequently radiates into the upper lumbar region. This pain often precedes intermittent jaundice.
- *Intermittent jaundice*: the jaundice is usually progressive, but may temporarily remit or even disappear as necrosis of the tumour occurs, allowing a transient escape of bile into the duodenum.
- *Diabetes*: glycosuria of recent onset in the elderly is suspicious.
- *Thrombophlebitis migrans* (Trousseau's sign*); the pathogenesis of this is unknown.
- *The general features of malignant disease*: anorexia and loss of weight.

Examination

The patient is frequently jaundiced, and half have a palpable gall bladder (Courvoisier's law). If the tumour is large, an epigastric mass may be palpable. The liver is frequently enlarged, either from the back-pressure of biliary obstruction or because of secondary deposits.

Special investigations

- *CT scan* may demonstrate the tumour mass. Fine-needle biopsy may be performed under imaging control.
- *Endoscopy* may visualize a peri-ampullary growth, which can then be biopsied.
- *Barium swallow* may show widening of the duodenal loop and a filling defect or irregularity of the duodenum resulting from invasion by the tumour.
- *Occult blood* may be present in the stools, especially from a periampullary tumour ulcerating into the duodenum. The stools are pale in the presence of jaundice, and may have a silvery appearance due to the peri-ampullary bleeding (the silvery stools of Ogilvie†).
- *Serum amylase* is rarely elevated.
- *Biochemical analysis* confirms the changes of obstructive jaundice (high bilirubin and alkaline phosphatase).

Differential diagnosis

This is from other causes of obstructive jaundice and from other causes of upper abdominal pain. Carcinoma of the body and tail of the pancreas, in which obstructive jaundice does not occur, is notoriously difficult to diagnose. Laboratory and X-ray investigations are usually negative.

Treatment

Treatment of carcinoma of the pancreas is usually symptomatic, and thus applicable to tumours of the head of pancreas, which present with obstructive jaundice and duodenal obstruction. Occasionally, curative

---

*Armand Trousseau (1801–67), Physician, Hôpital Ste Antoine and Hôpital, Dieu, Paris.

† Sir William Heneage Ogilvie (1887–1971), Surgeon, Guy's Hospital, London.

resection may be possible, otherwise palliation is more appropriate.

Curative surgical resections are possible where disease is confined to the peri-ampullary region. The procedure (Whipple's pancreatico-duodenectomy) involves removal of the duodenal C along with the pancreatic head and common bile duct; a gastro-enterostomy and biliary drainage using a Roux loop* of jejunum are fashioned to restore continuity, together with the implantation of the pancreatic duct into the jejunal loop. However, most tumours are inoperable, and those which are operable often have a poor long-term prognosis.

Palliative surgical bypass comprises a short circuit between the distended gall bladder and a loop of jejunum (cholecyst-jejunostomy), together with a duodenal bypass by a gastroenterostomy if duodenal obstruction is present.

Palliative intubation, by passage of a stent

---

*Cesar Roux (1857–1934), Professor of Surgery, Lausanne, Switzerland.

across the ampulla and through the obstructed common bile duct, is the other alternative to treat the obstructive jaundice. This may be performed either endoscopically (ERCP) or trans-hepatically (percutaneous transhepatic cholangiography).

Severe pain may be relieved by radiotherapy but usually requires management with opiates.

Prognosis

The outlook for patients with carcinoma of the pancreas itself is gloomy; even if the growth is resectable, the operation has a mortality of about 10% and only a small percentage survive for 5 years. Peri-ampullary growths, however, which present relatively early, have a reasonably good prognosis after resection, with about 25% 5-year survival.

Occasionally, a patient has a surprisingly prolonged survival after a palliative bypass operation. In such a case, the diagnosis was more likely to have been chronic pancreatitis mistaken for carcinoma.

CHAPTER 33

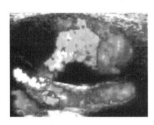

The Spleen

Splenomegaly

Physical signs

The spleen must be enlarged to about three times its normal size before it becomes clinically palpable. It then forms a swelling that descends below the left costal margin, moves on respiration, and has a firm lower margin, which may or may not be notched. The mass is dull to percussion, the dullness extending above the costal margin.

There are three important differential diagnoses.

1 An enlarged left kidney; unless this is enormous there is resonance over the swelling anteriorly, as it is covered by the gas-containing colon.

2 Carcinoma of the cardia or upper part of the body of the stomach; by the time such a tumour reaches palpable proportions there are usually symptoms of gastric obstruction, which suggest the site of the lesion.

3 An enlarged left lobe of liver.

Classification

It is essential to have a working classification of enlargements of the spleen.

1 *Infections*:
  (a) viruses—glandular fever;
  (b) bacterial — typhus, typhoid, septicaemia ('septic spleen');
  (c) protozoal — malaria, kala-azar, Egyptian splenomegaly (schistosomiasis);
  (d) parasitic—hydatid.

2 *Haemopoietic diseases*:
  (a) leukaemia — chronic myeloid and chronic lymphocytic;
  (b) lymphoma — Hodgkin's disease, non-Hodgkin's lymphoma;
  (c) myelofibrosis, idiopathic thrombocytopenia, polycythaemia rubra vera;
  (d) haemolytic anaemias—spherocytosis, β-thalassaemia.

3 *Portal hypertension.*

4 *Metabolic and collagen disease*:
  (a) amyloid — secondary to rheumatoid arthritis, collagen diseases, chronic sepsis;
  (b) storage diseases — Gaucher's disease, Niemann–Pick disease.

5 *Cysts, abscesses and tumours of the spleen*: all uncommon.

Massive splenomegaly in the UK is likely to be due to one of the following: chronic myeloid leukaemia, myelofibrosis, lymphoma, polycythaemia or portal hypertension.

If the spleen is palpable, special attention must be paid to detecting the presence of hepatomegaly and lymphadenopathy (see p. 278).

Splenectomy

Splenectomy is indicated under the following circumstances.
• *Rupture*: either from closed or open trauma or accidental damage during abdominal surgery.
• *Blood diseases*: haemolytic anaemia, thrombocytopenic purpura.
• *Tumours and cysts*.
• *Part of another operative procedure*, e.g. radical excision of carcinoma of the stomach, spleno-renal anastomosis for portal hypertension, distal pancreatectomy.

Complications of splenectomy
Gastric dilatation
Following splenectomy there is a gastric ileus. Swallowed air causes rapid dilatation of the stomach, which may tear ligatures on the small gastric vessels on the greater curve of the stomach, which are ligated during splenectomy; haemorrhage results. A naso-gastric tube is placed and regularly aspirated in all patients following splenectomy.

Thrombocytosis
Following splenectomy, the platelet count rises, often to a level of 1000×10^9/L (normal is $<400 \times 10^9$/L). In time, the count falls, but while high the patient is at a greater than normal risk of deep vein thrombosis and pulmonary embolus.

Post-splenectomy sepsis
One of the spleen's functions is to clear capsulated micro-organisms (such as *Pneumococcus*, *Meningococcus* and *Haemophilus influenza*) from the blood stream after they have been opsonized by the binding of host antibodies to their surface as part of the normal immune response. The spleen also has important phagocytic properties, as well as being the largest repository of lymphoid tissue in the body.

Removal of the spleen in splenectomy predisposes the patient, especially a child, to infection with organisms such as the *Pneumo-coccus*. The clinical course is of a fulminant bacterial infection, with shock and circulatory collapse, termed overwhelming post-splenectomy sepsis (OPSS).

Prophylactic immunization with pneumococcal, meningococcal and *Haemophilus influenza* type b vaccines should be administered, preoperatively where possible. In addition, children should have prophylactic daily low-dose penicillin until they reach adulthood. Adults should have penicillin for the first year after splenectomy, and longer if immunosuppressed.

Ruptured spleen

This is the commonest internal injury produced by non-penetrating trauma to the abdominal wall. It usually occurs alone, but may coexist with fractures of the ribs, rupture of the liver, the left kidney, the diaphragm or the tail of the pancreas.

Clinical features
Ruptures of the spleen fall into four groups.
1 *Massive bleeding with rapid death from shock.* This results from a complete shattering of the spleen or its avulsion from the splenic pedicle, and death may occur in a few minutes. Fortunately this is rare.
2 *Peritonism from progressive blood loss.* Following injury there are the symptoms and signs of progressive blood loss together with evidence of peritoneal irritation. Over a period of several hours after the accident the patient becomes increasingly pale, the pulse rises and the blood pressure falls. There is abdominal pain, which is either diffuse or confined to the left flank. The patient may complain of referred pain to the left shoulder tip or admit to this only on direct questioning.

On examination, the abdomen is generally tender, particularly on the left side. There may be marked generalized rigidity, or it may be confined to slight guarding of the left flank. The percussion note is impaired in the left flank due to the local collection of blood; this is a sign on which we have come to rely. Surprisingly enough, bruising of the abdominal wall is often absent or only slight.

3 *Delayed rupture.* This may occur from hours up to several days after trauma. There is the initial injury with concomitant pain, which soon settles. Then, following a completely asymptomatic interval, the signs and symptoms described above become manifest. This picture is produced by a subcapsular haematoma of the spleen, which increases in size and then ruptures the thin overlying peritoneal capsule with a resultant sudden, sharp haemorrhage.

4 *Spontaneous rupture.* A spleen diseased by, for example, malaria, glandular fever or leukaemia may rupture after only trivial trauma.

Special investigations

The diagnosis of a ruptured spleen is a clinical one, and in the face of massive haemorrhage the surgeon must proceed at once to laparotomy. In the less acute situation, the following investigations are useful.

• *Urinalysis* for blood: haematuria will suggest associated renal damage.

• *Chest X-ray* may reveal associated rib fractures, rupture of the diaphragm or injury to the left lung.

• *Abdominal X-ray*: the stomach bubble may be displaced to the right and there may be indentation of its gas shadow. The splenic flexure of the colon, if containing gas, may be seen to be displaced downwards by the haematoma.

• *Computed tomography (CT) scan* will often demonstrate the laceration of the spleen and the presence of intra-abdominal fluid, as well as identifying traumatic injuries to other organs.

Treatment

Resuscitation with blood replacement is commenced, and laparotomy performed. If the spleen is found to be avulsed or hopelessly pulped, emergency splenectomy is required. If there is minor laceration of the spleen, an attempt is made to preserve it, especially in children and young adults where there is a risk of post-splenectomy sepsis. This may be carried out by using fine sutures and haemostatic absorbable gauze.

Having controlled the bleeding, it is important to carry out a full examination to exclude injury to other organs.

CHAPTER 34

The Lymph Nodes and Lymphatics

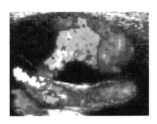

Enlarged lymph nodes are a common diagnostic problem. It is as well therefore to have a simple classification and clinical approach to this topic.

The lymphadenopathies

The lymphadenopathies are conveniently divided into those due to local and those due to generalized disease.

Classification

Localized

1 *Infective*:
   (a) acute, e.g. a cervical lymphadenopathy secondary to tonsillitis;
   (b) chronic, e.g. tuberculous nodes of neck.
2 *Neoplastic*: due to secondary spread of tumour.

Generalized

1 *Infective*:
   (a) acute, e.g. glandular fever (mononucleosis), septicaemia;
   (b) chronic, e.g. acquired immune deficiency syndrome (AIDS), secondary syphilis.
2 *The reticuloses*: Hodgkin's disease,* non-Hodgkin's lymphoma, chronic lymphocytic leukaemia.
3 *Sarcoidosis*.

*Thomas Hodgkin (1789–1866), Curator of Pathology, Guy's Hospital, London.

Clinical examination

The clinical examination of any patient with a lymph node enlargement is incomplete unless the following three requirements have been fulfilled.

1 The area drained by the involved lymph nodes has been searched for possible primary source of infection or malignant disease. There are four important points to remember.
   (a) *Cervical lymphadenopathy*. In addition to examining the skin of the head and neck, the inside of the oropharynx together with the larynx should be examined for chronic sepsis or malignant disease.
   (b) *Inguinal lymphadenopathy*. If a patient has an enlarged lymph node in the groin, the skin of the leg, buttock and lower abdominal wall below the level of the umbilicus must be scrutinized, together with the external genitalia and the anal canal.
   (c) *Testicular tumours* drain along their lymphatics, which pass with the testicular vessels to the para-aortic lymph nodes, and not to the inguinal lymph nodes.
   (d) *Virchow's node* is a prominent node in the left supraclavicular fossa arising from malignant disease below the diaphragm, e.g. gastric carcinoma, with secondaries ascending the thoracic duct to drain into the left subclavian vein. A supraclavicular node may also signify spread from intrathoracic or breast tumours.
2 The other lymph node areas have been examined, as enlarged lymph nodes elsewhere would suggest a generalized lymphadenopathy.

3 The liver and spleen have been carefully palpated; their enlargement will suggest a reticulosis, sarcoid or glandular fever.

Special investigations

In many instances the diagnosis of the cause of the lymphadenopathy will by now have become obvious. The following investigations may be required, however, in order to elucidate the diagnosis.

• *Examination of a blood film* may clinch the diagnosis of glandular fever or leukaemia.

• *Chest X-ray* may show evidence of enlarged mediastinal nodes or may reveal a primary occult tumour of the lung, which is the source of disseminated deposits.

• *Serological tests*: a human immunodeficiency virus (HIV) antibody test is performed if AIDS is suspected; syphilis may be confirmed by specific treponemal antigen tests.

• *X-ray of cervical nodes*: enlarged painless cervical lymph nodes should be X-rayed; tuberculous nodes often show typical spotty calcification.

• *Lymph node biopsy*: removal of one of the enlarged lymph nodes may be necessary for definite histological proof of the diagnosis. This is particularly so in Hodgkin's disease and non-Hodgkin's lymphoma.

Lymphoedema

Lymphoedema results from the obstruction of lymphatic flow, due to congenital abnormalities of the lymphatics, their obliteration by disease or their operative removal. It is characterized by an excessive accumulation of interstitial fluid. The causes of lymphoedema may be divided into congenital and acquired.

Congenital lymphoedema

Congenital or primary lymphoedema more commonly affects the lower limbs and is three times more common in females than males. It may be familial (Milroy's disease*). There are three principal pathological processes affecting the lymphatic channels in congenital lym-

---

A SWOLLEN LEG

Generalized disease
• Cardiac failure.
• Nephrotic syndrome.
• Liver failure.

Venous disease
• Venous thrombosis.*
• Deep venous insufficiency.
• Arterio-venous fistula,* e.g. Klippel–Trenaunay syndrome.

Lymphatic disease
• Primary lymphoedema.*
• Secondary lymphoedema,* e.g. filariasis, malignant infiltration, following surgery or irradiation to lymphatics.

* Also may cause unilateral upper limb swelling.

---

phoedema: aplasia, hypoplasia and varicose dilatation (megalymphatics).

Congenital lymphoedema has been characterized according to the typical time of onset:
• *lymphoedema congenita*, where lymphoedema is present from birth;
• *lymphoedema praecox*, where the condition develops at puberty;
• *lymphoedema tarda*, where the condition develops in adult life, is the most common presentation.

Acquired lymphoedema

• *Post-inflammatory*: the result of fibrosis obliterating the lymphatics following repeated attacks of streptococcal cellulitis, particularly where the lymphatic drainage is already compromised.

• *Filariasis*: *Filaria bancrofti* infects lymphatics; a chronic inflammatory reaction is set up with consequent lymphatic obstruction. There is gross lymphoedema, especially of the lower limbs and genitalia, often called elephantiasis.

• *Following radical surgery*, particularly after

*William Forsyth Milroy (1855–1942), Physician, Omaha, USA.

block dissection of the axilla, groin or neck in which extensive removal of lymphatics is performed.

• *Post-irradiation fibrosis.*

• *Malignant disease*: late oedema of the arm after axillary clearance and radical mastectomy is often indicative of massive recurrence of tumour in the axilla occluding the residual lymphatic pathways.

Special investigations

• *Lymphangiography* using radio-opaque contrast or radioactive isotope will confirm lymphatic obstruction, and contrast lymphangiography may demonstrate megalymphatics.

Differential diagnosis

The diagnosis of lymphoedema depends first of all on the exclusion of other causes of oedema, for instance venous obstruction, cardiac failure or renal disease, and second, the demonstration of one of the causes mentioned above. It was previously taught that lymphoedema could readily be differentiated from other forms of oedema on the simple physical sign of absence of pitting in the lymphoedematous limb. However, lymphoedema of acute onset will initially pit on pressure although it is true that when it becomes chronic the subcutaneous tissues become indurated from fibrous tissue replacement, and pitting will not then occur. However, oedema of any nature, if chronic, will have this characteristic.

Treatment of congenital lymphoedema
Conservative

Mild cases will respond to elevation and graduated elastic compression stockings.

Surgery

In severe cases surgery may be appropriate. Two approaches are possible. The first is to remove all the oedematous subcutaneous tissue down to the deep fascia with removal of the overlying skin as a split-skin graft and its re-application directly to the deep fascia. This leaves considerable scarring. The second approach is to provide alternative lymphatic drainage bypassing obstructions, such as by tunnelling a tongue of omentum down to the inguinal nodes, to provide drainage along mesenteric lymphatics to the thoracic duct, bypassing obstructed iliac nodes. Unfortunately the results are poor.

CHAPTER 35

The Breast

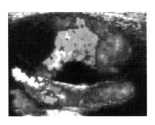

Developmental anomalies

Supernumerary nipples and breasts
Extra nipples or breasts may develop along the primitive milk line. These behave as the main breasts under the influence of circulating hormones, and may discharge during lactation.

Hypomastia
Hypomastia, almost complete failure of development of the breast, may be unilateral or bilateral. If bilateral it may be associated with ovarian failure or Turner's syndrome.

Nipple inversion
This may be primary, or secondary to duct ectasia or a carcinoma of the breast, when the process is more appropriately called nipple retraction. Primary indrawn nipples may cause problems during lactation but are of no other significance.

Symptoms of breast disease

There are three common symptoms of breast disease: a lump, bleeding or discharge from the nipple, and pain.

A lump in the breast
Ninety-five per cent of all lumps in the breast will be one of the four following:

1 carcinoma of the breast;
2 cyst;
3 fibroadenoma;
4 fibroadenosis (a localized area).

In addition, the following less common causes need to be considered.

1 *Traumatic:* fat necrosis.
2 *Other cysts:*
  (a) galactocele;
  (b) chronic abscess;
  (c) cystadenoma;
  (d) retention cyst of the glands of Montgomery.
3 *Other tumours:*
  (a) duct papilloma;
  (b) sarcoma (extremely rare).
4 *Chest wall swellings:*
  (a) lipoma;
  (b) thrombosis of superficial veins of breast or chest wall (Mondor's disease);

(c) tuberculosis or tumour of a rib;

(d) eroding aortic aneurysm;

(e) cold abscess (empyema necessitans).

Management

Although useful information can be derived about a lump in the breast by careful examination, it is a good clinical rule that any discrete lump in the breast must be excised for histological examination or aspirated for cytological examination: 'No woman should have a lump in the breast.'

If the lump is considered likely to be a cyst, it is safe practice to aspirate it to confirm the diagnosis. If it disappears, no further treatment is required. However, if no fluid is obtained, the lump should be surgically removed or submitted to fine-needle aspiration and cytological examination of the material obtained (see p. 284).

Discharge from the nipple

1 *Blood-stained*:

(a) duct papilloma, when blood arises from a single duct;

(b) intraduct carcinoma;

(c) Paget's disease;

(d) invasive carcinoma (unusual).

2 *Serous*: early pregnancy.

3 *Yellowish, brown or green*: fibroadenosis.

4 *Milky*: galactorrhoea may follow lactation but also can be drug induced or a manifestation of hyperprolactinaemia.

5 *Purulent*: breast abscess.

It is the first, the blood-stained discharge, that most alarms the patient. Its management is as follows.

Management

The patient is carefully examined; there may be one of the following possibilities.

Mass and discharge

A mass is discovered, pressure on which produces the discharge; the mass is excised and further treatment is based on the result of histological examination.

Discharge, no mass

If a mass is not discovered, it may be possible by pressing on one spot adjacent to the nipple to obtain a discharge. This segment of the breast is surgically explored and submitted for histological examination; again a limited or more extensive operation may be required, depending on the results of pathological examination. It is, however, very rare for a malignant condition to be present without a lump having been detected.

No mass, no discharge

If no mass can be felt and no discharge produced, a conservative approach is adopted; the patient is kept under supervision either until the site of discharge is located and excised, or the bleeding ceases; again, this is most unlikely to be the presentation of malignant disease of the breast.

Special investigations that may help are a *mammogram* and a '*ductogram*', performed by injecting contrast into the discharging duct.

Pain in the breast (mastalgia)

The possible causes of mastalgia to be considered are as follows.

• *Cyclical mastalgia*: typically the pain is present immediately before each period.

• *Fibroadenosis*: see later.

• *Breast abscess*.

• *Carcinoma of the breast*: this may give rise to heaviness or a 'pricking' pain.

• *Chest-wall lesions*, e.g. chondritis of the costal cartilage. This syndrome (Tietze's disease*) is of unknown aetiology, affects one or more of the second, third or fourth costo-chondral junctions and, left alone, resolves over a number of months.

Traumatic fat necrosis

Pathology

Disrupted fat cells released by trauma produce

---

*Alexander Tietze (1864–1927), Surgeon, Breslau, Germany.

a foreign-body giant-cell reaction with subsequent fibrosis and perhaps calcification.

Clinical features

Many women presenting with a lump in the breast attribute this to injury. A clinical diagnosis of fat necrosis should only be made when the trauma was sufficient to cause bruising of the breast and when the patient is obese. The lump itself may have become smaller in size and this again would suggest a non-malignant condition, in spite of the fact that clinically the lump may be tethered to the skin and accompanied by large axillary lymph nodes.

Treatment

This is excision, as it is impossible to be quite certain of the diagnosis without biopsy; a section through the lump reveals a pale, fibrous mass, which may contain central fluid fat or chalky material. Fine-needle aspiration cytology may also be diagnostic, but mammography may mislead and suggest a carcinoma.

Acute inflammation of the breast

Classification
- *Mastitis of the newborn* and *mastitis of puberty*: probably hormonal but may proceed to suppuration.
- *Mumps mastitis*: rare complication.
- *Traumatic* (due to the chafing of braces, etc.).
- *Subareolar*: from infection of one of the glands of Montgomery,* which are sebaceous-like glands around the areola.
- *Acute bacterial mastitis* and acute mammary abscess.

Acute bacterial mastitis

The commonest and most important acute inflammation of the breast. The majority occur during lactation, caused either by invasion by *Staphylococcus aureus* through an abrasion of

*William Fetherston Montgomery (1797–1859), Obstetrician, Dublin.

the nipple resulting in a circumareolar abscess, or along the milk ducts themselves, producing a deep intramammary infection. Typically, it affects mothers in the first month after their first pregnancy.

Non-lactational breast abscesses may also occur, but are a rarity after the menopause. They are often a manifestation of duct ectasia, and arise in the peri-areolar tissues. The common organisms include *Enterococcus* and *Bacteroides*, rather than the *Staphylococcus* of lactation.

Clinical features

The infection often occurs in a lactating mother. There may be a recent history of a cracked nipple. It commences as a cellulitis, which localizes into an abscess after several days.

Treatment
Cellulitis
If the patient is seen within the first 24 hours of the onset, when the condition is still a spreading cellulitis of the breast, infection may be aborted by antimicrobial chemotherapy, such as flucloxacillin or a cephalosporin.

Abscess
If the infection has been present for more than a day or two it is almost certain that a localized abscess will have begun to form. Once pus has formed, there is no place for antimicrobial chemotherapy alone, as this may result in chronic and recurrent abscesses burrowing through the breast. The classical treatment is to drain the abscess operatively, with antimicrobials continued until cellulitis has resolved. Occasionally, this may result in duct fistula.

More recently, daily ultrasound-guided aspiration of the abscess, combined with antimicrobial chemotherapy, has been advocated.

During treatment, the infant should be nursed on the contralateral breast, while milk engorgement of the affected side is relieved by manual expression or a breast pump. Suppression of lactation is no longer advocated.

Chronic abscess of the breast

Tuberculosis, gumma and actinomycosis of the breast are all very rare. The most likely chronic abscess of the breast is one following prolonged and misguided chemotherapy in the treatment of acute breast abscess ('antibioticoma' or 'penicillinoma').

Benign changes affect women from puberty to menopause, after which they only occur occasionally in the form of large cysts within the breast. By their nature the changes are frequently bilateral.

Aetiology

Any organ in the body that undergoes cyclical changes of proliferation and regression is prone to abnormalities of this process; examples are the prostate, thyroid and ovary as well as the breast. To reflect these changes the nomenclature of benign breast disease now refers to the processes as 'aberrations of normal development and involution' (ANDI). This nomenclature has the benefit of reclassifying the 'disease' into a disorder, and so acknowledges that its features are experienced by most women to a greater or lesser degree.

Presentations

The different manifestations of benign breast disease reflect the variations in activity of ductular and epithelial components under cyclical hormonal stimulation, with increasing activity followed by involution, together with perimenopausal involution. Within what was once variously called 'fibroadenosis', 'mammary dysplasia', 'chronic mastitis' and 'fibrocystic disease' are a number of different features, which may be present separately or in combination.

• *Cyclical mastalgia and nodularity*: a result of cyclical hormone changes.
• *Cyst formation*: aberration of lobular involution.

• *Sclerosing adenosis*: lobular involution.
• *Duct ectasia*: duct involution.
• *Fibroadenoma*: developmental aberration of lobular development.
• *Papilloma formation*: increased duct epithelial activity.

Examination

Examination may reveal diffuse lumpiness of both breasts or a mass confined to one sector of the breast, particularly the upper, outer quadrant. It is characteristic that this lumpiness is best defined by palpation between the index finger and the thumb, and it is more difficult to feel with the flat of the hand (in contrast to a carcinoma). This is because the segment of benign adenosis has almost the same consistency as the surrounding breast tissue.

Less commonly the patient presents with a local, smooth, spherical lump in the breast which may be of considerable size. It may be possible to elicit fluctuation or transillumination in such a lump, and then to be tolerably certain that the diagnosis is a cyst. Quite commonly, shotty nodes are palpable in the axilla.

Differential diagnosis

The differential diagnosis from an early carcinoma of the breast may be very difficult, indeed impossible; moreover, it is far from rare to find both conditions present within the same breast. The only pre-malignant condition is epithelial hyperplasia. It is sound practice therefore to *submit every localized mass in the breast to biopsy, either by needle aspiration, needle biopsy or excision.*

Special investigations

• *Fine-needle aspiration cytology*, in which an aspirate from the suspicious lesion is smeared onto a slide and examined microscopically, may suggest malignancy.
• *Needle core biopsy*: a core of tissue is removed using a Tru-Cut needle or similar device under local anaesthetic, and examined microscopically.
• *Ultrasound* will confirm a cystic lesion, and

may be helpful for guided aspiration of deep-seated cysts.

• *Mammogram*: a soft-tissue X-ray of the breast, which may reveal small carcinomas that typically show as an area of speckled calcification. It may also be helpful in reassuring the patient that a lesion is benign. Mammograms may reveal malignancies that are impalpable, but may mislead in some malignant lesions and infer a benign nature, and vice versa. Biopsy is the safest policy in any doubtful case.

Cyclical mastalgia

This describes breast pain and heaviness experienced a variable time before each period, and which generally declines with the onset of menstruation. It commonly presents in the mid-thirties, may be bilateral, and usually is felt in the upper outer quadrant of the breast. On examination the breasts are tender and engorged, with marked nodularity, particularly towards the axillary tail.

The aetiology of cyclical mastalgia is probably hormonal, with the engorgement being in part attributed to fluid retention. Treatment is difficult, and simple measures such as a firm supporting brassiere may help; essential fatty acids such as evening primrose oil, gonadotrophin antagonists (e.g. danazol) and dopamine agonists (e.g. bromocriptine) may all help. Tamoxifen, normally considered as an anti-tumour agent, has also been shown to decrease the pain at a low dose (10 mg/day).

Cyst formation

Cysts present as discrete lumps that may occur with a short history, and are often multiple and involve both breasts. In isolation, the lump may be perceived to be cancer by the patient, a fear that can be relieved by simple needle aspiration. The cysts represent aberrations of normal lobular change. They present in peri-menopausal women and may be painful. On palpation they are usually smooth and tense; occasionally, they may be fluctuant; if they develop deep within the breast, the normal consistency is masked. Needle aspiration reveals fluid that may be yellow, brown or green; blood-stained fluid is suspicious of malignancy. Simple cysts should disappear on aspiration. A blood-stained aspirate, the presence of a mass following aspiration and troublesome recurrence of the cyst (more than once) are indications for biopsy of the area.

Sclerosing adenosis

This may present as a firm, mobile breast lump, or as mastalgia. It affects women in the mid-thirties to the menopause. It is characterized by lobular enlargement with proliferation of small ductules and acini in a fibrous stroma on microscopy. In addition to causing a lump and pain, the lesion may also calcify and mimic carcinoma on mammography.

Duct ectasia

Duct ectasia, also called 'plasma-cell mastitis' and 'granulomatous mastitis', results from abnormal dilatation of large peri-areolar lactiferous ducts. The dilated ducts fill with secretions producing a stagnant collection of creamy or green material of toothpaste consistency. A chronic inflammatory response to this collection results, termed periductal mastitis, amongst which plasma cells are prominent (hence the old term plasma cell mastitis). The end result of the dilatation, stagnation and inflammatory response may be fibrosis, nipple retraction and nipple discharge. There may be recurrent breast abscesses, which are usually peri-areolar. The process is usually bilateral, but the cause of the dilatation in the first place is unclear.

Treatment of breast lumps

The golden rule is that 'no woman is allowed to have a lump in her breast without a diagnosis'.

Needle aspiration

A discrete lump that may be a cyst is subjected to immediate aspiration under local anaesthetic in the out-patient clinic. If clear fluid is obtained and the lump completely disappears, one can be certain that it is a simple cyst. The rare condition of a carcinoma in the wall of a cyst (cystadenocarcinoma) will yield blood-stained fluid on aspiration and a persistent lump can still be felt; urgent excision biopsy is then necessary. Cytology of the aspirate may also confirm malignancy.

Excision biopsy

If no fluid is obtained, or cytology is equivocal, a tissue diagnosis must be made. This is per-formed either by excision biopsy or by fine-needle aspiration and cytological examination. Should this prove to be an area of benign change, the patient is reassured and suitable follow-up arranged. If a fibroadenoma is confirmed, local excision is all that is necessary. If the biopsy proves to be a carcinoma, further treatment is discussed on page 290.

Mammography

The patients who are not submitted to surgery are the large group of women with diffuse granularity of one or, more usually, both breasts with no localized mass. A mammogram is helpful (see above), particularly in post-menopausal women, but usually the patient can be reassured that there is no evidence of malig-nant disease and kept under supervision in the out-patient clinic. Monthly self-examination can also be taught and the patient advised to report if she finds any discrete lump.

Tumours

Classification
Benign
- Fibroadenoma.
- Intraduct papilloma.

Malignant
1 *Primary:*
  (a) carcinoma;
  (b) intraduct carcinoma;
  (c) Paget's disease of the nipple;
  (d) fibrosarcoma.
2 *Secondary:*

  (a) direct invasion from tumours of the chest wall;
  (b) metastatic deposits from melanoma.

Fibroadenoma
Pathology
This is a firm, encapsulated, benign tumour with a whorled appearance on cut surface. Microscopically, it comprises fibrous tissue surrounding epithelial duct proliferation. Fibroadenomas represent aberrations of lobular development.

Clinical features
Fibroadenomas occur after the age of puberty, commonly in young women, and may be multiple. They are highly mobile 'breast mice' which are not attached to the skin. Rarely, in middle-aged or elderly women a very large lobular fibroadenoma (phylloides tumour) may be found, which may even ulcerate the overlying skin by pressure necrosis (serocystic disease of Brodie*). The majority of these remain benign, but a few may undergo sarcomatous change.

Treatment
Fine-needle aspiration cytology may confirm the diagnosis, but most women are best reas-sured by excision and histological confirmation of the diagnosis.

Duct papilloma
This is a result of hyperplasia of the duct epithelial lining. It may be part of a generalized hyperplasia (previously called papillomatosis or epitheliosis) or may occur as a solitary entity.

Generalized hyperplasia is associated with malignant change, and extreme examples are often termed ductal carcinoma-*in-situ*. Duct hyperplasia is the only form of benign breast disease that may predispose to malignancy.

A solitary duct papilloma is usually situated

---

*Sir Benjamin Brodie (1783–1862), Surgeon, St George's Hospital, London. He also described chronic abscess of bone.

in one of the 15–20 ducts near the nipple in a young woman. The patient complains of bleeding from the nipple and the examiner may either find a small elliptical swelling adjacent to the nipple, pressure on which produces this discharge, or that merely pressure on one spot causes blood to emerge from the mouth of the duct.

An X-ray 'ductogram' may define the lesion.

Treatment
The lump should be excised with, of course, histological examination of the specimen, or, if no lump can be felt, excision of the small segment of breast tissue from which the discharge can be expressed.

Carcinoma
This is an immensely important subject — the commonest malignant disease of women in the Western world, with 30 000 new cases and about 15 000 deaths annually in the UK; 1 in 9 women will develop breast cancer during their life. Any age may be affected, but it is rare below the age of 30 years.

Aetiology
There is an increased incidence of breast cancer with age. In addition there are several proven risk factors, and several other factors that are thought to be associated with increased risk but where the evidence is equivocal. The following are identified risk factors.

Genetic factors
• *Family history*: two- to threefold increased incidence in first-degree relatives.
• *Gene carriage*: the genes BRCA1 and BRCA2 have been identified as significant risk factors. BRCA1 carriage (1 in 300 women) gives an 85% chance of developing breast cancer by the age of 80 years; many of the tumours occur in young women.
• *Previous breast cancer*: there is an increased risk of developing a second (metachronous) cancer, perhaps reflecting a field change.

Hormonal factors
Increased exposure to oestrogens is a significant risk factor.
• *Sex*: females are 100 times more likely to have a breast carcinoma than men.
• *Menarche and menopause*: early age at menarche (11 years and under) and late menopause (51 years and over) are associated with a higher risk.
• *Parity*: nulliparous women have higher risk than multiparous women; later age at first pregnancy increases risk compared with younger age.
• *Exogenous steroids*: oral contraceptive pill and hormone-replacement therapy may slightly increase the incidence of breast cancer, particularly if taken for more than 8 years and with high oestrogen preparations.

Other factors
High socio-economic status, heavy alcohol intake and previous colonic or ovarian carcinomas are also risk factors.

Only duct hyperplasia (epitheliosis, papillomatosis), of all the benign breast diseases, is associated with an increased risk of carcinoma.

Pathology
Clinical and macroscopic types
• *Scirrhous (75%)*: stellate, hard and encapsulated; the cut surface is grey, concave, gritty and with white spots, resembling an unripe pear.
• *Atrophic scirrhous*: scar-like tumour occurring in the shrivelled breast of the elderly.
• *Papillary*: intraduct or intracystic.
• *Inflammatory*: a fulminating form, sometimes occurring in or after pregnancy ('mastitis carcinomatosa'), characterized by dermal lymphatic involvement resulting in erythema and a peau d'orange appearance.
• *Paget's disease of the nipple* (see p. 291).

Microscopic classification
The classification of malignant breast disease has seen as many changes in terminology as

that of benign breast disease. The importance of any terminology is to be able to identify any types of specific prognostic or therapeutic importance. Breast carcinoma may be either derived from ductal (90%) or lobular (10%) epithelium. Pre-invasive *in situ* forms of each exist, but the majority are invasive.

1 Duct carcinoma.

(a) *Invasive duct carcinoma* (non-specific): the majority of duct carcinomas have no specific histological features.

(b) *Medullary carcinoma* (5%): well-circumscribed tumour often with a pseudo-capsule. There is typically a prominent lymphocytic infiltrate, a host response that probably accounts for the slightly better prognosis of this type of duct carcinoma.

(c) *Tubular carcinoma* (3%): a well-differentiated cancer characterized by the presence of tubular structures. It is similar in appearance to sclerosing adenosis, both histologically and on mammography. It has a much better prognosis, with a 10-year survival of around 75%, and distant metastases are uncommon.

(d) *Mucoid (or colloid) carcinoma (3%):* excessive mucus production is a feature; it also has a relatively good prognosis.

(e) *Papillary carcinoma (2%):* usually well-circumscribed with characteristic papillary formation; invasion across the basement membrane distinguishes it from the *in situ* form.

(f) *Paget's disease:* intra-epithelial neoplasia with underlying duct carcinoma.

2 Lobular carcinoma.

(a) *Invasive lobular carcinoma:* characterized by small monotonous cell pattern, sometimes in Indian file and sometimes arranged like targets in concentric circles.

(b) *Lobular carcinoma-in-situ:* a pre-malignant condition, often present in both breasts.

Spread

Direct extension. Involvement of skin and subcutaneous tissues leads to skin dimpling,

retraction of the nipple and eventually ulceration. Extension deeply involves pectoralis major, serratus anterior and eventually the chest wall.

Lymphatic. Blockage of dermal lymphatics leads to cutaneous oedema pitted by the orifices of the sweat ducts, giving the appearance of peau d'orange. Dermal lymphatic invasion produces daughter skin nodules and eventually 'cancer *en cuirasse*', the whole chest wall becoming a firm mass of tumour tissue. The main lymph channels pass directly to the axillary and internal thoracic lymph nodes (Fig. 35.1). Later, spread occurs to the supraclavicular, abdominal, mediastinal, groin and opposite axillary nodes.

Blood stream. Blood-borne spread is most commonly to lungs, liver and bones (at the sites of red bone marrow, i.e. skull, vertebrae, pelvis, ribs, sternum, upper end of femur and upper end of humerus). The brain, ovaries and suprarenals are also frequent foci of deposits.

Trans-coelomic. Pleural and peritoneal seeding occurs commonly in advanced disease, accompanied by pleural effusion and ascites respectively.

Staging

Manchester staging. The following clinical staging is in common use (Fig. 35.2).

I The lump is confined to the breast, with or without some degree of skin fixation to it or with indrawing of the nipple.

II As above, but in addition the axillary lymph nodes are enlarged and quite mobile.

III The tumour and/or the nodes are fixed superficially and/or deeply.

IV Distant metastases are present.

There is a high degree of clinical error, about 25% in fact, in estimating whether a tumour is stage I or II — axillary lymph nodes may be involved, although they cannot be felt; conversely axillary nodes that are palpable

LYMPHATIC DRAINAGE

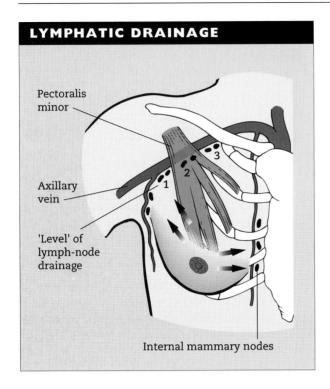

Pectoralis minor

Axillary vein

'Level' of lymph-node drainage

Internal mammary nodes

Fig. 35.1 The lymphatic drainage of the breast.

may prove free from tumour. However, the classification is of great practical importance, as patients with stage I and II lesions are usually submitted to 'curative' surgery, whereas those in stages III and IV are only suitable for palliative treatment (see section on treatment below).

Clinical features

The patient may present with local symptoms, usually a painless lump in the breast (although occasionally she may complain of a pricking discomfort). Sometimes the principal complaint is of recent indrawing of the nipple or of blood-stained discharge. In addition, a small percentage of patients present with symptoms produced by secondaries, e.g. backache, pathological fracture, or dyspnoea from lung and pleural involvement.

Examination of a patient with a lump in the breast must be carried out in an orderly manner, as follows.

Inspection

The breasts are inspected for evidence of nipple elevation or retraction, or of skin fixation to the underlying tumour; the latter is then checked by gently moving the lump within the breast. Recent nipple retraction is very suggestive of malignant disease, but the nipple may have been indrawn since birth or following a previous acute infection. Skin fixation is also strong supporting evidence of carcinoma, although it may be seen rarely over an area of fibroadenosis and may accompany fat necrosis or follow chronic abscess.

Palpation

Palpation commences first with the normal breast. The diseased breast is then examined, the clinical features of the lump being determined with particular reference to skin attachment and deep fixation. The axillary nodes and then all the other lymph node areas are palpated. A search is made of the other foci of

BREAST CANCER

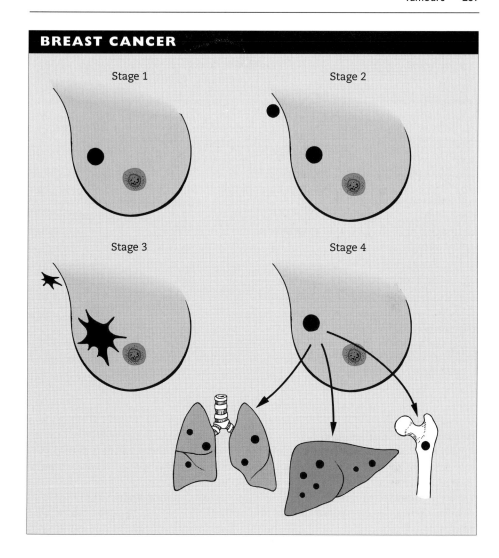

Stage 1

Stage 2

Stage 3

Stage 4

Fig. 35.2 The clinical staging of breast cancer.

possible distant spread; examine the chest, palpate the liver, test for the presence of ascites and examine the pelvis.

Special investigations
Diagnostic investigations
Confirmation of the diagnosis may be achieved by a combination of the following.
• *Mammography*: characteristic appearances

are of a dense opacity with an irregular outline, spiculations radiating from its centre, micro-calcification (like grains of salt) in the centre and skin tethering.
• *Fine-needle aspiration*: to distinguish solid from cystic, and cytological examination to confirm malignancy.
• *Needle core biopsy* (e.g. Tru-Cut): may be performed under local anaesthetic in the clinic. Histological diagnosis prior to surgery avoids the need for intraoperative frozen section, and allows the patient to be fully informed prior to surgery.

• *Excision biopsy*: remains the gold standard, and should be combined with 'sampling' of the ipsilateral axillary lymph nodes.

Staging investigations

To seek secondary deposits.
• *Chest X-ray*.
• *Bone scan*.
• *Liver ultrasound*.
• *Full blood count*: anaemia and leucopenia suggest widespread bone-marrow involvement.

Treatment

One of the biggest changes in surgery in the last 30 years has been the realization that the results from relatively conservative surgery are as good as the results achieved by the mutilating surgery advocated by Halsted.* Halsted believed that tumours spread by permeation through surrounding tissue. By widely excising breast tissue, including removal of the pectoral muscles, cure could be achieved. However, in breast cancer, spread probably occurs by microembolization, and in many cases treated by radical mastectomy microscopic metastases will already have occurred; evidence of dissemination may become manifest months or years after the primary tumour has been removed. More recently, the controversy regarding the optimal treatment has subsided with the advent of properly conducted prospective randomized clinical trials.

Stages I and II

When the disease is clinically confined to the breast tissue alone or has only involved the axillary lymph nodes with no evidence of either spread into adjacent tissues, or of widespread dissemination, the surgeon hopes to be able to eradicate the disease and achieve a 'cure'.

Current opinion favours a relatively conservative approach. Most surgeons perform either a wide local excision of the tumour ('lumpectomy'), with a 1-cm margin, together with axil-

*William Stewart Halsted (1852–1922), Professor of Surgery at Johns Hopkins, Baltimore, USA.

lary lymph node sampling (at least four nodes) or clearance. Post-operative radiotherapy is given. If the excision margins are involved, a further excision, or simple mastectomy is performed.

The other treatment option is simple mastectomy, although this is more mutilating. Radiotherapy is given if the nodes are involved.

Because of the relatively poor prognosis in advanced stage II disease (those with extensive lymph node involvement), suggesting that in 60% of these patients occult dissemination of tumour has already occurred at the time of presentation, there is particular interest in the trials in progress on the value of adjuvant cytotoxic or hormonal therapy in this group.

Stage III cases

Surgical clearance of the disease is now impossible. Local radiotherapy often produces useful palliative results, although a 'toilet' operation is often required to remove a fungating and ulcerating local lesion.

Stage IV and recurrences after previous mastectomy

A solitary distant deposit, e.g. in one bone, or local recurrence in the scar following mastectomy, is best treated by local radiotherapy.

Topical injection of a cytotoxic may be used in the treatment of malignant ascites or pleural effusion after preliminary aspiration of the fluid.

Adjuvant therapy

Where dissemination is widespread or suspected, adjuvant therapy is used. This involves the use of anti-oestrogen therapy (e.g. tamoxifen). About 30% of all breast tumours are hormone dependent. The tumour oestrogen receptor (ER) assay, at present only performed at special referral centres, is helpful in predicting the likelihood of response. ER-positive tumours respond to hormone therapy in 60% of cases, whereas ER-negative tumours are rarely hormone dependent (10%).

There are several methods of hormone therapy available. Tamoxifen, a potent anti-oestrogen, has a low incidence of side-effects and should be the first line of treatment in both pre- and post-menopausal patients.

For patients who do not respond to tamoxifen the following should be instituted.

- *Pre-menopausal or early post-menopausal*: ovarian ablation, either by oöphorectomy or radiotherapy.
- *Post-menopausal women*: either stilboestrol or ethinyl oestradiol.
- *'Pharmacological adrenalectomy'*, by means of aminoglutethimide, which inhibits synthesis of cortisol and suprarenal androgen and oestrogen. This has replaced bilateral adrenalectomy and hypophysectomy.

In patients with widespread disease not responding to hormone therapy, temporary regression may be effected by means of cytotoxic drugs, particularly in the form of combination therapy.

Pregnancy and breast cancer

Fortunately, carcinoma of the breast occurs rarely during pregnancy and lactation. The disease process, presumably because of hormonal effects, may be considerably accelerated, often with the appearance of an inflammatory type of lesion, the so-called mastitis carcinomatosa. In most cases, however, the tumour behaves like a cancer of the same stage in a non-pregnant woman.

Although the prognosis is serious it is not necessarily hopeless. Treatment is carried out along the lines already indicated according to the stage at which the disease presents. Most surgeons advise termination of the pregnancy in the first trimester, but later pregnancies are allowed to run to term after which adjuvant radiotherapy and chemotherapy may be administered.

Prognosis

The 5-year survival rate in stage I tumours is approximately 80%, but only 50% at 10 years. Stage II lesions have a 5-year survival rate of approximately 50%. A small number of stage III and IV growths may also have prolonged survival, especially if slow growing or hormonally dependent.

In addition to the staging of the tumour, histological grading is also of great importance; the less differentiated the tumour, the worse the prognosis.

Carcinoma of the male breast

This accounts for fewer than 1% of all cases of breast cancer. In men, breast cancer affects an older age group, with a peak incidence at 60 years.

Clinically, it usually presents as a firm, painless subareolar lump, although gynaecomastia, breast tenderness and nipple discharge may also be present. Microscopically, it is usually a ductal carcinoma, and is quite advanced at presentation.

Treatment consists an extended mastectomy with lymph node sampling. As so little skin is available it is often necessary to carry out a skin graft to the cover the resulting cutaneous defect. For *in situ* disease simple mastectomy will suffice.

The prognosis is worse than in the female, probably because of the sparse amount of breast tissue present, which allows rapid dissemination of the growth into the regional lymphatics.

Post-operative radiotherapy reduces the incidence of local recurrence, but does not affect overall survival; most tumours respond to tamoxifen, which is therefore given as adjuvant therapy. For advanced disseminated disease, chemotherapy can produce reasonable palliation.

Paget's disease of the nipple

Paget* described diseases of bone, penis and nipple, all of which bear his name.

---

*Sir James Paget (1814–99), Surgeon, St Bartholomew's Hospital, London. He also described disease of bone and penis, and discovered the parasite of trichinosis in humans while a first-year medical student.

Pathology

The nipple lesion occurs in middle-aged and elderly women. It presents as a unilateral red, bleeding, eczematous lesion of the nipple, which is eventually destroyed. It is associated with a carcinoma of the underlying breast, which may or may not form a palpable mass.

Microscopic appearance

The epithelium of the nipple is thickened with prolongations of the rete pegs. The deeper layers of the epithelium contain multiple clear Paget cells with small dark-staining nuclei; these are hydropic malignant cells. The underlying dermis contains an inflammatory cellular infiltration.

Careful search of the breast after mastectomy usually reveals the presence of an associated intraduct carcinoma, often at some distance from the nipple, even if this was clinically impalpable.

Aetiology

Paget's disease probably represents the invasion of the nipple by malignant cells arising in a duct that also gave origin to the associated breast tumour.

Treatment

Mastectomy or local excision are required with post-operative radiotherapy. In the absence of a palpable mass the prognosis is excellent. When a mass is present the prognosis resembles carcinoma of the breast in general and depends on the stage of the tumour and its histological grade.

Breast screening

Because micrometastases are frequently present when only a small lump can be detected by palpation, much effort has been devoted to discover breast cancer before there is a lump. A nationwide mammography breast screening is now in progress in the UK. All women between 50 and 65 years of age are offered mammography every 3 years. A suspicious lesion on X-ray that cannot be felt has to be localized by three-dimensional radiography and a wire inserted into the radiologically abnormal tissue so that the surgeon can remove the area by local excision and confirm that the specimen is the correct portion of breast by repeat X-ray of the specimen. Histological examination of the specimen will establish the diagnosis. If carcinoma is found, management is as for stage I tumours outlined above. Early data from screen trials indicate a pickup of one suspicious mammogram in 1000 and of these selected cases 50% are malignant. It is hoped that this early detection will be rewarded by a significant improvement in survival and that the expensive screening process does not in itself cause harm from the radiation exposure.

CHAPTER 36

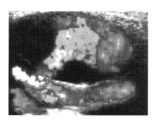

The Neck

The thyroid gland is considered separately in Chapter 37, and the parathyroids in Chapter 38.

Branchial cyst and sinus

Anatomy

There are six arches and five clefts in the branchial system. The first arch forms the lower face, its external cleft the external auditory meatus, and its internal cleft the Eustachian tube. The second arch grows down over the third and fourth arches to form the skin of the neck. Normally there is no external cleft, while the internal cleft forms the tonsillar fossa.

Aetiology

Persistence of remnants of the second branchial arch may lead to formation of a branchial cyst, sinus or fistula. The external cleft remnants open just anterior to the sternocleidomastoid, at the junction of the upper one-third and lower two-thirds. A sinus or fistula represent a patent second branchial arch sinus, which passes between internal and external carotid artery to the tonsillar fossa.

Clinical features

The *branchial cyst* usually presents in early adult life and forms a soft swelling 'like a half-filled hot water bottle', which bulges forward from beneath the anterior border of the sternocleidomastoid. It is lined by squamous epithelium and contains pus-like material, which is in fact cholesterol. It often presents following an upper respiratory tract infection. Clinical diagnosis can be clinched by aspirating a few drops of this fluid from the cyst and demonstrating cholesterol crystals under the microscope. Occasionally, the cyst may become infected.

Differential diagnosis is from a tuberculous gland of neck or from an acute lymphadenitis.

The rare *first branchial arch cyst* may present just below the external auditory meatus at the angle of the jaw, with extension closely related to the VII nerve.

The *branchial sinus* presents as a small orifice, discharging mucus, which opens over the anterior border of sternocleidomastoid in the lower part of the neck. The majority are present at birth but a secondary branchial sinus may form if an infected branchial cyst ruptures. The sinus extends upwards between the internal and external carotid arteries to the side wall of the pharynx. It may open into the tonsillar fossa (which represents the second internal cleft) to form a branchial fistula.

Treatment

Surgical excision is required.

A LUMP IN THE SIDE OF THE NECK

When considering the swellings that may arise in any anatomical region, one enumerates the anatomical structures lying therein and then the pathological swellings that may arise from them. The side of the neck is an excellent example of this exercise.

Skin and superficial fascia
• Sebaceous cyst.
• Lipoma.

Lymph nodes
• Infective.
• Malignant.
• The lymphomas, lymphatic leukaemia (see p. 277).

Lymphatics
• Cystic hygroma.

Artery
• Carotid body tumour.
• Carotid artery aneurysm.

Salivary glands
• Submandibular salivary tumours or sialectasis.
• Tumours in the lower pole of the parotid gland.

Pharynx
• Pharyngeal pouch.

Branchial arch remnant
• Branchial cyst.

Tuberculous cervical adenitis

With a general decline in tuberculosis, this once common lesion (mainly of children) is now relatively rarely seen in this country, except in the aged, sufferers from acquired immune deficiency syndrome (AIDS) and in immigrants from Asia. Cervical nodes are usually secondarily involved from a tonsillar primary focus, although the adenoids or even the dental roots may occasionally be the primary source of infection. The organisms may be human or bovine and occasionally the disease is secondary to active pulmonary infection. The upper jugular chain of nodes is most commonly affected.

Clinical features
At first the nodes are small and discrete; then, as they enlarge, they become matted together, caseate, and the abscess so formed eventually bursts through the deep fascia into the subcutaneous tissues, producing a 'collar stud' abscess. Left untreated, this discharges onto the skin, resulting in a chronic tuberculous sinus.

Differential diagnosis
Solid nodes must be differentiated from acute lymphadenitis, one of the lymphomas or secondary deposits. The breaking-down abscess must be differentiated from a branchial cyst (see above).

Diagnosis is assisted by an X-ray of the neck; usually the chronic tuberculous nodes show flecks of calcification.

Treatment
A full course of anti-tuberculous chemotherapy is given. Small nodes are treated conservatively and the patient is kept under observation. If the nodes enlarge, e.g. 1 cm or more in diameter, they should be excised. If the patient presents with a 'collar stud' abscess, the pus is evacuated, a search made for the hole penetrating through the deep fascia and the underlying caseating gland evacuated by curettage.

It is not usually necessary to treat the infected tonsils or adenoids, as the infection resolves with the chemotherapy.

Carotid body tumour (chemodectoma)

Pathology
A slow-growing tumour that arises from the chemoreceptor cells in the carotid body at the

carotid bifurcation. Most behave in a benign fashion; in a few patients the tumour becomes locally invasive and may metastasize. There is a familial tendency to development of the tumour.

Macroscopically, it is a lobulated, yellowish tumour closely adherent to the major arterial trunks.

Microscopically, it is made up of large chromaffin polyhedral cells in a vascular fibrous stroma.

Clinical features

The tumour presents as a slowly enlarging mass in a patient over the age of 30 years, which transmits the carotid pulsation. The mass itself may be so highly vascular that it too demonstrates pulsation with a bruit on auscultation. Occasionally, pressure on the carotid sinus from the tumour produces attacks of faintness. Extension of the tumour may lead to cranial nerve palsies (VII, IX, X, XI and XII), resulting in dysphagia and hoarseness.

Special investigations

• *Duplex ultrasound* gives precise localization of the tumour and its relation to the carotid and its bifurcation.
• *Arteriography* shows the carotid bifurcation to be splayed open by the mass and the rich vascularity of the tumour is demonstrated.
• *Magnetic resonance imaging and computed tomography scanning* show the tumour and its relation to the carotid artery.

Treatment

It is often possible to dissect the tumour away from the carotid sheath. If the carotid vessels are firmly involved, resection can be performed with graft replacement of the artery.

In the elderly, these slow-growing tumours can be left untreated.

CHAPTER 37

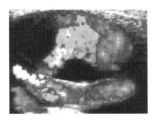

The Thyroid

Congenital anomalies

Embryology

The thyroid gland forms as a diverticulum originating in the floor of the pharynx, and descends through the tongue, past the hyoid, to its position in the neck. The diverticulum usually closes, leaving a pit at the base of the tongue (the foramen caecum, which lies in the midline at the junction of the anterior two-thirds and the posterior third of the tongue). Failure of the thyroid to descend or incomplete descent of the track may result in ectopic thyroid tissue (Fig. 37.1). Incomplete obliteration of the track may result in fistula or sinus formation. In all cases of unexplained midline nodules in the neck, thyroid tissue should be suspected. A radio-iodine scan should be performed to ensure that there is normal thyroid tissue present in the correct place before the lump is removed.

Lingual thyroid

Rarely, the thyroid fails to descend into the neck. Such a patient presents with a lump at the foramen caecum of the tongue. This is termed a lingual thyroid, and may represent the sum total of thyroid tissue, or may be a remnant that failed to descend. If such a swelling is removed, the patient may have no other functioning thyroid tissue.

Thyroglossal cyst

A thyroglossal cyst forms in the embryological remnants of the thyroid and presents as a fluctuant swelling in the midline of the neck. It is diagnosed by its characteristic physical signs: it moves upwards when the patient protrudes the tongue (because of its attachment to the tract of the thyroid descent), and also moves on swallowing (because of its attachment to the larynx by the pretracheal fascia).

Treatment

Such cysts should be removed surgically, together with remnants of the thyroglossal tract and the body of the hyoid bone.

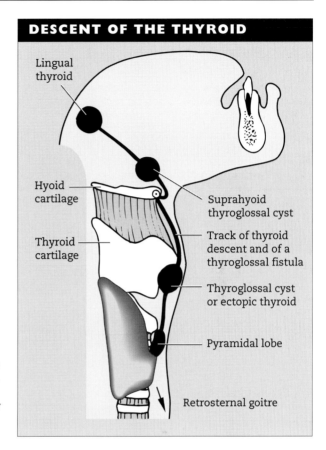

DESCENT OF THE THYROID

Lingual thyroid

Hyoid cartilage

Thyroid cartilage

Suprahyoid thyroglossal cyst

Track of thyroid descent and of a thyroglossal fistula

Thyroglossal cyst or ectopic thyroid

Pyramidal lobe

Retrosternal goitre

Fig. 37.1 The descent of the thyroid, showing possible sites of ectopic thyroid tissue or thyroglossal cysts, and also the course of a thyroglossal fistula. (The arrow shows the further descent of the thyroid that may take place retrosternally into the superior mediastinum.)

Thyroglossal fistula

This presents as an opening onto the skin in the line of the thyroid descent, in the midline of the neck. It may discharge thin, glairy fluid and attacks of infection can occur.

Treatment

The treatment is to excise the fistula, and this excision must be complete. The track runs in close relationship to the body of the hyoid, therefore this should be removed in addition to the fistula; dissection is continued up to the region of the foramen caecum of the tongue.

Thyroid physiology

The thyroid gland is concerned with the syn-

thesis of the iodine-containing hormones thyroxine (tetra-iodothyronine, T4) and tri-iodothyronine (T3), which control the metabolic rate of the body; T3 is the active hormone, and T4 is converted to T3 in the periphery. The thyroid gland also secretes calcitonin from the parafollicular C cells, which reduces the level of serum calcium and is therefore antagonistic to parathormone.

Iodine in the diet is absorbed into the blood stream as iodide, which is taken up by the thyroid gland. After entering the follicle, the iodide is converted into organic iodine, which is then bound with the tyrosine radicals of thyroglobulin to form the precursors of the thyroid hormones. The colloid within the thyroid vesicles is composed of thyroglobulin, synthesized in the follicular cells, and T3 and T4.

These hormones are released into the blood stream after being separated from thyroglobulin within the follicular cells. In the general circulation, about 99% of T3 and T4 is bound to protein and it is the minute amount of unbound 'free' thyroid hormones in the circulating blood that produces the endocrine effects of the thyroid gland.

Physiological control of secretion

The immediate control of synthesis and liberation of T3 and T4 is by thyroid-stimulating hormone (TSH) produced by the anterior pituitary. TSH is secreted in response to the level of thyroid hormones in the blood by a negative-feedback mechanism. The secretion of TSH is also under the influence of the hypothalamic thyrotrophin-releasing hormone (TRH).

Pharmacological control of secretion

The production of thyroid hormones can be inhibited by the thiouracils and carbimazole, which block the binding of iodine but do not interfere with the uptake of iodide by the gland. Although less T3 and T4 are produced, the thyroid gland tends to become large and vascular with treatment by these drugs.

High doses of iodide given to patients with excessive thyroid hormone production result in an increase in the amount of iodine-rich colloid, and a diminished liberation of thyroid hormones; the gland also becomes less vascular. The effects of iodide treatment are maximal after 2 weeks of treatment and then diminish.

Lack of iodine in the diet prevents the formation of thyroid hormones, and excess pituitary TSH is produced, which may result in an iodine-deficient goitre. Thiocyanates prevent the thyroid gland from taking up iodide.

Pathology of goitre

A goitre is synonymous with an enlargement of the thyroid gland, and by itself the word conveys no information about the nature of the enlargement.

Nodular goitre

Like the breast, ovary and prostate, the thyroid gland undergoes periods of activity and regression at different times. There is excessive thyroid activity at puberty and during pregnancy (producing a 'physiological' goitre) and a fall in activity after the menopause. The commonest cause of enlargement of the thyroid gland in the UK is a nodular goitre, and this has similarities with the commonest pathological conditions of the breast and prostate, namely fibroadenosis and benign hyperplasia. In a nodular goitre, the gland is enlarged, irregular and partly cystic.

There is an excessive degree of activity and regression resulting in a varied appearance of the gland. Some vesicles are lined with hyperactive epithelium and others with flattened atrophic cells. Some contain no colloid, others an excessive amount. The thyroid interstitium is excessive with a certain amount of fibrosis and mononuclear cell infiltration. Nodular goitres may produce a normal amount of T4, but sometimes excessive T4 production results in hyperthyroidism in this condition ('secondary thyrotoxicosis').

Complications

• Tracheal displacement or compression.
• Haemorrhage into a cyst (which may produce urgent tracheal compression).
• Toxic change.
• Malignant change (rare).

Colloid goitre (endemic goitre)

All diseases of the thyroid are commoner in geographical locations in which the water and diet are low in iodine. In the UK the most notorious district was Derbyshire and the frequency of goitres in this region gave rise to the term 'Derbyshire neck'. Iodination of table salt has all but abolished this state of affairs. Switzerland, Nepal, Ethiopia and Peru are also areas where natural iodine is very scarce in the diet and water, and thyroid disease is common.

The commonest lesion of the thyroid gland due to iodine deficiency is the colloid goitre in which the gland is enlarged and the acini are atrophic with a large amount of colloid. As has been mentioned, this accumulation of colloid is probably due to over-secretion of TSH from the anterior pituitary, acting on the thyroid, which is unable to produce T4.

Hyperplasia

In primary Graves' disease the thyroid is uniformly enlarged and there is hyperactivity of the acinar cells with reduplication and infolding of the epithelium. The gland is very vascular and there is little colloid to be seen. Lymphocyte infiltration is usually a predominant feature.

Clinical features in thyroid disease

Patients may present complaining of a lump in the neck and/or with symptoms due to excessive or diminished amounts of circulating T4.

The thyroid swelling

The characteristics of an enlarged thyroid are a mass in the neck on one or both sides of the trachea, which moves on swallowing, since it is attached to the larynx by the pre-tracheal fascia. The draining lymph nodes lie adjacent in the anterior triangle of the neck.

Retrosternal goitre

Evidence of retrosternal enlargement of the thyroid should be sought by palpation with the neck fully extended. A retrosternal thyroid can block the venous return to the superior vena cava and result in engorgement of the jugular veins and their tributaries and in oedema of the upper part of the body—a cause of the superior mediastinal syndrome. In such cases, X-rays of the thoracic inlet should be taken; the enlarged thyroid will be shown as a radio-opaque mass in the retrosternal position.

Tracheal displacement

The trachea should be examined to determine displacement or compression by the thyroid enlargement; the patient should be asked to take a deep breath, when stridor may become apparent.

Vocal cord integrity

The vocal cords should be examined by indirect laryngoscopy, as thyroid carcinoma may infiltrate the recurrent laryngeal nerves causing vocal cord paralysis. If surgery is contemplated it is important to know whether or not the cords are functioning normally before operation.

Hyperthyroidism

Clinical features of hyperthyroidism are determined by examination of the eyes and the hands, as well as from the history and examination of the neck. T4 potentiates the actions of adrenaline, and many of the features of hyperthyroidism represent increased activity of the sympathetic nervous system.

History

The patient is irritable and nervous, and cannot keep still. The appetite is increased and yet there is a loss of weight. Diarrhoea is occasionally a feature. The patient prefers cold environments rather than warm. Palpitations due to tachycardia or atrial fibrillation may occur.

Examination
The thyroid gland

This is usually smoothly enlarged but not invariably so. It may be highly vascular and demonstrate a bruit and thrill.

The eyes

A number of eye signs are present in thyrotoxicosis.

• *Exophthalmos* is present in most patients with thyrotoxicosis of Graves' disease, due to oedema and infiltration of mononuclear cells of the orbital fat and extrinsic muscles of the eye.

• *Lid retraction*: the innervation of the levator palpebrae superioris is partly under sympathetic control. In thyrotoxicosis it is tonically active, retracting the upper lid, giving the appearance that the patient is staring.

• *Lid lag*: ask the patient to follow your finger as you move it from over the head downwards — the upper lid does not immediately drop, revealing the white sclera above the cornea.

• *Dilated pupils* due to sympathetic pupil dilator tone.

• *Double vision* following the examiner's finger to the upper outer quadrant. This is due to infiltration of the extrinsic muscles of the eye causing exophthalmic ophthalmoplegia.

The hands

• *Sweating*: the hands are warm and moist.

• *Tachycardia*: a rapid pulse is almost invariable and typically the sleeping pulse is also raised. There may be atrial fibrillation and indeed the patient may present with heart failure.

• *Onycholysis*: the nail lifts off the nail bed, a condition also seen in psoriasis and with some fungal infections.

• *Finger clubbing*, more accurately termed thyroid acropathy.

• *Fine tremor* of the outstretched hands is present and reflects the increased sympathetic activity.

The simplest and most reliable clinical test of hyperthyroidism is the *sleeping pulse rate*: the greatest difficulty in the clinical diagnosis of hyperthyroidism is its differentiation from an acute anxiety state. However, such patients when sleeping will have a normal pulse rate, whereas in patients with hyperthyroidism the sleeping pulse will remain elevated.

The exophthalmos is an extremely distressing condition for the patient and, if severe, the patient is unable to close the eyelids; the eyes are then liable to corneal ulceration and eventual blindness. This condition is difficult to treat, but may respond to high-dosage corticosteroids; surgical decompression of the orbit with suture of the eyelids across the eyeball (tarsorrhaphy) may be required.

A rare clinical feature of hyperthyroidism is thickening of the subcutaneous tissues in front of the tibia, the so-called '*pre-tibial myxoedema*'.

Aetiology

Patients with hyperthyroidism fall into two groups, primary (Graves' disease[*]) and secondary.

Primary hyperthyroidism (Graves' disease)

This occurs usually in young women with no preceding history of goitre. The gland is smoothly enlarged and exophthalmos is a common feature. Symptoms are primarily those of irritability and tremor; exophthalmos and ophthalmoplegia are often quite marked. Primary hyperthyroidism is due to the action of stimulatory autoantibodies directed at the thyroid gland and mimicking the action of TSH; one such antibody is the 'long-acting thyroid stimulator' (LATS).

Secondary hyperthyroidism

Secondary hyperthyroidism is over-activity developing in an already diseased and hyperplastic gland. It is a disease of middle-age, occurring in patients with a pre-existing non-toxic goitre. The gland is nodular and there are no eye changes. Symptoms fall more on the cardiovascular system, the patient often presenting in heart failure with atrial fibrillation, although nervousness, irritability and tremor may also be present.

Hypothyroidism

Congenital hypothyroidism

Congenital hypothyroidism or cretinism is a condition in which the child is born with little or no functioning thyroid. The infant is stunted and mentally defective, with puffy lips, a large tongue and protuberant abdomen, often surmounted by an umbilical hernia.

Adult hypothyroidism

In adults, hypothyroidism (or myxoedema)

[*]Robert Graves (1796–1863), Physician, Meath Hospital, Dublin, Ireland.

usually affects women, and most often occurs in the middle-aged or elderly. These patients have a slow, deep voice and are usually overweight and apathetic, with a dry, coarse skin and thin hair, especially in the lateral third of the eyebrows. In contrast with hyperthyroidism, myxoedematous patients usually feel cold in hot weather, have a bradycardia and are constipated. They are often anaemic and may suffer from heart failure due to myxoedematous infiltration of the heart.

Investigations in thyroid disease

• *Serum free T4 and free T3.* Measurement of the biologically active unbound fraction is more accurate than measurement of total T3 and T4; elevation suggests hyperthyroidism.
• *TSH level*: raised in myxoedema; suppressed in hyperthyroidism, the gland secreting T4 autonomously.
• *Thyroid scintogram*: radio-iodine studies of the thyroid gland provide very useful information. A small tracer dose of γ-ray emitting ^{131}I is injected intravenously and the gland scanned with a γ-ray detector to map areas of high uptake reflecting high activity. A nodule in the thyroid gland that is hyperactive can be pinpointed by this method, a so-called '*hot nodule*'. Similarly, a nodule that is not producing T4 will not take up the radio-iodine, e.g. a cyst or tumour ('*cold nodule*').
• *Thyroid antibodies*, against the globulin or microsomal components of the gland, indicate an autoimmune pathology such as Hashimoto's thyroiditis, or Graves' disease.
• *Ultrasound* gives valuable information as to whether a mass is solid or cystic.
• *Fine-needle aspiration* allows material to be obtained for cytological examination. It is now the principal investigation for all solitary nodules, often under ultrasound guidance.
• *Serum cholesterol* is usually raised in myxoedema and may be normal or a little low in hyperthyroidism.
• *Electrocardiogram (ECG)*: in myxoedema cardiac involvement will show low electrical activity with small complexes. Atrial fibrillation complicating hyperthyroidism will be confirmed.

Clinical classification of thyroid swellings

The clinical assessment of a patient with a thyroid swelling has two components.
1 *The physical characteristics of the gland itself.* Is it smoothly enlarged? Is there a single nodule present? Is it multinodular?
2 *The endocrine state of the patient.* Is the patient euthyroid, hyperthyroid or hypothyroid?
    A synthesis of these two observations gives a simple clinical classification of the vast majority of thyroid swellings, as follows:
• *Smooth, euthyroid enlargement of the thyroid gland*: this is the 'physiological' goitre, which tends to occur at puberty and pregnancy.
• *Nodular, euthyroid gland*: this is the common nodular goitre, there being either a solitary nodule or multiple nodules.
• *Smooth, toxic goitre*: primary hyperthyroidism or Graves' disease.
• *Nodular toxic goitre*: secondary hyperthyroidism.
The less common findings are as follows:
• *Smooth, firm enlargement with myxoedema*: Hashimoto's disease (p. 306). Usually in a middle-aged woman, and the gland is sometimes asymmetrical and irregular.
• *Invasive enlargement, hard*: carcinoma
Riedel's thyroiditis and acute thyroiditis are uncommon (p. 306).

Outline of treatment of goitre

Euthyroid nodular enlargement
Multinodular goitre
Thyroidectomy is advised in patients with an enlarged, non-toxic, nodular goitre when there are symptoms of tracheal compression and dyspnoea. In addition, in younger patients, it is reasonable to advise operation because of the

danger of haemorrhage into a thyroid cyst with the risks of acute tracheal compression, and because of the small risk of toxic or malignant change in the gland. The patient may also be concerned with the cosmetic appearance of the swollen neck.

In elderly patients with a long-standing goitre that is symptomless, it is good practice to leave well alone.

T4 replacement may be effective by reducing TSH secretion, and so suppressing further enlargement. It should also be given following thyroidectomy to suppress enlargement of the remaining gland tissue.

Single euthyroid nodule
In the patient with a single nodule in the thyroid this may be a solitary benign adenoma, a malignant tumour, or most likely of all, a cyst in a thyroid showing the histological changes of a nodular goitre. Half of all solitary nodules are in fact prominent areas of multinodular goitres.

Traditionally, all solitary nodules were excised to make a diagnosis. Nowadays, fine-needle aspiration combined with isotope and ultrasound scans can usually differentiate nodules that should be excised from benign cysts. Cysts are aspirated, and checked at an interval to ensure that they do not re-collect. Cytology cannot distinguish benign adenomas from carcinomas, so these should all be excised.

Hyperthyroidism
The available therapy comprises:
- anti-thyroid drugs, of which carbimazole is the drug of choice;
- β-adrenergic blocking drugs;
- anti-thyroid drugs combined with subsequent thyroidectomy;
- radioactive iodine.

Carbimazole
This is given in a dosage of 10 mg t.d.s. and is combined with sedation and bed rest in the acute phase of hyperthyroidism. There is rapid regression of toxic symptoms, the patient beginning to feel better and to gain weight with reduction of tachycardia within a week or two. Treatment is continued for 12 months. If symptoms recur, a further 6 months' treatment is given, after which surgery is advised. Unfortunately, a high relapse rate (up to 60%) occurs after terminating the treatment, even if this is prolonged for 2 or more years. Medical treatment alone is therefore usually confined to the treatment of primary hyperthyroidism in children and adolescents.

The toxic effects of carbimazole include a drug rash, fever, arthropathy, lymphadenopathy and agranulocytosis; the last is the dangerous complication which is potentially lethal, but occurs in well under 1% of patients. The first symptom is a sore throat and patients on carbimazole must be warned to discontinue treatment immediately if this occurs and to report to hospital. Granulocyte colony-stimulating factor (G-CSF) may be required.

Beta-adrenergic blocking drugs
In patients with severe hyperthyroidism, propranolol induces rapid symptomatic improvement of the cardiovascular features due to sympathetic over-activity, while the hyperthyroidism comes under control with specific anti-thyroid therapy.

Drugs and surgery combined
The majority of adult patients in the UK are treated with preliminary carbimazole until euthyroid and are then submitted to subtotal thyroidectomy.

Radioactive iodine
From the patient's point of view this is the most pleasant treatment, as all the patient has to do is swallow a glass of water containing the radio-iodine. There is no need for prolonged treatment with drugs nor the risk of operation; it is particularly useful in recurrence of hyperthyroidism after thyroidectomy. It usually takes 2 or 3 months before the patient is rendered euthyroid. Anti-thyroid drugs, with or without a β-blocker, may be used to control symptoms during this time.

There is a theoretical risk of malignant change in the irradiated gland, although there has been no report of this occurring in humans. It is, however, current practice not to use radio-iodine in patients under the age 45 years and, in addition, not to employ it in young women who may become pregnant during treatment, as there is a very real danger of affecting the infant's thyroid. Another disadvantage of this treatment is the high incidence of late hypothyroidism, which rises to near 30% after 10 years and which requires replacement therapy with T4.

Complications of thyroidectomy

In addition to the hazards of any surgical operation there are special complications to consider following thyroidectomy. These can be divided into hormonal disturbances (the thyroid itself and the adjacent parathyroid glands) and injury to closely related anatomical structures.

1 *Hormonal*:
   (a) tetany (parathyroid removal or bruising);
   (b) thyroid crisis;
   (c) hypothyroidism (due to extensive removal of thyroid tissue);
   (d) late recurrence of hyperthyroidism (inadequate operation in the toxic gland).
2 *Damage to related anatomical structures*:
   (a) recurrent laryngeal nerve;
   (b) injury to trachea;
   (c) pneumothorax;
3 *The complications of any operation, especially*:
   (a) haemorrhage;
   (b) sepsis;
   (c) post-operative chest infection;
   (d) hypertrophic scarring (keloid).
   Some of these complications require further consideration here.

Hypoparathyroidism
This may result from inadvertent removal of the parathyroids or their injury during opera-

tion. The patient may develop tetany (p. 307) a few days post-operatively with typical carpopedal spasms, which may be induced by tourniquet around the arm (Trousseau's sign, p. 307), and a positive Chvostek's sign (p. 307); this is elicited by tapping lightly over the zygoma when the facial muscles will be seen to contract. The serum calcium falls to below 1.5 mmol/L.

Treatment
Treatment consists of giving 10 ml of 10% calcium gluconate intravenously followed by oral calcium together with vitamin D derivatives (ergocalciferol or alfacalcidol). Often the tetany is transient and the injured parathyroids recover; in other cases, permanent treatment with alfacalcidol is required. Parathormone is not used.

In addition to frank tetany, which occurs in about 1% of cases, milder degrees of hypoparathyroidism may occur and may present with mental changes (depression or anxiety neurosis), skin rashes and bilateral cataracts. A low post-operative calcium is treated by the administration of oral calcium and/or vitamin D daily by mouth.

Thyroid crisis
An acute exacerbation of hyperthyroidism seen immediately post-operatively is now extremely rare because of the careful preoperative preparation of these cases. It is, however, a frightening phenomenon with mania, hyperpyrexia and marked tachycardia which may lead to death from heart failure. The cause is not fully understood, but it may be due to a massive release of T4 from the hyperactive gland during the operation.

Treatment
Treatment comprises heavy sedation with barbiturates, propranolol, intravenous iodine and cooling by means of ice packs.

Recurrent laryngeal nerve injury
The recurrent laryngeal nerve lies in the groove between the oesophagus and trachea in

close relationship to the inferior thyroid artery. Here it is at risk of division, injury from stretching, or compression by oedema or blood clot.

If one nerve alone is damaged, the patient may have little in the way of symptoms apart from slight hoarseness because the opposite vocal cord compensates by passing across the midline during phonation. However, if both recurrent nerves are damaged there is almost complete loss of voice and serious narrowing of the airway; a permanent tracheostomy may be required, although an incomplete injury may recover in time. It is estimated that the nerve is injured in about 2–3% of thyroidectomies.

Haemorrhage

This occurring shortly after thyroidectomy is a dangerous condition, as bleeding into the thyroid bed may compress the trachea already softened by pressure from the thyroid swelling. The neck becomes distended with blood; there is acute dyspnoea and stridor, as well as shock from blood loss.

Treatment

This may be an extreme emergency and must be dealt with at once by decompressing the neck in the ward. The skin and the subcutaneous sutures are removed, the wound is opened and the blood clot expressed. The patient can then be transferred to theatre, anaesthetized, bleeding points secured and the wound resutured.

Thyroid tumours

Classification
Benign
• Adenoma.

Malignant
1 *Primary* (five main types):
   (a) papillary adenocarcinoma;
   (b) follicular adenocarcinoma;
   (c) anaplastic;
   (d) medullary carcinoma;
   (e) lymphoma (rare).
2 *Secondary*:
   (a) direct invasion from adjacent structures, e.g. oesophagus;
   (b) very rare site for blood-borne deposits.

Benign adenoma

Although benign encapsulated nodules in the thyroid gland are common, the majority are part of a nodular colloid goitre. A small percentage represent true benign adenomas.

Thyroid carcinoma
Pathology

Thyroid carcinoma affects females twice as often as males, often arising in pre-existing goitres, and has been reported following radiation of the neck in childhood. There are two groups of thyroid carcinoma:
1 the well-differentiated adenocarcinomas (papillary, follicular and medullary);
2 anaplastic spheroidal cell carcinoma.

Such important differences occur between these two groups that they might almost be considered separate disease entities.

Papillary carcinoma

This is the commonest type of thyroid cancer, comprising 60% of thyroid cancers. It occurs in young adults, adolescents or even children. It is a slow-growing tumour and lymphatic spread occurs late. Deposits in the regional lymph nodes may be solitary and in the past have been mistakenly regarded as lateral aberrant thyroid tissue. However, a careful search of the thyroid gland will reveal a well-differentiated tumour in the homolateral lobe.

Follicular carcinoma

This occurs in young and middle-aged adults, and is commoner in areas where endemic goitres are common. It has a tendency to blood-stream spread and therefore a worsened prognosis; lymph-node spread is uncommon.

Medullary carcinoma

This arises from the parafollicular C cells and may secrete calcitonin. It may occur at any age and, unlike other thyroid tumours, has a roughly equal sex distribution. It may be familial and may be associated with other cancers in the multiple endocrine neoplasia syndrome (type II, associated with phaeochromocytoma and either parathyroid tumours or neuro-fibromas, see p. 308). Familial forms can be identified by a marker on chromosome 10, potentially useful for screening members of affected families; calcitonin can be used as a marker of the tumour. The characteristic finding is deposits of amyloid between the nests of tumour cells.

Anaplastic carcinoma

This occurs in the elderly, thus reversing the usual state of affairs, in that the more malignant tumours of the thyroid occur in the older age group. Rapid local spread takes place with compression and invasion of the trachea. There is early dissemination to the regional lymphatics and blood-stream spread to the lungs, skeleton and brain.

Clinical features

Tumours may present like other goitres as a lump in the neck, often more rapidly growing. Dysphagia is uncommon, and suggestive of an anaplastic tumour; more common is the complaint that swallowing is uncomfortable. Pain may occur with local infiltration, and hoarseness is suggestive of infiltration of the recurrent laryngeal nerve. Deep cervical lymph nodes may be palpably enlarged. The patients are usually euthyroid.

Treatment

Well-differentiated tumours can be treated by a combination of surgery, thyroid suppression by T4, and radio-iodine.

Papillary carcinoma

The extent of surgical treatment advocated varies between removal of the affected lobe (total thyroid lobectomy) to removal of both lobes (total thyroidectomy); in both cases, affected nodes should be treated by block dis-section of the affected side. Occasionally, the tumour can be multifocal, and advocates of total thyroidectomy recommend the more aggressive treatment to cover this possibility. In either case, the patient is subsequently started on T4 to suppress the TSH completely, and so take away the drive to remaining thyroid tissue, which, being well differentiated, is usually responsive to TSH.

Many of these well-differentiated tumours take up radioactive iodine, and it is possible to treat recurrences or metastases by ^{131}I therapy. A tracer dose of radioactive iodine will give evidence of the suitability of isotope therapy by confirming uptake of the radio-iodine in the secondary deposits.

Follicular carcinoma

Follicular carcinoma is usually treated by total lobectomy. However, if there is evidence of more aggressive behaviour with vascular and capsular invasion, total thyroidectomy should be performed, even if this means early re-operation. In these cases, surgery is usually followed by radio-iodine treatment. T4 replacement therapy is then indicated.

Medullary carcinoma

The tumour is often multicentric, and total thy-roidectomy is indicated. Metastatic disease in the lymph nodes is common on presentation, so clearance is required, extending from the hyoid above to the brachio-cephalic veins below.

Anaplastic carcinoma

The anaplastic carcinomas may be treated by radical thyroidectomy but frequently these patients present with an already inoperable mass in the neck. Palliative radiotherapy may give temporary relief and tracheostomy may be required for the obstructed airway.

Prognosis

This is very different in the two groups of cases; the well-differentiated tumours are often associated with long survival, even in the presence of lymph node deposits, whereas patients with anaplastic tumours are usually dead within a year, either from local invasion or widespread dissemination.

Hashimoto's disease

Hashimoto's disease* is an uncommon thyroid disease that has received considerable attention, as it was the first of the autoimmune diseases to be elucidated. The patient is usually a middle-aged woman with clinical evidence of hypothyroidism. The gland is uniformly enlarged and firm, although it may occasionally be asymmetrical and irregular.

Macroscopically, its cut surface is lobulated and greyish yellow. Microscopically, there is diffuse infiltration with lymphocytes, increased fibrous tissue and diminished colloid. It is considered to be an autoimmune disease in which the patient has developed circulating antibodies to her own thyroid. Such antibodies, which react against thyroglobulin, can be demonstrated in about 90% of cases.

It is important to diagnose the condition correctly by demonstrating the presence of thyroid antibodies and, if necessary, by biopsy, because thyroidectomy will precipitate severe hypothyroidism in these cases. Occasionally, lymphoma occurs in such glands.

*Hakaru Hashimoto (1881–1934), Surgeon in private practice, Japan.

Treatment

T4 replacement therapy up to 0.3 mg/day will shrink the gland and the symptoms of myxoedema should disappear.

Riedel's thyroiditis

Riedel's thyroiditis† is an extremely rare disease of the thyroid in which the gland may be only slightly enlarged but is woody hard with infiltration of adjacent tissues. The cause of this condition is not known, but it may represent a late stage of Hashimoto's disease or possibly be inflammatory in origin.

It is mistaken clinically for a thyroid carcinoma, but histologically the gland is replaced by fibrous tissue containing chronic inflammatory cells. It is associated with other conditions such as retroperitoneal fibrosis, sclerosing cholangitis and fibrosing mediastinitis.

A wedge resection of a portion of the gland may be required if symptoms of tracheal compression develop.

De Quervain's thyroiditis

De Quervain's thyroiditis‡ is a rare condition usually affecting young women. It usually follows a viral infection of the upper respiratory tract. The gland is slightly enlarged, firm and tender. It is generally self-limiting, and rarely leads to hypothyroidism.

†Bernhard Riedel (1846–1916), Professor of Surgery, Jena, Germany.
‡Fritz de Quervain (1868–1940), Professor of Surgery, Berne, Switzerland.

CHAPTER 38

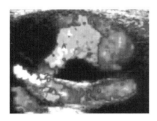

The Parathyroids

Anatomy and development

The parathyroids are four endocrine glands (sometimes three or five) about the size of split peas, which usually lie in two pairs behind the lateral lobes of the thyroid gland. The superior parathyroids arise from the *fourth* branchial pouch, and the inferior glands from the *third* pouch in association with the developing thymus. The inferior parathyroids may lie almost anywhere in the neck and also in the superior mediastinum in relationship to the thymus gland.

Physiology

The parathyroids produce parathormone (PTH), which has profound influence on calcium and phosphate metabolism. The exact mechanisms of its action are not known, but there appear to be two main effects.

1 It increases the excretion of phosphate from the kidney by inhibiting its tubular reabsorption (phosphaturic effect); tubular reabsorption of calcium is reciprocally increased.

2 It stimulates osteoclastic activity in the bones resulting in the decalcification and liberation of excessive amounts of calcium and phosphorus in the blood.

Effects of increased PTH production

• A raised serum calcium and a lowered serum phosphate, as these substances are related reciprocally.

• An increased excretion of phosphate in the urine (phosphaturic effect of PTH).

• An increased excretion of calcium in the urine. The large amount of calcium filtered (due to the hypercalcaemia) exceeds the tubules' capacity to resorb it all, so increased calcium excretion occurs.

• Osteoclasis, with a raised serum alkaline phosphatase associated with decalcification of the bones.

Hypoparathyroidism

Lack of PTH results in a low serum calcium and hyperirritability of skeletal muscle with carpo-pedal spasms, the syndrome being called *tetany*. The most common cause of this is removal or bruising of the parathyroids in thyroidectomy (see p. 303). Tetany is liable to occur if the serum calcium falls below 1.5 mmol/L.

Clinical features

Spasms may affect any part of the body, but typically the hands and feet. The wrists flex and the fingers are drawn together in extension, the so-called '*main d'accoucheur*'. This spasm may be induced by placing a tourniquet around the arm for a few minutes (Trousseau's sign[*]). Hyperirritability of the facial muscles may be demonstrated by tapping over the facial

---

[*]Armand Trousseau (1801–67), Physician, Hôpital Necker, Paris. Allso described thrombophlebitis migrans associated with cancer.

MULTIPLE ENDOCRINE NEOPLASIA (MEN) SYNDROMES

These syndromes are characterized by the development of a number of endocrine adenomas, or adenocarcinomas, in the same patient. Some, such as medullary carcinoma of the thyroid, may be familial.

MEN type I
• Pancreatic tumour: islet-cell tumours except β-cell tumours (insulinoma).
• Parathyroid tumour.

• Pituitary tumour, e.g. prolactinoma.
• Adreno-cortical tumour.

MEN type II
• Medullary carcinoma of the thyroid.
• Phaeochromocytoma.
• Parathyroid tumour—only in type IIA (Sipple's syndrome).
• Neurofibromas of tongue, lips and eyelids—only in type IIB.

---

nerve which results in spasm (Chvostek's sign*).

Note that clinical tetany may occur with a normal level of serum calcium in alkalosis (e.g. over-breathing, excessive prolonged vomiting) because of a compensatory shift of ionized calcium to the un-ionized form in the serum.

Tumours

Pathology
These are usually single. The lower glands are affected more commonly than the upper ones. The tumours are soft, encapsulated and a brown–grey colour. Most are benign adenomas, and carcinoma of the parathyroid is rare.

The tumour may coexist with other endocrine tumours such as pancreatic islet-cell tumour, anterior pituitary adenoma, thyroid medullary carcinoma and phaeochromocytoma, as part of the multiple endocrine neoplasia (MEN) syndrome.

Hyperparathyroidism
There are four distinct types of pathologically increased PTH secretion.

1 *Primary hyperparathyroidism*: increased secretion due to a solitary parathyroid adenoma; the

*Frantisek Chvostek (1835–84), Physician at Josefsakademie, Vienna.

remaining parathyroid glands are suppressed by the high circulating calcium.

2 *Secondary hyperparathyroidism*: in some 10% of patients with hyperparathyroidism, the condition is found to be due to a hyperplasia of all four parathyroid glands. This occurs most commonly in patients with renal failure maintained by dialysis, in whom renal conversion of 25-hydroxycholecalciferol (calcidol) to 1,25-dihydroxycholecalciferol (calcitrol) is impaired. This active form of vitamin D is required for absorption of calcium from the gut; deficiency results in hypocalcaemia, which chronically stimulates PTH production. The parathyroid glands undergo hyperplasia in response. This can be prevented by administering 1α-hydroxycholecalciferol (alfacalcidol), so bypassing the renal 1α-hydroxylase step.

3 *Tertiary hyperparathyroidism*: prolonged secondary hyperparathyroidism leads to autonomous PTH production, which continues even after renal transplantation replaces the deficient vitamin D conversion step. Parathyroidectomy is required.

4 *Ectopic PTH*: hyperparathyroidism is occasionally due to ectopic PTH production by tumours, such as squamous carcinoma of the bronchus.

Clinical features
These depend on the results of excessive production of PTH by the tumour (see

above). Presenting symptoms may include the following.

• *Bone changes*: spontaneous fractures or pain in the bones. X-ray will show decalcification of the bones with cyst formation. The weakened bones may be deformed; this condition is known as osteitis fibrosa cystica or Von Recklinghausen's disease* of bone. There may be metastatic calcification in soft tissues, arterial walls and the kidneys.

• *Renal effects*: renal stones, infection associated with renal calculi, calcification in the renal substance or uraemia. It is important to remember that chronic renal disease with impaired excretion of phosphate may result in secondary hyperplasia of the parathyroid glands with features similar to those of a primary adenoma of the parathyroid.

• *Abdominal pain*: constipation is common. Dyspepsia or frank duodenal ulceration is also sometimes associated with parathyroid adenoma, as is pancreatitis. If ulcer symptoms persist after treatment of the adenoma, the presence of a gastrinoma should be excluded by serum gastrin assay (MEN syndrome association).

• *Vague ill health associated with high serum calcium*: the patient very often complains of lassitude, weakness, anorexia and loss of weight. Thirst and polyuria are common.

The main effects are summarized as: 'stones, bones, abdominal groans'.

Special investigations

• *Serum calcium* is usually raised to above 2.75 mmol/L (corrected for serum albumin concentration). Other causes of raised serum calcium include metastatic cancer, multiple myeloma and sarcoidosis; in all these the serum calcium falls if a 10-day course of corticosteroids is given, but no significant change takes place in true hyperparathyroidism (*the cortisone suppression test*).

• *Serum PTH level* is raised.

• *Excretion of calcium by the kidneys*: the urinary excretion of a standard calcium intake is increased.

• *Serum phosphate* is low.

• *Serum alkaline phosphatase* is raised.

• *X-rays of the bones* may show subperiosteal decalcification and cyst formation.

• *Abdominal X-rays and IVU* may show renal stones or nephrocalcinosis.

• *Subtraction scanning*: a technetium scan is taken up by the thyroid; this is followed by a thallium scan, taken up by both the thyroid and parathyroid. Subtraction of the first from the second reveals a 'hot spot' denoting a functioning parathyroid tumour.

• *Magnetic resonance imaging* may localize a tumour particularly if it is in the superior mediastinum.

• *Venous sampling*, where blood samples are taken from the great veins at varying locations around the neck and assayed for PTH, may help localize occult adenomas.

Treatment

Treatment is by removal of the parathyroid adenoma. This may be rather difficult to find as often quite small tumours can produce gross metabolic disturbances. The neck is very carefully explored, first of all in the usual sites of the parathyroid glands and, if no tumour is found, then more extensive dissection is made into the neck and into the superior mediastinum.

---

*Frederick von Recklinghausen (1833–1910), Professor of Pathology, Strasbourg. Also described neurofibromatosis.

CHAPTER 39

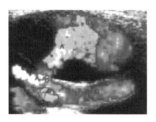

The Thymus

The thymus gland controls the development of T lymphocytes in the embryo and neonate.

In adult life the thymus is a fat infiltrated remnant, but to the surgeon it is of importance in having an ill-understood connection with myasthenia gravis and of being a rather rare site of mediastinal tumour.

Tumours

Tumours of the thymus are of complex pathology; they may arise from either the epithelium (Hassall's corpuscles) or lymphoid tissue, or from a mixture of both. They may be benign (occasionally cystic) or malignant and rapidly invasive. Peak incidence is in the sixth and seventh decades.

Clinical features
There are three modes of presentation:
1 a mediastinal mass;
2 associated with myasthenia gravis;
3 associated with immune deficiency states.

Treatment
Treatment is by thymectomy via median sternotomy, combined with radiotherapy if malignant to prevent mediastinal recurrence.

Early invasion, with no more than pleural and mediastinal fat involvement, carries a good prognosis (90% at 5 years); involvement of the pericardium, great vessels or lung has a poor prognosis.

Myasthenia gravis

This is a condition of muscle weakness apparently due to a defect at the neuromuscular junction in which the motor end plate becomes refractory to the action of acetylcholine due to the presence of circulating antibodies to the acetyl choline receptor. About 10% of cases are associated with a tumour of the thymus, and thymic hyperplasia is present in most of the remaining cases.

Clinical features
Females are twice as commonly affected as males, and the disease usually commences in early adult life. The extrinsic ocular muscles are most often affected and may indeed be the only ones involved, with ptosis, diplopia and squint. The affected muscles become weak with use and recover, partially or completely, after rest. The voice is weak and death may eventually occur from respiratory muscle failure.

Treatment
The majority of cases are controlled by choline esterase inhibitors, e.g. pyridostigmine.

Thymectomy is indicated if the disease is progressive and the prognosis is best in young females (under the age of 40 years) with a history of 5 years or less. The results are not as good in those cases associated with a thymic tumour.

CHAPTER 40

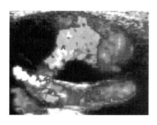

The Suprarenal Gland

The suprarenal (adrenal) glands are paired glands situated above and medial to the upper pole of each kidney. The cortex derives from the mesoderm of the urogenital ridge, while the medulla derives from neural crest ectoderm. This different origin accounts for the different physiology of medulla and cortex, and the different pathology encountered surgically.

Physiology
Cortex
The suprarenal cortex secretes three groups of steroids:

1 *glucocorticoids*, which regulate carbohydrate metabolism, protein breakdown and fat mobilization;
2 *androgenic corticoids*, which are virilizing;
3 *mineralocorticoids*, which regulate mineral and water metabolism. Aldosterone acts to retain sodium and water and to excrete potassium.

Glucocorticoids and androgens are under hypothalamic control via adrenocorticotrophic hormone (ACTH) secreted by the anterior pituitary gland; mineralocorticoids are under the control of the renin–angiotensin system (p. 70). As the steroids share a similar biochemical structure, it is not surprising that there is some overlap in actions; thus, hydrocortisone (cortisol), a glucocorticoid, also affects salt and water metabolism and has sex steroid effects (acne, hirsutism) if given in large amounts.

Suprarenal medulla
The suprarenal medulla is richly innervated, and produces the catecholamines adrenaline and noradrenaline in response to autonomic stimulation.

Pathology
The main pathologies affecting the suprarenal gland are increased function, due to tumour or hyperplasia, decreased function, due to atrophy, infarction or removal, or abnormal function due to enzyme disorders.

Increased function
• *Glucocorticoids* (Cushing's syndrome): adreno-cortical adenoma; ACTH-producing pituitary adenoma; ectopic ACTH production (paraneoplastic).
• *Androgenic corticoids*: virilism (the adreno-genital syndrome).
• *Mineralocorticoids*: primary hyperaldosteronism (Conn's syndrome).
• *Catecholamines*: phaeochromocytoma.

Decreased function
Hypoadrenalism is most commonly a sequel of a prolonged steroid therapy, in which endogenous steroid production is suppressed, fol-

lowed by abrupt steroid withdrawal. It may also due to:

- congenital suprarenal hypoplasia;
- autoimmune destruction — Addison's disease;*
- suprarenal infarction, a rare consequence of stress or sepsis (notably meningococcal sepsis);
- bilateral adrenalectomy, intentionally (to treat Cushing's syndrome) or secondary to bilateral nephrectomy;
- suprarenal infiltration by secondary tumours from primaries in bronchus and breast.

Enzyme disorders

Congenital suprarenal hyperplasia, the collective description for the suprarenal hyperplasia resulting from increased ACTH secretion, may result from certain enzyme disorders. ACTH is produced in excess because glucocorticoids, the end point in the pathway of steroid hormone synthesis, are not produced due to one of many possible enzyme deficiencies. Instead, all the substrate synthesized is turned into an intermediate hormone, such as an androgen.

Cushing's syndrome

Cushing's syndrome† is produced by increased circulating corticosteroids. Excepting therapeutic exogenous steroid administration, the majority of cases result from pituitary adenoma producing ACTH resulting in hyperplasia of the suprarenal cortex (the disease that Cushing first decribed); about 10% are due to benign or malignant adrenocortical tumours or, rarely, ectopic ACTH production by a distant tumour, e.g. carcinoma of the lung.

*Thomas Addison (1773–1860), Physician, Guy's Hospital, London.
†Harvey Cushing (1869–1939), Professor of Surgery, Harvard Medical School, Boston, USA.

Clinical features

The syndrome usually affects young adults (occasionally children); females more often than males. The appearance is characteristic; adiposity with central distribution, abdominal striae, a red moon face and diabetes. There may be osteoporosis, leading to vertebral collapse. Associated mineral and androgenic corticoid over-secretion produce varying degrees of hypertension, hirsutism and acne, with amenorrhoea in the female or impotence in the male.

Special investigations

These may be thought of as investigations to confirm the diagnosis, and investigations to identify the cause.

- Urinary 24-hour cortisol level is raised; but may also be raised in the obese and in patients under stress.
- Plasma cortisol: raised levels, and loss of the normal diurnal variation (low at night, up in the morning) is suggestive.
- Dexamethasone suppression test, in which the steroid dexamethasone is administered over a period of days and at different doses, and the plasma cortisol is measured; suppression of cortisol occurs with high-dose dexamethasone in the presence of pituitary tumours; ectopic ACTH and suprarenal tumours do not suppress.
- Plasma ACTH is raised in the presence of ectopic or pituitary ACTH-driven disease; its secretion is suppressed by autonomous suprarenal tumours.
- Computed tomography (CT) scan of the abdomen may demonstrate the tumour in the suprarenal gland.

Treatment

If due to bilateral hyperplasia, bilateral adrenalectomy is performed and the patient placed on a maintenance dose of cortisone. Removal of the affected suprarenal gland is carried out in cases of adenoma or carcinoma.

Cases due to basophil adenoma of the pituitary respond to hypophysectomy.

Primary hyperaldosteronism (Conn's syndrome)

Conn's syndrome* is a rare syndrome produced by an aldosterone-secreting adenoma of the suprarenal cortex. Characteristically, there is a low serum potassium (which results in episodes of muscle weakness or paralysis), raised serum sodium and alkalosis together with hypertension. There may also be polyuria and polydipsia.

The condition is interesting because, although rare, it represents a curable cause of hypertension.

Special investigations
• *Plasma aldosterone.* The diagnosis is confirmed by demonstration of excess aldosterone in the plasma.
• *Abdominal CT scan* may demonstrate the tumour, which is often small.
• *Selective angiography* may be needed to delineate the lesion.

Treatment
The involved suprarenal is explored and the tumour (which is usually small) removed.

The adreno-genital syndromes

These rare syndromes result from the hypersecretion of adreno-cortical androgens, due either to a defect in the enzyme pathway of steroid production, commonly 21-hydroxylase deficiency (the congenital form), or due to an autonomous tumour producing androgens (the acquired form).

Congenital adreno-genital syndrome
Also known as congenital suprarenal hyperplasia, this is due to an inborn defect of normal steroid synthesis (especially hydrocortisone) by the suprarenal cortex. Excessive ACTH pro-

*Jerome Conn (1907–94), Physician, University of Michigan, USA.

duction by the pituitary then occurs with resulting hyperplasia of the cortex and hypersecretion of cortical androgens.

Acquired adreno-genital syndrome
In children it is always due to an adreno-cortical tumour, which is usually malignant. In young adults the condition may be due either to a tumour or to cortical hyperplasia in cases of Cushing's syndrome where androgen production is excessive.

Clinical features
These are conveniently divided into three varieties depending on age of onset.

Infancy
In the congenital variety of the adreno-genital syndrome, the new-born female has a large clitoris and is often mistaken for male (female pseudo-hermaphrodite). Growth is initially rapid, but the epiphyses fuse early so that the final result is a stunted child. There may be episodes of acute adreno-cortical insufficiency, especially with stress or infection.

Childhood
Virilization occurs in the female and precocious sexual development, particularly of the penis, in the male. This can be well summarized as 'little girls become little boys and little boys become little men'.

Adults
Amenorrhoea, hirsutism and breast atrophy in the female, often associated with other features of Cushing's syndrome. In the male, feminization is seen, but this is extremely rare.

Differential diagnosis
The diagnosis is based on detecting the excessive amount of steroid precursors, such as 17α-hydroxyprogesterone, which is raised in the commonest congenital form, 21-hydroxylase deficiency.

Differentiation must be made from the masculinizing tumour of ovary, in which the

17-ketosteroid urinary excretion is normal, and also the common condition of simple hirsutism in the female.

Treatment

Bilateral cortical hyperplasia in infancy is treated by suppressing the excess ACTH secretion with exogenous steroids (e.g. hydrocortisone); on this regimen the virilizing features clear, and growth progresses normally. In the acquired variety, the tumour is treated by removal, and hyperplasia is treated by bilateral adrenalectomy with hydrocortisone maintenance treatment.

Non-functioning tumours of the suprarenal cortex

Small non-secreting adenomas of the suprarenal cortex are common post-mortem findings that are of no significance, and that are increasingly detected by modern cross-sectional imaging techniques such as CT and magnetic resonance imaging (MRI). Non-functioning carcinomas of the suprarenal cortex are rare; they resemble renal carcinoma in appearance (hence the original hypothesis that the hypernephroma was of suprarenal origin). They are highly malignant and frequently invade the subjacent kidney.

Adreno-medullary tumours

Classification
Primary
• Neuroblastoma.
• Phaeochromocytoma.
• Ganglioneuroma.

Secondary
A common site, especially from breast and bronchus.

Neuroblastoma

A highly malignant tumour of sympathetic cells occurring in children under the age of 5 years,

and the commonest malignant tumour in neonates and infants under 1 year old. It may be bilateral, and up to 80% are associated with chromosomal abnormalities.

Macroscopically, it varies from a small nodular tumour to a large retroperitoneal mass, containing areas of haemorrhage and necrosis. Microscopically, it arises from neuroblasts of the adrenal medulla, or within any cells of neuro-ectodermal origin along the spine.

Capsular invasion occurs early with spread to adjacent tissues, the regional nodes and by the blood to bones and the liver.

Special investigations
• *CT, MRI, ultrasound and bone scan* are all used to stage the disease.
• *Neurone-specific enolase* is a sensitive marker of disseminated disease, and can be used as a tumour marker following treatment.

Treatment

A combined approach with surgical removal of local disease followed by chemotherapy and/or radiotherapy is necessary.

Prognosis

Early disease, localized to the area of origin and in the absence of distant or lymph-node spread, carries a favourable prognosis, as do absence of chromosome abnormalities, and age under 1 year old together with histologically well-differentiated tumour.

Phaeochromocytoma

A physiologically active tumour of chromaffin cells, which secretes noradrenaline and adrenaline in varying proportions. Ten per cent are malignant and 10% are multiple; 10% occur outside the suprarenal gland in the sympathetic chain or the organ of Zuckerkandl near the aortic bifurcation; 10% are familial (the '10% tumour').

Any age may be affected, but the tumour is particularly found in young adults. The sexes are equally affected.

Clinical features

These are produced by excess circulating

adrenaline and noradrenaline. There is hypertension, which is paroxysmal or sustained, and which may be accompanied by palpitations, headache, blurred vision, fits, papilloedema and episodes of pallor and sweating. There may be hyperglycaemia with glycosuria. Attacks may be infrequent, or occur several times a day.

The diagnostic triad, with high specificity and sensitivity is said to be:
• *headache*, sudden in onset, and pounding;
• *tachycardia* and/or palpitations;
• *sweating*.

Occasionally, the tumour may coexist with neurofibromas and café-au-lait spots, medullary carcinoma of the thyroid or a parathyroid adenoma (multiple endocrine neoplasia syndrome, see p. 308).

Special investigations
Diagnosing the presence of a phaeochromocytoma
• *Urinary catecholamines*, particularly vanillylmandelic acid (VMA) collected over a 24-hour period, are usually raised, particularly during an acute hypertensive attack.

Locating a phaeochromocytoma
• *CT or MRI* may demonstrate the site and size of the tumour.
• *131I-MIBG scan*: m-iodobenzylguanidine (MIBG) is a structural analogue of noradrenaline, which is taken up by chromaffin cells of the suprarenal medulla and concentrated in adrenergic granules; it is also taken up by phaeochromocytomas and is useful both in localizing occult primaries and detecting secondary spread.
• *Selective catheterization* of the suprarenal veins with blood sampling for catecholamine estimation; a raised value in the blood obtained from the inferior vena cava at this level is useful confirmatory evidence of the presence of a tumour in the absence of abnormality on scanning.

Treatment
Surgical excision is performed. Prior to surgery, the patient receives both α- (e.g. phenoxybenzamine) and β- (e.g. propranolol) adrenergic blockade, as manipulation of the tumour during the operation may cause release of catecholamines and cause gross hypertension.

Patients with phaeochromocytomas are relatively volume depleted, and immediately following removal of the tumour the blood pressure may fall to unrecordable levels; this is countered by volume replacement, although a noradrenaline infusion is sometimes required.

Ganglioneuroma
A benign, slow-growing tumour of sympathetic ganglion cells, which only becomes clinically manifest if it reaches a large size. Only about 15% arise in the suprarenal; the rest elsewhere along the sympathetic chain.

CHAPTER 41

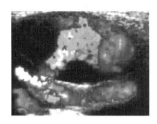

The Kidney and Ureter

Congenital anomalies

Embryology (Fig. 41.1)

The embryology of the kidney involves three separate stages. Initially, a pronephros develops in the posterior wall of the coelomic cavity. This is replaced by the mesonephric system, which comprises a long ridge of mesoderm, the mesonephros, with its duct, the mesonephric (Wolffian*) duct. The mesonephros itself then disappears except that, in the male, some of its ducts become the efferent tubules of the testis. At the lower end of the mesonephric duct a diverticulum develops. This diverticulum becomes the metanephric duct, on top of which develops a cap of tissue, the metanephros. The metanephros gives rise to the glomeruli and the proximal part of the renal duct system. The metanephric duct forms the ureter, renal pelvis, calyces and distal ducts. The mesonephric duct atrophies in the female, the remnant being called the epoöphron, and in the male it gives rise to the epididymis and the vas deferens.

*Kaspar Friedrich Wolff (1733–94), Born in Berlin, Germany, Professor of Anatomy, St Petersburg, Russia.

The kidney originally develops in the pelvis of the embryo and then migrates cranially, acquiring a progressively more proximal arterial blood supply as it does so. This complex developmental process explains the high frequency with which congenital anomalies of the kidney, the ureter and the renal blood supply are found.

Common renal anomalies

• *Pelvic kidney*: due to failure of cranial migration of the developing kidney.

• *Horse-shoe kidney*: produced by fusion of the two metanephric masses across the midline (see below).

• *Duplex system*: double ureters and/or kidneys due to duplication of the metanephric bud.

• *Congenital absence* of one kidney (1 in every 2500 subjects). Congenital absence of a kidney is extremely rare, but should be borne in mind whenever the possibility of nephrectomy arises, for instance after kidney trauma.

• *Polycystic kidneys*: possibly due to failure of linkage between the metanephric duct system and the metanephros (see below).

• *Congenital hydronephrosis*: produced by neuromuscular inco-ordination at the pelvi-ureteric junction.

EMBRYOLOGY OF THE KIDNEY

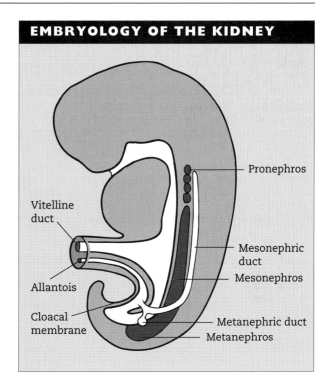

Fig. 41.1 Development of the pro-, meso- and metanephric systems (after Langman).

- *Aberrant renal arteries*: one or more arteries supplying the upper or lower pole of the kidneys are very common; they represent the persistence of aortic branches that pass to the kidney in its lower embryonic position.

Polycystic disease, the various types of re-duplication of the renal pelvis and the abnormal fusions are all associated with an increased incidence of infection when compared with kidneys that are anatomically normal.

Horseshoe kidney

During the kidneys' ascent from their position as the metanephros in the embryo, they may fuse. The commonest example is fusion of the lower poles across the midline, forming one large horseshoe-shaped kidney. The linked lower ends of the kidneys usually lie in front of the aorta in the region of the fourth or fifth lumbar vertebra and the ureters descend from the front of the fused kidneys.

Clinically, horseshoe kidneys may present as a firm mass in the pelvis, or with recurrent urinary tract infection. An intravenous urogram (IVU) will show rotation of the two renal pelvises with the ureters arising close to the midline. Usually, the renal pelvises are directed laterally.

The main surgical importance of horseshoe kidneys is as the differential diagnosis of a lump in the pelvis since the consequences of removing such renal tissue as an undiagnosed 'mass' are disastrous.

Duplex system

Instead of a single metanephric mass draining via a single ureter into the bladder, part of the system may be duplicated. Most common is separation of the renal pelvis into a double pelvis draining the upper and lower pole separately. This may extend distally as a bifid ureter, which unites to form a single ureter in its distal third, entering the bladder by a common ostium. Occasionally, a second diverticulum grows from the mesonephric duct producing a double ureter. In this circumstance the lower pole ureter always enters the bladder in the normal position, while the upper pole ureter enters in an ectopic position, either in the bladder, or rarely directly into the urethra below the external sphincter in the male, or onto the perineum in the female.

Duplex anomalies are usually asymptomatic, but may present as a cause of hydronephrosis (p. 321) or urinary tract infection. Ectopic ureters often present with infection due to reflux up the abnormal ureteric orifice resulting in chronic pyelonephritis of the upper pole. Ectopic ureters opening into the urethra or onto the perineum are a cause of dribbling incontinence.

Polycystic disease
Pathology
This may arise from failure of fusion of the metanephros with its duct; the result is multiple cysts throughout the renal substance, nearly always in both kidneys. These cysts are surrounded by attenuated renal tissue. The condition is either inherited as an autosomal recessive form, presenting in childhood with renal failure, or the more common autosomal dominant form presenting in middle age. Genetically, the dominant form may result from a number of different gene mutations, the commonest being in the *PKD1* gene (chromosome 16p31).

There may be associated multiple cysts in other viscera, particularly the liver (30%), lungs, spleen or pancreas (10%). In addition there is a strong association with intracranial berry aneurysms.

Presentation of adult polycystic kidney disease
Polycystic kidney disease presents between 30 and 60 years of age with one of the following.
• *Abdominal mass*: symptomless, bilateral, lobulated renal swellings found on routine examination.
• *Haematuria*.
• *Loin pain*, usually aching.

• *Urinary tract infection*.
• *Renal failure*: presenting with headache, lassitude, vomiting and a refractory anaemia.
• *Hypertension*.
• *Intracranial haemorrhage*, as a result of hypertension or 'berry' aneurysm.

On examination the enlarged lobulated kidneys are usually readily palpable. There may be the clinical features of chronic uraemia, and the blood pressure is often raised.

Special investigations
• *Ultrasonography* is very accurate in detecting the multiple cysts in adults, but is less so in children because of the smaller size of the cysts.
• *Urea and creatinine* are often raised because of the impaired renal function.
• *IVU* demonstrates the typical elongated spidery calyces stretched out, and indented by the cysts.

Treatment
Left untreated, many patients may survive in reasonable health well past middle age. Medical treatment is required in the management of the complicating hypertension and renal failure (dialysis and transplantation). Nephrectomy is performed for uncontrollable hypertension, recurrent pain, infection or haematuria, and, with very large kidneys, to provide enough room in the iliac fossa to accommodate a renal transplant.

Renal cysts
Simple unilocular cysts of the kidney are quite common. A simple cyst may be small or may reach a very large size. Several cysts may be present and both kidneys may be affected. The cause is unknown, but may relate to tubular dilatation. The incidence increases with age.

Clinical features
The cyst may be symptomless and may be found as a mass on routine clinical examination. If very large, it may present as an aching pain in the loin. Haematuria is absent, and this is an important point in differentiation from a renal carcinoma.

Special investigations
• *Urine* is clear, even on microscopic examination.
• *Ultrasonography* confirms a cystic mass.
• *IVU* demonstrates a round filling defect, which displaces but does not invade the calyces.
• *Computed tomography (CT) scan* shows one (or more) fluid-filled cysts, which do not enhance with intravenous contrast.

Treatment
The cyst can be aspirated under ultrasound control. Clear serous fluid is obtained. Occasionally, surgical exploration is indicated if a firm diagnosis cannot be made between cyst and tumour. Simple decapping of the cyst is all that is required, leaving the base of the cyst attached to the kidney.

Haematuria

Classification
Two useful rules:
1 when considering the causes of bleeding from any orifice in the body, always remember the general causes due to bleeding diatheses;
2 when considering any local cause of symptoms in the genito-urinary tract, always think of the whole tract from the kidneys to the urethra.
Haematuria is an excellent example of these two general rules and the causes can be classified as follows (Fig. 41.2).

General
• *Bleeding diatheses*, e.g. anticoagulant drugs, thrombocytopenic purpura.

Local
• *Kidney*: trauma, polycystic disease, glomerulonephritis, tuberculosis, infarction (from emboli in mitral stenosis or infective endocarditis), stone and tumour.
• *Ureter*: stone and tumour.
• *Bladder*: trauma, cystitis, stone, tumour and bilharzia.

• *Prostate*: 'varices' in benign prostatic enlargement.
• *Urethra*: trauma, stone and tumour.

Management
Blood in the urine is an alarming symptom and usually brings the patient rapidly to the doctor. It should always be taken seriously and requires full history, examination and appropriate special investigations.

History
Haematuria accompanied by pain in one or other loin suggests renal origin, and colicky pain indicates a stone in the renal pelvis or ureter, or partial ureteric obstruction by clot. Terminal bleeding with severe pain and frequency indicates bladder calculus. Dribbling of blood from the urethra independent of micturition is typical of a urethral origin for the blood. Completely painless and otherwise symptomless haematuria is suggestive of a tumour in the urinary tract.

A history of recent sore throat, especially in a child, would make a diagnosis of acute nephritis a possibility. Always check whether the patient is on anticoagulant therapy or if there is a history of bleeding tendencies; haematuria while on anticoagulation is still more commonly due to a renal pathology, which the anticoagulation has made symptomatic — full investigation is warranted.

Examination
One or other kidneys may be palpable, a carcinoma of the bladder may be felt on bimanual examination. An enlarged prostate, particularly if the patient is hypertensive, suggests prostatic 'varices', although other causes must be excluded before this diagnosis is finally made.

Special investigations
• *Urine microscopy*. The presence of red cells will exclude haemoglobinuria and beeturia (following ingestion of beetroot). The presence of casts will indicate nephritis; pus cells and organisms suggests and infection.

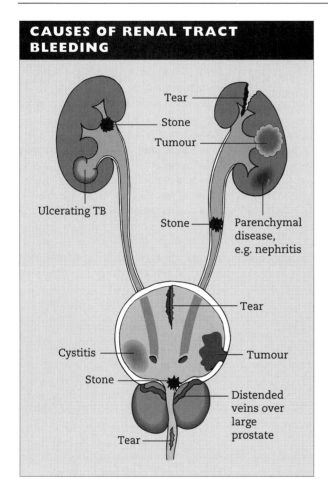

CAUSES OF RENAL TRACT BLEEDING

Tear

Stone

Tumour

Ulcerating TB

Stone — Parenchymal disease, e.g. nephritis

Tear

Cystitis

Tumour

Stone

Distended veins over large prostate

Tear

Fig. 41.2 Some important causes of bleeding in the urinary tract.

• *IVU* may reveal a localized renal lesion or may show a filling defect in the ureter or bladder. Stones in the urinary tract will be displayed on this investigation; look for them carefully on the preliminary plain films, as they are obscured by contrast in the urogram. Upper tract (ureter and renal pelvis) urothelial tumours are usually demonstrated as filling defects in the contrast.

• *Cystoscopy* will show any intravesical lesion in addition to bleeding from the prostate or blood emerging from one or other ureter. Cystoscopy is best performed immediately after presentation with haematuria.

These are the minimum investigations required for anyone with haematuria. Other investigations such as ultrasonography, CT and selective renal angiography may be required in some cases.

Injury to the kidney

The kidney may be injured by a direct blow in the loin or occasionally by a penetrating wound. The degree of damage varies from slight subcapsular bruising to complete rupture and fragmentation of the kidney or its avulsion from its vascular pedicle.

Clinical features

Clinically, there is usually local pain and tenderness and haematuria is a common finding. Retroperitoneal   haematoma   may   cause abdominal distension due to ileus. There may be associated injury to other viscera, especially the spleen.

Special investigations
- *Urine*: macroscopic haematuria is usual.
- *IVU*: damage to the kidney may be shown by extravasation of contrast medium outside the renal outline or distortion or rupture of the renal calyces. This examination will also determine whether or not there is a normal kidney on the other side.
- *Ultrasound examination* can delineate a renal tear as well as indicating injury to other solid viscera, the liver and spleen. Views may be obscured, however, if there is considerable intra-abdominal gas.
- *CT scan*: particularly useful in defining solid visceral injuries and is not affected by distended loops of bowel. The rapid data acquisition time and clarity of view of modern scanners make contrast-enhanced CT the investigation of choice in patients with multiple trauma.

Treatment
Associated injuries and shock will require appropriate treatment.

In practice, most cases fortunately resolve with conservative management, namely bed rest, serial observations of the urine to determine whether or not the haematuria is clearing, and careful clinical charting of blood pressure and pulse rate.

Nephrectomy is required in renal trauma in the following circumstances:
- *continued bleeding*, which threatens life;
- *severe hypertension* persisting after renal injury;
- *lack of function* in the affected kidney after several months, but only if symptomatic (e.g. recurrent infections, stone formation).

Hydronephrosis

Pathology
Hydronephrosis is a dilatation of the renal pelvis and calyces due to partial or complete obstruction to the out-flow of urine. It may result from congenital neuromuscular inco-ordination at the pelvi-ureteric junction or from obstruction of the urinary outflow. This obstruction may be unilateral, e.g. due to a stone or tumour in the ureter, or the block may involve the urethra, e.g. prostatic hypertrophy, urethral stricture, posterior urethral valve (newborn) with resultant bilateral hydronephrosis.

Aberrant renal vessels were considered to be a common cause of hydronephrosis, because they frequently cross the dilated renal pelvis at its junction with the ureter. It is probably unusual for these aberrant vessels actually to initiate the hydronephrosis; more likely they snare the congenitally dilated pelvis and merely act as a secondary constrictive factor.

Complications
- *Infection*: resulting in pyonephrosis (p. 326).
- *Stone formation*: calculi readily deposit in the infected stagnant urine.
- *Hypertension*: secondary to renal ischaemia.
- *Renal failure*: where there is extensive bilateral destruction of renal tissue.
- *Traumatic rupture* of the hydronephrotic pelvis.

Clinical features
An uncomplicated hydronephrosis on one side may be symptomless or may produce a dull, aching pain in the loin often mistaken for 'lumbago' or 'rheumatism'. Occasionally, there may be acute attacks of pain resembling ureteric colic, particularly after drinking large volumes of fluid (most notably beer).

Associated infection may present with fever, pyuria, rigors and severe loin pain. Bilateral hydronephrosis may present with the clinical features of uraemia. Very often it is the underlying cause, e.g. the ureteric calculus, the enlarged prostate or the urethral stricture, that manifests itself clinically.

On examination, the enlarged kidney may be palpable. The size of this may vary according to the state of distension of the renal pelvis.

Special investigations

- *Ultrasound* shows a dilated collecting system (calyces and pelvis).
- *IVU* confirms the diagnosis, demonstrating an enlarged renal pelvis and swollen, dilated club-like calyces. If renal function is severely impaired, the kidney may not secrete contrast.
- *Retrograde pyelogram*, via a catheter inserted up the ureter at cystoscopy, may be required to show the exact anatomy of the hydronephrosis and to demonstrate any obstructive cause in the ureter.

Treatment

This is directed at removal of any underlying obstructive cause of the hydronephrosis. Where the cause is a neuromuscular inco-ordination, an operation to widen the pelvi-ureteric junction (pyeloplasty) may save the kidney from progressive damage. A completely useless (particularly an infected) kidney is an indication for nephrectomy provided the other kidney has reasonable function.

Hydronephrosis in a solitary kidney is an indication for emergency drainage, either by percutaneous nephrostomy or retrograde passage of a double J ureteric stent.

Urinary tract calculi

Aetiology

Knowledge of stone formation within the urinary tract is still inadequate and many stones form without apparent explanation. Predisposing factors may be classified into three main groups:

1 inadequate drainage;
2 excess of normal constituents in the urine;
3 presence of abnormal constituents in the urine.

Inadequate drainage

Calculi may form whenever urine stagnates, e.g. within a hydronephrosis or in a diverticulum of the bladder.

Excess of normal constituents

Increased concentration of solutes in the urine, either due to a low urine volume or an increased excretion, may result in precipitation from a supersaturated solution.

- *Inadequate urine volume*: renal stones are particularly common in people from temperate climates who go to live in the tropics, where dehydration produces extremely concentrated urine.
- *Increased excretion of calcium*, hypercalciuria, may be secondary to hypercalcaemia, or, more commonly, idiopathic. Common causes of an increase in serum calcium are hyperparathyroidism (see p. 308) and prolonged immobilization (e.g. an orthopaedic patient on traction or a paraplegic person confined to bed).
- *Increased uric acid* in the serum may be accompanied by uric acid stone formation. The commonest cause is gout, but it may also occur following chemotherapy for leukaemia, lymphoma or polycythaemia.
- *Increased oxalate excretion* results from increased dietary intake, with strawberries, rhubarb, leafy vegetables and tea being amongst the culprits. Hyperoxaluria is also a complication of loss of the terminal ileum (e.g. in Crohn's disease or after surgical resection).

Presence of abnormal constituents

- *Urinary infection*, particularly in the presence of obstruction, e.g. hydronephrosis or chronic retention, produces epithelial sloughs upon which calculi may deposit. In addition, infection may alter the urine pH favouring precipitation of certain solutes. A high pH, brought about by the presence of urea-splitting organisms such as *Proteus*, favours calcium phosphate stone formation, for example.
- *Foreign bodies*, such as non-absorbable sutures inserted at operation, ureteric stents, sloughed necrotic renal papilla or a fragment of broken urinary catheter, may act as a nidus for stone formation.
- *Vitamin A deficiency*, which may occur in primitive communities, results in hyperkera-

tosis of the urinary epithelium, which again provides the debris upon which stones may form.

• *Cystinuria* (resulting from an inborn error of amino-acid metabolism) may result in cystine stone deposition.

Composition of urinary calculi

The three common stones are oxalate, phosphate and urate.

• *Oxalate stones* (calcium oxalate) are the most common (60%). They are hard with a sharp, spiky surface, which traumatizes the urinary epithelium; the resultant bleeding usually colours the stone a dark brown or black.

• *Phosphate stones* (33%) are composed of a mixture of calcium, ammonium and magnesium phosphate ('triple phosphate stone'). They are hard, white and chalky. They are nearly always found in an infected urine and produce the large 'stag-horn' calculus deposited within a pyonephrosis.

• *Uric acid and urate stones* (5%) are moderately hard and brown in colour with a smooth surface. Pure uric acid stones are radio-translucent but, fortunately for diagnosis, most contain enough calcium to render them opaque to X-rays.

• *Cystine stones* account for about 1% of urinary calculi.

Note that a stone found in the lower urinary tract may have arisen there primarily or it may have migrated there from a primary source within the kidney.

Clinical features (Fig. 41.3)

Pain is the presenting feature of the great majority of kidney stones, but if the calculus is embedded within the solid substance of the kidney it may be entirely symptom-free. Within the minor or major calyx system the stone produces a dull loin pain. Impaction of the stone at the pelvi-ureteric junction, or migration down the ureter itself, produces the dreadful agony of ureteric colic; the pain radiates from loin to groin, is of great severity and is accompanied by typical restlessness of the patient, who is quite unable to lie still in

bed. Unlike the usual textbook description, the pain is not usually intermittent, but is continuous, although quite often with sharp exacerbations on a background of continued pain. There is often accompanying vomiting and sweating.

Haematuria, which may be microscopic or macroscopic, is frequently present so that detection of blood in the urine is an extremely helpful means of confirming the clinical diagnosis.

Special investigations

These are usefully divided into investigations to confirm the diagnosis, and others to elucidate the aetiology of the stone.

Diagnostic investigations

• *Urine* is tested for the presence of blood.

• *Plain abdominal X-ray* specifically looking at kidneys, ureters and bladder (more accurately termed a KUB), will show the presence of stone in 90% of cases.

• *IVU* will demonstrate the exact anatomy of the renal system, e.g. the presence of associated hydronephrosis, although a completely obstructed kidney may show no function whatsoever.

There is an important catch for the unwary; a small stone within the kidney may be completely obscured by the contrast of the pyelogram. Never state that a kidney is free from stones without first carefully inspecting a plain X-ray of the renal area.

Investigation of the underlying cause

• *Urine microscopy and culture*: the urine is cultured for bacteria and examined microscopically for the presence of cystine crystals.

• *Analysis of the stone*, whether passed spontaneously or removed surgically, should be performed.

• *Uric acid* estimation. The serum uric acid is raised in gout with its associated uric acid stones.

• *Serum calcium* estimation is carried out. Hypercalcaemia (a value above 2.75 mmol/L) is suspicious of the presence of a parathyroid

URINARY CALCULI

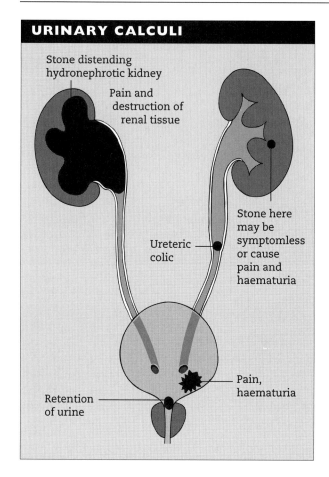

Stone distending hydronephrotic kidney

Pain and destruction of renal tissue

Ureteric colic

Stone here may be symptomless or cause pain and haematuria

Pain, haematuria

Retention of urine

Fig. 41.3 Diagram of the effects of urinary calculi.

tumour, although the incidence of stones due to this cause is low.

Complications
• *Hydronephrosis*: see page 321.
• *Infection*: pyelonephritis, pyonephrosis.
• *Anuria* due either to impaction of calculi in the ureter on each side, or blockage of the ureter in a remaining solitary kidney.

Treatment
Acute ureteric colic
Analgesia, either repeated injections of pethidine or rectal diclofenac, is given to relieve the severe pain. The great majority of small stones within the ureter (up to the size and shape of a date stone) pass spontaneously. These ureteric

stones tend to lodge at one of three places: (i) the pelvi-ureteric junction; (ii) the point at which the ureter crosses the pelvic brim; and (iii) the entrance of the ureter into the bladder. The lower the stone, the more likely it is to pass spontaneously.

Ureteric calculi
If the stone remains in the ureter following an episode of acute colic and cannot or will not pass spontaneously, intervention is necessary. This can normally be achieved endoscopically with the aid of a Dormia stone basket or electrohydraulic lithotriptor. If non-invasive methods fail, the stone may have to be removed by open operation (*ureterolithotomy*).

Renal calculi

A small calculus lodged in the solid substance of the kidney without symptoms can be left alone but kept under periodic survey. Larger renal stones require removal. This may be performed percutaneously by nephroscopy. Large stones may be shattered using either an ultrasonic or electrohydrolic lithotriptor.

Extracorporeal lithotripsy can be employed to shatter the stone without any open surgery. Ultrasonic shock waves are focused onto the calculus and cause it to shatter. The small fragments are passed spontaneously, often resulting in acute colic.

Only occasionally now is it necessary to perform open surgery simply to remove the stone, either through the kidney substance (*nephrolithotomy*) or, wherever possible, through its pelvis (*pyelolithotomy*). Where the kidney is grossly and irreparably damaged, nephrectomy should be performed.

Acute calculus anuria

This may be due to blockage of both ureters by stone, or obstruction of a solitary kidney. It is treated by catheterizing the ureters or, if the ureteric catheter cannot be passed beyond the obstruction, the impacted stone must be removed, and, if necessary, drainage of the renal pelvis is carried out via a nephrostomy. If the patient is uraemic, the general condition is first improved by haemo- or peritoneal dialysis and nephrostomy, before definitive surgery.

Treatment of the cause

In every case of renal stone an attempt is made to determine the underlying cause and eliminate it. Thus, renal infection is dealt with and surgical correction of any obstructive lesion performed. A small percentage of recurrent and bilateral stones are found to be due to parathyroid tumour (see p. 308), removal of which will prevent further recurrences. In every case of renal calculus disease, the patient should be instructed to drink liberal quantities of fluid in order to encourage the production of a dilute urine.

Urinary tract infections

The urinary tract may be divided into the upper tract, comprising ureter and kidney, and the lower tract, comprising bladder and urethra. Lower tract infections arise from ascending infection up the urethra. Upper tract infection may be either due to haematogenous infection of the kidney, or an ascending infection from the lower urinary tract.

Cystitis

Cystitis is usually an ascending infection, which, because of the short urethra, is more common in women, often as a sequela of copulation. In men it is commonly the consequence of urethral or prostatic obstruction. Urethral catheterization invariably results in bacterial colonization of the bladder.

The principal symptoms are of a stinging/burning pain on passing urine (dysuria), with increased frequency and urgency. Haematuria may be present, and examination confirms a low-grade pyrexia and suprapubic tenderness. Loin pain suggests ascending infection.

Special investigations

In the female, recurrent infections are an indication for full investigation. In men and children, a single episode is unusual and merits investigation.

- *Urine microscopy and culture* to identify the causative organism (invariably bowel flora, usually *Escherichia coli*). The presence of pus cells with no growth is a feature of bladder cancer.
- *Ultrasound scan* of the bladder and kidneys may reveal dilatation of the upper tracts. A post-micturition ultrasound scan may demonstrate a large residual volume of urine within the bladder suggesting obstruction or atony.
- *Plain abdominal X-ray* to exclude a bladder stone as a source of recurrent infection.
- *Cystoscopy*: bladder diverticula and other structural defects should be sought.

Treatment

Antibiotics are given according to sensitivity of the infecting organism. A high oral fluid intake is encouraged. Alkalinizing the urine with potassium citrate, and drinking cranberry juice is helpful. Recurrent post-coital cystitis is an indication for prophylactic antibiotic therapy. Any underlying cause, e.g. calculus or prostatic obstruction, must be dealt with.

Chronic pyelonephritis

Chronic pyelonephritis describes the effect of recurrent infections, which result in shrunken, scarred kidneys. It is more common in childhood, as the growing kidney seems most susceptible, and chronic pyelonephritis accounts for almost 20% of chronic renal failure in adults. In childhood, it is due to a combination of two factors: vesico-ureteric reflux and intrarenal reflux.

Vesico-ureteric reflux

Where the normal valve mechanism at the vesico-ureteric junction is deficient, such as with an ectopic ureter in a duplex system, urine can pass back up the ureter during bladder contraction.

Intrarenal reflux

The collecting duct enters the calyx of the kidney, leaving the renal papilla. The ducts normally open obliquely, such that, as the pressure within the calyx increases, the ducts close preventing urine from refluxing into the kidney (intrarenal reflux). If the ducts do not open obliquely, as is seen in compound papillae, intrarenal reflux may occur. If the urine is infected, the resultant inflammation leaves a permanent scar and loss of nephrons. Repeated episodes of infection result in major damage and loss of function.

Clinical features

While the typical features of urinary infection, namely dysuria, frequency and pyrexia, may be present, subclinical infection, often only signified by urinary incontinence at night, is common, particularly in children.

Special investigations

- *Micturating cystogram*: contrast is first introduced into the bladder; the patient voids, and reflux of urine during voiding can be recorded.
- *IVU* may show scarring, with a thin cortex overlying a distorted calyx, particularly at the upper and lower pole. The normal cupping of the calyces is reversed, and is termed clubbing.

Treatment

The cause of the chronic pyelonephritis should be treated when identified. Long-term low-dose antibiotic prophylaxis is given to patients with asymptomatic or frequent infections.

Pyonephrosis

This is an infected hydronephrosis in which the kidney becomes no more than a bag of pus. If the ureter is obstructed there may be little to find on examining the urine, although more commonly pyuria is a marked feature. Usually the enlarged tender kidney is easily palpable.

Special investigations

- *IVU* shows little or no function and an enlarged renal shadow.
- *Dimercaptosuccinate (DMSA) scintigraphy* will quantify the residual function in the kidney after treatment.

Treatment

There should be urgent drainage by percutaneous nephrostomy. If there is no residual renal function, nephrectomy is required.

Carbuncle of the kidney

This is better termed cortical abscess of the kidney and represents a haematogenous infection, usually *Staphylococcus aureus*, coming from a primary focus such as a cutaneous boil.

Clinical features

There is pyrexia, toxaemia, pain and tenderness in the loin, and the kidney may be palpable.

Special investigations

- *Urine* is frequently sterile unless the abscess bursts into the calyceal system.
- *Full blood count*: there is a leucocytosis.
- *IVU* shows distortion of the calyces but often the oedematous kidney excretes poorly.

Treatment

Treatment consists of surgical drainage, together with antibiotics.

Perinephric abscess

Infection of the perinephric space is usually secondary to rupture of a carbuncle of the kidney. Rarely, it may complicate a pyonephrosis or infection of a traumatic peri-renal haematoma.

Clinical features

There is the constitutional evidence of acute infection and in addition a diffuse tender bulge in the affected loin. This is particularly well seen when the back is carefully inspected with the patient lying prone.

Special investigations

- *Abdominal X-ray (a KUB)* may show loss of the psoas shadow due to retroperitoneal oedema.
- *IVU* may be normal or may show the features of a renal cortical abscess or a pyonephrosis.
- *CT scan* will enable accurate localization of the abscess.

Treatment

Surgical drainage through a flank incision.

Renal tuberculosis

Pathology

The kidney may be involved either as part of a generalized miliary spread of tuberculosis or more commonly as a focal lesion representing haematogenous spread from a distant site in the lungs (25% of cases have pulmonary tuberculosis), the bone or gut. The original focus may be quiescent at the time of active renal disease.

Early lesions are found near the junction of the cortex and medulla. These enlarge, caseate and then rupture into a calyx, eventually producing extensive destruction of renal substance. The ureter becomes infiltrated and thickened; its obstruction leads to tuberculous pyonephrosis. Rarely a pyonephrosis becomes completely walled off as a symptomless, caseous and calcified mass ('autonephrectomy').

Spread of infected urine down the ureter frequently produces a tuberculous cystitis and may result in infection of the epididymis and seminal vesicles.

Untreated, the contralateral kidney often becomes involved, but this probably represents a separate haematogenous spread.

Clinical features

The patient is usually a young adult, often with a present or previous history of tuberculosis elsewhere. In the UK, the patient is likely to be an immigrant from Asia. Symptoms in the early stages are mild and indeed may be entirely absent. There may be dysuria, frequency, pyuria or haematuria, which may be gross but is more usually slight or only microscopic. There may be loin pain on the affected side.

In more advanced cases the dysuria and frequency become intense because of extensive involvement of the bladder, and then constitutional symptoms of tuberculosis, with fever, night sweats, loss of weight and anaemia, may be present.

In some cases a tuberculous epididymitis is the presenting feature (see p. 360).

Examination is usually negative, but the kidney may be tender and palpable. The epididymis and seminal vesicles may be enlarged and thickened if involved. The epididymis often feels craggy due to calcification.

Special investigations

• *Urine* is commonly sterile to ordinary culture but contains pus cells and is acid in reaction ('sterile acid pyuria') as well as protein and usually red cells. Acid-fast bacilli may be present on containing Ziehl–Neelson staining of a spun deposit from an early morning specimen of urine. Three early morning specimens of urine are sent for culture which takes 6 weeks.

• *IVU* may show failure of calyceal filling, irregularity of calyces and patchy calcification.

• *Chest X-ray* may show a primary lung focus.

• *Cystoscopy* may reveal a decreased capacity of the bladder, an oedematous mucosa on which tubercles may be seen and perhaps a 'golf-hole' ureteric orifice, the ureter being held rigidly open by surrounding fibrosis.

Treatment

Anti-tuberculous therapy should not be commenced until the diagnosis has been confirmed, as, once undertaken, treatment must be prolonged. Treatment usually involves isoniazid, and rifampicin supplemented by pyrazinamide. Healing occurs with the production of fibrous tissue, which in early cases merely produces a small scar. In advanced disease this fibrous tissue may lead to stricture formation at the neck of a calyx or at the pelvi-ureteric junction with a secondary hydronephrosis. Similar scarring of the heavily involved bladder may produce gross contraction on healing.

Surgery is only indicated in a minority of patients with advanced disease or where complications occur.

Renal failure

Acute renal failure

Acute renal failure is characterized by a reduced glomerular filtration rate (GFR), retention of nitrogenous waste (urea and creatinine rise), impaired acid–base balance (acidosis develops) and, usually, a reduced urine output.

An absence of urine production is termed anuria, while production of less than 400 ml/day in the adult is oliguria.

Aetiology

In the surgical context, acute renal failure may be a consequence of surgery, or be due to a surgically treatable lesion.

The causes of acute renal failure may be usefully divided into pre-renal, renal, and post-renal, in a similar way to the causes of jaundice relative to the liver. The presence of two kidneys means that the pathology must affect both kidneys in order to manifest, unless one kidney has previously failed or been removed.

Pre-renal causes

Pre-renal factors involve reduction in the blood flow to the kidney resulting in a decreased glomerular filtration rate.

1 *Fluid loss:*
   (a) blood loss, e.g. haemorrhage;
   (b) plasma loss, e.g. burns, generalized peritonitis;
   (c) electrolyte loss, e.g. vomiting, diarrhoea, fistula, inadequate replacement.

2 *Impaired circulation:*
   (a) General factors, e.g. hypotension due to sepsis, cardiac failure;
   (b) local factors, e.g. aortic dissection where the renal arteries are excluded from the circulation.

Renal perfusion is maintained in the presence of mild hypoperfusion by a number of regulatory mechanisms; vasoconstriction of splanchnic, muscular and cutaneous vascular beds, and alteration of afferent and efferent renal arteriolar tone. The GFR is normally maintained even if the mean arterial pressure falls to 60–80 mmHg. In hypertensive patients, the elderly, and patients with pre-existing renal disease (e.g. diabetic nephropathy), autoregulation may be impaired and the GFR maintained only at higher mean pressures. Some drugs, particularly non-steroidal anti-inflammatory drugs (NSAIDs) and angiotensin-converting enzyme (ACE) inhibitors, also impair the normal compensatory mechanisms and make the kidney more sensitive to hypovolaemia.

Renal causes

Renal causes of acute renal failure include factors directly acting upon the glomerular apparatus and tubules:
• acute tubular necrosis (ATN);
• acute cortical necrosis, due to severe ischaemia;
• myoglobin, released following a crush injury, or reperfusion of an ischaemic limb;
• drugs, e.g. antibiotics such as gentamicin, NSAIDs such as diclofenac;
• acute nephritis — interstitial nephritis or glomerulonephritis.

Post-renal, or obstructive, causes

An obstruction lesion occurring at any level from the tubules to the urethra may cause renal impairment. Only in patients with a solitary kidney will an upper tract obstruction cause acute renal failure; otherwise the obstruction is likely to be in the lower tracts and affect both kidneys.

Clinical features

The majority of cases of acute renal failure are pre-renal in aetiology, which means that the kidneys will recover as soon as the circulation is restored. The diagnosis is usually clear; the patient has failed to pass urine and bladder catheterization reveals no urine, or a mere trickle. The most common 'cause' of apparent oliguria while catheterized, i.e. a blocked catheter, should always be excluded.

Special investigations

Initial investigation should be rapidly performed, since rapid treatment may prevent life-threatening sequelae, and the shorter the period of failure the more quickly renal function will be restored.
• *Serum electrolytes*: urea and creatinine are raised; potassium may be very high and demands immediate treatment (see below).
• *Renal tract Doppler ultrasound*: are there two

kidneys, and are they perfused? Are they normal size, or is one small, suggesting prior renal disease? Is there evidence of hydronephrosis/hydro-ureter? Is the bladder full, or empty? If obstruction is documented it should be rapidly relieved, and this may require bladder catheterization or even nephrostomy.
• *Urine microscopy and stick test* for blood and protein. Some blood may be present as a consequence of urethral catheterization. Rhabdomyolysis is suggested by a postive stick test for blood without red cells on microscopy. Acute nephritis should be considered when blood and protein are present.

Management

Replenish the intravascular volume

Initial management requires a clinical assessment of the intravascular volume to determine the extent of volume depletion. The best signs are the following.
• *Jugular venous pressure* (JVP)—is it visible and is it raised?
• *Postural hypotension*: is there a fall in blood pressure when the patient stands up? (If the patient cannot stand, it should be measured lying and sitting up in bed.)

Depletion of intravascular volume is suggested by a postural fall in blood pressure and a low (not visible) JVP. Treatment requires rapid infusion of a fluid that remains in the intravascular compartment (blood, colloid or saline, but not dextrose). Infusion is continued until the JVP is visible and postural hypotension corrected. Until a diuresis is established, potassium additives should not be given, as patients are likely to be hyperkalaemic.

A *central venous catheter* may be inserted at this stage to measure accurately the central venous pressure (CVP); the target pressure is $10\,cmH_2O$ measured relative to the axilla. In septic patients or those with cardiac disease, a pulmonary artery catheter (Swann–Ganz) may be helpful, both for measurement of the pulmonary capillary wedge pressure and to determine systemic vascular resistance and so indicate the requirement for inotropes such as noradrenaline.

Once volume repletion is achieved, the infusion is stopped until the urine output picks up. Further infusion would result in fluid overload, and would require dialysis to remove in the absence of renal function.

Dopamine and diuretics

If rehydration is unsuccessful in inducing a diuresis, low-dose dopamine infusion (1 μg/kg/min) may help, and a bolus of frusemide (100–500 mg over 15 minutes) should be given.

If these measures fail to induce a diuresis, it is likely that either acute tubular necrosis, or, less commonly, acute cortical necrosis has occurred.

Hyperkalaemia

A potassium over 6.5 mmol/L should be treated immediately to avoid life-threatening ventricular arrhythmias. The electrocardiogram (ECG) changes with increasing potassium; first the T waves become peaked (tenting); next the P waves disappear and finally the ECG becomes sinusoidal. Resolution of these appearances can be monitored with treatment.

Calcium gluconate (10 ml of 10% i.v.) should be given over a few minutes, to stabilize the myocardium. Insulin and dextrose (15 units of soluble insulin in 50 ml of 50% dextrose) is given as an infusion over 10–20 minutes. This drives potassium into the cells, and lowers serum potassium by 1–2 mmol/L. Because these measures do not remove potassium from the body, a more definitive treatment is necessary before the potassium rises once more. This is best achieved by establishing a diuresis, but, if this fails, urgent dialysis is indicated. Potassium exchange resins (e.g. calcium resonium), taken by mouth or given by enema, may give good interim potassium control. However, they tend to cause constipation, so a laxative (e.g. lactulose 10–20 ml b.d.) should also be prescribed.

Acute tubular necrosis

Persistence of acute renal failure after correction of hypovolaemia is usually due to the development of acute tubular necrosis (ATN). This is characterized by a prolonged period of oliguria lasting anywhere from a few days to 3–6 weeks.

Pathology

The condition usually follows ischaemia to the kidneys. Different parts of the nephron are more sensitive to ischaemia than others, so that while the glomerular apparatus is usually preserved, the tubules, especially the proximal tubules, suffer patchy ischaemic damage. The kidneys become enlarged and oedematous. As this damage recovers, renal function returns.

Clinical features

The features are of a persistent oliguria, unresponsive to replenishment of the intravascular circulating volume. The symptoms are those of acute renal failure described above.

Treatment

If ATN is established, the patient should be managed by regular dialysis until function returns. Recovery of function is characterized by a stepwise increase in urine output, although there may be a short polyuric phase during which maintenance of fluid balance can be difficult.

If function fails to return, it is more likely that acute cortical necrosis occurred with necrosis of glomeruli in addition to tubules.

Chronic renal failure

Chronic renal failure may be classified into three groups, like acute renal failure. Most causes are non-surgical, but some surgically correctable causes are given below.

1 *Pre-renal*: renal artery stenosis.
2 *Post-renal (obstructive)*:
   (a) congenital posterior urethral valves;
   (b) prostatic hypertrophy/carcinoma, which causes chronic retention and upper tract dilatation;

(c) urethral stricture;

(d) cervical carcinoma, infiltrating the ureters;

(e) urothelial tumour affecting bladder base or both ureters.

Symptoms are of malaise, weakness, confusion, hiccoughs with pallor, hypertension and fluid overload (e.g. pulmonary oedema, ankle oedema) on examination. The investigations are those of acute renal failure, and are directed at finding a treatable cause such as prostatic hypertrophy. In the absence of a treatable lesion, established renal failure is managed by renal replacement therapy with either peritoneal or haemodialysis, with a view to renal transplantation in the future.

Renal tumours

Tumours of the kidney are divided into those arising from the kidney substance itself and those originating from the renal pelvis.

Classification
Of the kidney itself
1 Benign:
(a) adenoma (small and symptomless);
(b) haemangioma (a rare cause of haematuria).
2 Malignant.
(a) Primary: nephroblastoma, adenocarcinoma.
(b) Secondary: the kidney is an uncommon site for deposits of carcinoma although it may be involved in advanced cases of lymphoma and leukaemia, as well as tumours of breast and bronchus.

Of the renal pelvis
- Papilloma.
- Transitional carcinoma.
- Squamous carcinoma.

The two principal tumours of the kidney are the nephroblastoma, which usually occurs in children under the age of 4 years, and adenocarcinoma, which usually occurs over the age of 40 years.

Nephroblastoma (Wilms' tumour*)
Pathology
This is an extremely anaplastic tumour, which usually arises in children under the age of 5 years, although it occasionally affects older children and adolescents. It probably originates from embryonic mesodermal tissue. Bilateral tumours are present in 5–10% of cases, and there is an association with congenital anomalies (aniridia, hemihypertrophy, macroglossia) in a few patients.

Macroscopically, the tumours are large and may be difficult to distinguish from neuroblastoma (see p. 314). They are pale on cut section, and contain areas of haemorrhage.

Microscopically, there is a mixture of mesenchymal and epithelial components, with spindle cells, epithelial tubules and smooth or striated muscle fibres.

The regional lymph nodes are soon invaded, and spread occurs by the blood stream to the lungs and liver.

Clinical features
Rapid growth produces a large mass in the loin, although involvement of the renal pelvis is late and therefore haematuria relatively uncommon. Other features include weight loss and anorexia, fever and hypertension. Children may also present on account of metastases, which occasionally involve bone.

Special investigations
- *Ultrasonography* may distinguish the solid tumour from a cystic or hydronephrotic mass.
- *CT scan* is useful for staging and preoperative assessment, in particular to look at the contralateral kidney.

*Max Wilm (1867–1918), Professor of Surgery, first in Basle, Switzerland, and then Heidelberg, Germany.

Treatment

Where possible nephrectomy is performed. In early disease, with no residual tumour following surgery, cytotoxic chemotherapy alone will give prolonged survival. For more extensive disease, radiotherapy is given. Where the tumour is unresectable, chemotherapy is given and nephrectomy performed once the tumour regresses.

This intensive therapy has improved the prognosis of a condition that previously could seldom be cured. Overall prognosis is 80% 5-year survival, with cure of early disease.

Adenocarcinoma (hypernephroma or Grawitz's tumour*)

Pathology

This tumour accounts for 80% of all renal tumours. Males are affected twice as often as females. The patients are usually 40 years of age or over. It may be associated with familial conditions such as tuberose sclerosis and von Hippel–Lindau disease, and can be bilateral.

Macroscopically, the tumour appears as a large, vascular, golden yellow mass, usually in one or other pole of the kidney (hence its earlier name hypernephroma).

Microscopically, the tumour cells are typically large with an abundant foamy cytoplasm and a small central densely staining nucleus.

The tumour originates from the renal tubules and not from suprarenal rests as was postulated by Grawitz.

Spread

• *Directly* thoughout the renal substance with invasion of the perinephric tissues.
• *Via lymphatics* to the para-aortic lymph nodes.
• *Via blood stream* with growth along the renal vein into the inferior vena cava (IVC), from which it may shower emboli. Metastases in the lung, bones and brain are common. Occlusion of the IVC results in a typical appearance with bilateral leg oedema.

*Paul Grawitz (1850–1932), Pathologist, Grefswald, Germany.

The adenocarcinoma of the kidney is a tumour that may occasionally produce a solitary blood-borne deposit, so that removal of the primary together with this deposit has been followed in some instances by prolonged survival.

Clinical features

The patient may present with either symptoms of local disease, or of one of the paraneoplastic syndromes with which it may be associated.

Local disease

The triad of symptoms of a renal cell carcinoma are:

1 haematuria, present in half the cases—it may produce clot colic;
2 loin pain, aching, present in 40%;
3 loin mass presenting in 25%.

Rarely, a left varicocele may occur (1%) as a consequence of tumour spread along the left renal vein occluding the confluence with the testicular vein on that side.

General features

In addition to local symptoms the patient may present with the general features of malignancy, namely anaemia, loss of weight and occasionally as a pyrexia of unknown origin (PUO), or as a consequence of secondary deposits, e.g. a pathological fracture.

Paraneoplastic syndromes

A number of hormones may be released from renal adenocarcinomas. Amongst the results are hypertension (renin production), polycythaemia (erythropoietin) and hypercalcaemia (ectopic parathormone production).

On examination the diseased kidney may be palpable.

Special investigations

• *Urine* nearly always contains either macroscopic or microscopic blood.
• *IVU* reveals distortion of the calyces by a polar tumour which may occasionally show flecks of calcification.
• *Ultrasonography and CT scanning* provide

accurate visualization of the tumour and can indicate spread to lymph nodes and caval invasion.

• *Angiography* is valuable to demonstrate a typical tumour circulation, and differentiates the avascular filling defect of a renal cyst.

Treatment

Radical nephrectomy is performed. Radio-therapy is indicated if the tumour has the surrounding perinephric fat. Post-operative treatment with progestagens may be worth-while in some patients with disseminated disease.

The 5-year survival rate after successful resection is about 50%, but metastases may occur many years after nephrectomy. Poor prognostic factors include perinephric invasion and lymphatic invasion.

Tumours of the renal pelvis

Transitional cell tumours of the renal pelvis vary in malignancy from benign papillomas to highly anaplastic transitional cell carcinomas.

A squamous carcinoma of the renal pelvis may occur when there has been squamous metaplasia of the epithelium; one-third of these cases are associated with renal calculus.

Clinical features

Patients present usually either with haema-turia or with hydronephrosis due to ureteric obstruction. The tumour may seed down the ureter and even involve the bladder.

Treatment

Treatment is nephro-ureterectomy or, if feasible, local wide excision and plastic reconstruction.

CHAPTER 42

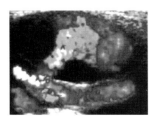

The Bladder

Urachal anomalies

Urachal defects may result from anomalies of the primitive urachal connection. There are three principal anomalies.

1 *Urachal fistula*: a persistent urachal tract, resulting in a urinary discharge at the umbilicus.

2 *Urachal diverticulum*, an out-pouching of the bladder, the urachal equivalent of a Meckel's diverticulum and the vitello-intestinal duct.

3 *Urachal cyst*: if the urachus persists but is closed above and below. The cyst often becomes infected in later life, presenting with peri-umbilical pain and inflammation.

Treatment
In all cases treatment is excision.

Bladder exstrophy (ectopia vesicae)

Failure of fusion of the structures forming the anterior abdominal wall may cause a number of anomalies. Lower urinary tract changes include bladder exstrophy, where the ureters together with the bladder trigone open directly onto the anterior abdominal wall below the umbilicus. This is usually associated with a failure of fusion of the pubic bones, and, in the male, there is an associated epispadias. Typically there is a widened pelvis with a waddling gait.

The infant is completely incontinent of urine, with excoriation of the abdominal skin and a permanent unpleasant ammoniacal smell of infected urine. If the condition is untreated the child may die of pyelonephritis or else frequently develops a carcinoma of the bladder rudiment after initial metaplastic change.

Treatment
Traditional treatment is reimplantation of the ureters either into the colon or into an ileal loop (uretero-ileostomy) combined with excision of the bladder itself as a prophylaxis against malignant change. More recently, complex reconstructive operations to refashion a new bladder have been tried. They are best performed soon after birth, and are unsuitable if there is only a small bladder remnant.

Rupture of the bladder

The bladder may rupture either intraperitoneally or extraperitoneally.

Intraperitoneal rupture
This follows a penetrating wound (e.g. a bullet wound) or crush injury to the pelvis when the bladder is distended. Occasionally, it is consequent upon instrumentation of the bladder, either surgically or during self-catheterization;

rarely, the over-distended bladder of retention may rupture spontaneously.

Extraperitoneal rupture

More common; the bladder may be torn by a spicule of bone in a pelvic fracture or occasionally may be wounded during a hernia operation or repair of a cystocele.

Clinical features

Intraperitoneal rupture produces the typical picture of peritonitis with generalized abdominal pain, marked rigidity and a silent abdomen. *Extraperitoneal rupture* is associated with extraperitoneal extravasation of blood and urine producing a painful swelling that arises out of the pelvis. In this case, differentiation must be made from rupture of the membranous urethra (see p. 348), although this may not be possible until surgical exploration is carried out. Typically, however, a urethral tear is accompanied by anterior displacement of the prostate, which can be detected on rectal examination.

Diagnosis is confirmed by intravenous urogram (IVU) or cystogram, but the latter should be withheld if a urethral injury is possible, as it involves urethral catheterization.

Treatment

Treatment is invariably surgical. The intraperitoneal rupture is sutured and the bladder drained by means of an indwelling urethral (Foley) catheter. It may be possible to suture the extraperitoneal rupture, but if this is inaccessible at the base of the bladder drainage by a suprapubic catheter will suffice to allow healing to occur. The retropubic space is drained and the patient given antibiotic therapy.

Diverticulum of the bladder

The vast majority of diverticula of the bladder are secondary to bladder out-flow obstruction, although a small number are congenital in origin. As it is usually the male bladder which becomes obstructed, 95% of diverticula occur in men.

Pathology

The muscle of the bladder wall hypertrophies as a result of obstruction, and becomes trabeculated. Out-pouches of mucosa occur between the bands of muscle fibres. One or more of these sacs may increase in size to form a fully developed diverticulum, which, because it is devoid of practically all muscle in its wall, is unable to empty and undergoes progressive distension.

Complications

• *Urinary infection* because of urinary stagnation.

• *Calculus formation:* because of a combination of infection and stasis.

• *Malignant change* may occur in its wall.

• *Hydronephrosis* may rarely occur due to pressure of the diverticulum against the adjacent ureter.

Clinical features

The majority of diverticula remain silent unless they undergo one of the complications listed above. Some are found incidentally during investigation of the underlying obstructive lesion, e.g. a prostatic hypertrophy or urethral stricture. Occasionally, a large, uninfected diverticulum gives the strange symptom of double micturition ('*pis en deux*'). In this circumstance, the patient empties his bladder but a substantial amount of the urine passes into the distensible diverticulum. No sooner does micturition end than the diverticulum passively empties again into the bladder, giving the surprised patient the desire once again to empty his bladder.

Special investigations

• *IVU:* contrast medium enters the diverticulum.

• *Cystoscopy:* the mouth of the diverticulum can be visualized.

Treatment

Although small diverticula can be left alone, larger examples must be excised at the time of definitive treatment of the underlying obstructive lesion. Unless excised they become the source of persistent post-operative infection.

Bladder stone

The varieties of bladder calculi are the same as renal stones, namely phosphate, oxalate, urate and rarely cystine.

Aetiology

Bladder stones either originate in the kidney, pass down the ureter into the bladder where they remain and grow, or they originate *de novo* in the bladder. Stones that arise in the bladder are due to:

• *Stasis and infection*: bladder stones commonly arise as a consequence of out-flow obstruction (e.g. urethral stricture or prostatic enlargement). They may be secondary to an atonic bladder in a paraplegic person, and may have arisen first within a bladder diverticulum.
• *Foreign body*: a calculus will deposit on a long-term indwelling catheter or on any foreign body inserted into the bladder.

Clinical features

The typical triad of symptoms of bladder stone are frequency, pain and haematuria. In addition, patients sometimes complain of intermittent stopping of the urinary flow as the stone blocks the internal urinary meatus like a ball valve, and occasionally actual retention of urine may occur if the stone impacts in the urethra.

• *Frequency* is more troublesome during the day than at night, probably because in the upright position the stone lies over, and irritates, the bladder trigone.
• *Pain* is felt in the suprapubic region, in the perineum and the tip of the penis; it particularly occurs at the end of micturition, when the bladder contracts down upon the calculus.

• *Haematuria* tends to occur as the last few drops of urine are passed.

Special investigations

• *Plain abdominal X-ray* (specifically a KUB): the majority of bladder stones are radio-opaque and are readily visible
• *Cystoscopy* allows stones to be seen as well as to be fragmented and retrieved.

Treatment

Unless the stone is very small, when there is a possibility that it will pass spontaneously, it should be removed either by means of crushing with an endoscopic lithotrite under direct vision, by disintegration in a shock-wave lithotripter (if available) or by open cystotomy through a suprapubic incision. At this operation any underlying cause, e.g. a diverticulum or urethral obstruction, must be dealt with or a stone will rapidly recur.

Tumours

Pathology

Bladder tumours may be classified as follows, together with their relative incidence.

Benign
• Transitional cell papilloma (<1%).

Malignant
1 *Primary*:
   (a) transitional cell carcinoma (90%);
   (b) squamous carcinoma arising in an area of metaplasia (7%);
   (c) adenocarcinoma (uncommon, but may occur in urachal remnants) (2%);
   (d) sarcomas (rare)
2 *Secondary*: direct invasion from adjacent tumours, i.e. colonic, renal, ovarian, uterine, prostatic tumours.

Transitional cell papilloma

Transitional cell papillomas grade imperceptibly into malignant tumours, and many pathologists regard them as low-grade carcinomas, especially because they have a tendency to recur after treatment, to seed elsewhere in the bladder and to undergo frank malignant change.

Transitional cell carcinoma
These are commonly found in middle-aged and elderly patients. Males are far more frequently affected than females.

Aetiology
Risk factors include cigarette smoking (twofold increase in incidence), and workers in the aniline dye and rubber industry because of the excretion of carcinogens such as β-naphthylamine in the urine. The manufacture of many of the more dangerous dyes and chemicals has been abolished in this country. There is a high incidence of malignant change in the exposed bladder mucosa of ectopia vesicae (p. 334), in diverticula of the bladder and in the bladder infected with schistosomiasis; in these cases, characterized by chronic inflammation, squamous carcinoma is common.

Pathology
Although any part of the bladder may be involved, growths are particularly common at the base, trigone and around the ureteric orifices. They are often multiple, signifying a field change throughout the transitional urothelium with the tendency for tumours to develop anywhere from the renal pelvis to the urethra.

Macroscopic appearance
The well-differentiated papillomas form fine fronds, which resemble seaweed floating in the urine. The more malignant tumours are sessile, solid growths, which infiltrate the bladder wall, then ulcerate, often with marked surrounding cystitis.

Microscopic appearance
The papillomas have a connective tissue core and no involvement of the stem. The carcinomas may be well- or poorly differentiated transitional cell tumours but, rarely, keratinizing squamous cell tumours or adenocarcinomas may be seen.

Spread
• *Local*, with infiltration of the bladder wall, the prostate, urethra, sigmoid colon and rectum, or, in the female, the pelvic viscera. The ureteric orifices may be occluded, producing hydronephrosis and ultimately renal failure. The pelvic skeleton may be directly invaded.
• *Lymphatic*, to the iliac and para-aortic lymph nodes.
• *Blood-borne* spread occurs late to the liver and the lungs.
• *Implantation* may take place into the scar if open operation is performed.

Clinical features
Bladder tumours usually present with painless haematuria. A malignant tumour that ulcerates and invades may also produce dysuria, frequency and urgency of micturition. Occasionally, the patient may present with hydronephrosis due to ureteric obstruction or with retention of urine due either to clot, or to growth involving the urethra. In late cases there may be severe pain from pelvic invasion or uraemia from bilateral ureteric obstruction.

Examination is usually negative in benign papilloma, but a malignant tumour is quite frequently palpable on bimanual examination, best performed at the time of cystoscopy.

Special investigations
• *Urine examination* usually reveals blood, either to the naked eye or microscopically. Cytological examination may detect malignant cells.
• *IVU* may demonstrate a filling defect and perhaps ureteric obstruction or hydronephrosis. At the same time the presence of pelvic bony secondaries may be revealed.
• *Cystoscopy* is the most valuable investigation since the exact nature of the tumour can be determined and a biopsy obtained.

Staging

Staging is generally according to the TNM system. The local staging (T) involves both bimanual palpation and histological examination to ascertain the depth of invasion through the bladder wall.

Treatment

The management of bladder carcinoma is difficult and the results are often poor. Factors to be taken into consideration are the degree of differentiation of the tumour (information obtained by endoscopic biopsy), the extent of local spread, evidence of dissemination and the general condition of the patient.

Papilloma

Most benign papillomas can be controlled by fulguration or resection via an operating cystoscope. Once the patient has developed a papilloma there is a high risk of further lesions occurring, and the patient should be supervised by regular cystoscopic examinations.

Superficial cancers (T1 and T2)

Tumours that do not penetrate the bladder wall (T1 and T2) may be removed by endoscopic resection followed by regular cystoscopic review. Seventy per cent will have recurrent tumour, which can usually be treated either by cystoscopic coagulation or further endoscopic removal. Poorly differentiated T2 tumours should best be treated as if they were T3.

Deeply invasive cancers (T3 and T4)

If the bladder wall has been breached (T3) or the pelvic wall or prostate actually invaded (T4), radiotherapy is used, often preceded by a preliminary debulking of the tumour by transurethral resection. Endoscopic follow-up at frequent intervals is necessary. If the tumour recurs, or fails to respond to radiotherapy, then, in the absence of metastatic disease, total cystectomy should be performed (salvage cystectomy).

At cystectomy, the bladder and distal ureters are removed, along with the prostate or gynaecological organs, with implantation of the ureters into a tube of ileum brought out as a stoma (an ileal conduit). Alternatively, implantation of the ureters into the sigmoid colon can be performed, but there is a high incidence of ascending infection, and hyperchloraemic acidosis due to the resorption of chloride from the colon.

Total cystectomy may also be indicated where there is extensive papillomatosis that cannot be controlled by diathermy, or to remove a seriously damaged post-irradiation bladder that is grossly fibrosed or subject to persistent haematuria as a result of post-radiotherapy telangiectasia.

CHAPTER 43

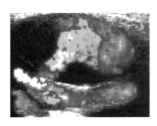

The Prostate

There are two common conditions of the prostate that require consideration: benign enlargement and carcinoma.

Benign enlargement

Pathology

Some degree of enlargement of the prostate is extremely common from the age of 45 years onwards, but this enlargement often produces either no, or only minor, symptoms. Seventy per cent of men have benign hyperplasia by the age of 70 years.

The prostate, like the breast and thyroid, is composed of glandular tissue and stroma, which have periods of activity and involution throughout life under the influences of a changing milieu of hormones. Associated with these periods, the gland may become enlarged, with excessive proliferation of both fibrous and epithelial tissue.

Enlargement of the prostate results in encroachment on the prostatic urethra. The median lobe may also enlarge, a rounded swelling overlying the posterior aspect of the internal urinary meatus. The three lobes may then obstruct the urethral lumen, impeding the passage of urine.

Pathological consequences of out-flow obstruction

• *Trabeculation of the bladder:* as a result of the obstruction, the bladder hypertrophies and the thickened muscle bands produce trabeculation.

• *Bladder diverticula* form from saccules between muscle bands.

• *Bladder stones* form as a consequence of urinary stasis, particularly in diverticula.

• *Urinary infection* may occur (especially after catheterization).

• *Hydronephrosis* results from back pressure on the ureters, which may result in renal failure.

• *Renal failure*, due to progressive hydronephrosis, resulting in anaemia and uraemia. It is commonly referred to as obstructive nephropathy.

Clinical features

There are three types of symptoms that result from prostatic hypertrophy: *obstructive symptoms* consequent upon bladder out-flow impedance, *irritative symptoms* due to the muscular instability of the bladder (detrusor instability), and the *symptoms of the sequelae* such as infection or renal failure.

Obstructive symptoms

The narrowing of the prostatic urethra and the possible median lobe enlargement cause the patient's difficulty in passing urine, with a poor and intermittent stream. There may be difficulty starting (hesitancy), and dribbling at the end of micturition (terminal dribbling).

Associated with the prostatic enlargement, there may be partial obstruction and congestion of the prostatic plexus of veins, which may produce haematuria, which usually occurs at the end of micturition when the bladder contracts around the enlarged intravesical part of the prostate. As a cause of haematuria, bleeding from distended veins should only be diagnosed after exclusion of intravesical and upper tract tumours.

Eventually, the bladder is likely to fail to overcome the obstruction and this results in retention of urine. This may be *acute*, with sudden onset and severe pain, or *chronic*, in which the bladder gradually becomes distended and the patient develops dribbling overflow incontinence, with little or no pain. It is in the latter group that uraemia is likely to occur. In some instances a complete obstruction then supervenes ('*acute on chronic obstruction*').

Symptoms of detrusor instability

Involuntary contractions of the distended bladder result in frequency, urgency and nocturia. Urinary tract infection may exacerbate the symptoms, or precipitate acute retention (see below).

Symptoms of renal failure

The obstruction to the out-flow of the bladder may result in renal failure with drowsiness, headache and impairment of intellect due to uraemia. It is therefore always wise to examine the bladder for enlargement and to determine the blood urea on an elderly man with inexplicable behavioural changes.

Examination

The patient with an enlarged prostate, if uraemic, is likely to be pale and wasted, with a dry, furred tongue; he may be mentally confused. Examination of the abdomen may reveal a large bladder, which may reach to the umbilicus or even above. The swelling has the typical globular shape of the bladder arising from the pelvis, and dull to percussion. If there is acute obstruction the bladder will be tender to palpation.

On rectal examination the prostate will be enlarged. Typically, in benign enlargement the lateral lobes are enlarged and a sulcus is palpable between them in the midline posteriorly. This is in contrast to carcinoma, which usually involves the posterior part of the gland and obliterates the sulcus with a craggy, hard mass. The size of the prostate may appear to be larger than it really is if the bladder is grossly enlarged and pushes the prostate down towards the examining finger. The gland should therefore be palpated again after catheterization and before operation.

Special investigations

• *Serum urea and creatinine* to identify renal failure.

• *Prostate-specific antigen* is a sensitive indicator of prostatic carcinoma, and has superceded measurement of acid phosphatase.

• *Haemoglobin* is estimated, since uraemia inhibits the bone marrow and leads to anaemia.

• *Urine culture* on a mid-stream specimen (MSU): an infected renal tract severely complicates prostatic disease. Most of the patients with prostatic disease do not have an infected urine until the bladder and urethra have been instrumented.

• *Ultrasound scan* will demonstrate bladder enlargement, hydronephrosis and hydro-ureter. Following voiding it can be used to estimate the amount of residual urine in the bladder. Normally there is none; however, in the presence of bladder out-flow obstruction the bladder cannot be completely emptied. Ultrasound has replaced the intravenous urogram (IVU) in the routine investigation of patients with out-flow obstruction.

• *IVU* will give useful evidence of renal function; normally contrast medium should be visible after 5 minutes. More specifically, the pyelogram will show evidence of back pressure of the kidneys (namely hydronephrosis and hydro-ureter), enlargement of the bladder with chronic retention, or residual urine due to inability to empty the bladder completely. Bladder diverticula may be demonstrated. Intravesical enlargement of the prostate is shown by a globular filling defect at the base of the bladder and acute hooking of the terminations of the ureters due to the enlarged prostate pushing up the trigone of the bladder. The films of the lumbar spine and bony pelvis should be scrutinized for evidence of secondary deposits (present in about 25% of malignant prostates).

Complications of prostatic hypertrophy

These are classified as follows.

1 *Prostatic complications*:
   (a) acute retention;
   (b) chronic retention;
   (c) haemorrhage.
2 *Bladder complications*:
   (a) diverticula;
   (b) urinary infection;
   (c) stone formation.
3 *Renal complications*:
   (a) hydronephrosis;
   (b) uraemia.

Treatment

This depends on whether the patient is an elective case, with troublesome prostatic symptoms, especially marked nocturnal frequency, or whether he presents urgently with retention (see p. 344).

Medical therapy

Attempts to manipulate prostatic growth pharmacologically are generally short lived. Two principal agents have had some success:

1 *finasteride*, which inhibits the enzyme 5α-reductase, blocks the conversion of testosterone to its active metabolite dihydrotestosterone in the prostate;

2 *prazosin* and other α-adrenergic receptor antagonists, inhibit the bladder and bladder neck muscular contraction.

Both classes of drug give some improvement in urinary flow rates, but with some side-effects (e.g. drowsiness, postural hypotension with prazosin).

Cure is invariably dependent on carrying out some type of prostatectomy.

Endoscopic prostatectomy: trans-urethral resection (TUR)

The prostate can be removed endoscopically by means of an operating cystoscope, using a diathermy cutting loop or laser fibre. It is useful in dealing with fibrotic and malignant prostatic obstruction but it is also used routinely for benign enlargement. The mortality and morbidity in skilled hands are very low, and this technique is now the treatment of choice in all but very enlarged prostates. Removal of too little of the gland results in the recurrence of the patient's symptoms, while removing too much may damage the urethral sphincteric mechanism.

Open prostatectomy

If the prostate is very large or if there is some coexistent intravesical pathology, such as a large diverticulum or tumour that requires removal at the same time, an open operation may be necessary. This is performed either by the trans-vesical route or by the retropubic approach.

Complications of prostatectomy

Trans-urethral prostatectomy has a low morbidity and mortality, particulary in view of the elderly population in which it is usually performed.

• *Haemorrhage*: primary haemorrhage is more common with malignant glands, with large resections, and in patients on aspirin, which should therefore be stopped pre-operatively. Post-operative irrigation and warming the patient are important in stopping fibrinolysis.

• *TUR syndrome*: absorption of large volumes of the irrigating fluid through the open prostatic veins may result in hyponatraemia and confusion.

• *Retrograde ejaculation* is almost certain after TUR. It does not alter potency.

• *Bladder neck stenosis*, due to stricturing of the bladder neck following resection, may occur and presents with out-flow obstruction.

• *Urinary incontinence* is uncommon but may

occur if the resection is extended below the verumontanum with damage to the urethral sphincter.

• Recurrent 'prostatism': failure to resect enough prostate may lead to early recurrence of symptoms. Late recurrence is due to either regrowth of an adenoma, or malignant change.

Carcinoma

Pathology
This is a relatively common tumour in elderly males but is rare below the age of 50 years. Many prostates with apparent benign hypertrophy have a malignant focus on careful histological examination of the resected gland.

Macroscopic appearance
The tumour is usually situated in the posterior part of the prostate beneath its capsule and appears as an infiltrating, hard, pale area.

Fig. 43.1   The clinical stages of prostatic carcinoma: (a) a hard nodule in the prostate; (b) a mass obliterating the median sulcus; (c) infiltration outside the prostatic capsule.

Microscopic appearance
An adenocarcinoma, usually well differentiated but occasionally anaplastic.

Spread
• Local: there is invasion of the periprostatic tissues and adjacent organs (i.e. the bladder, urethra, seminal vesicles) and, rarely, invasion around and ulceration into the rectum.
• Lymphatic: to the iliac and para-aortic nodes.
• Blood-borne: especially to the pelvis, spine and skull, usually as osteosclerotic lesions. Secondaries may also be found in the liver and lung.

Clinical features
The symptoms of carcinoma of the prostate may be identical to those of benign enlarge-ment, but in addition the patient may present with symptoms of secondary deposits, par-ticularly with pain in the back from involvement of the vertebrae. As with cancer anywhere, the patient's general condition is likely to be poor, with weight loss and anaemia.

As the tumour enlarges locally, three stages can be recognized on rectal examination (Fig. 43.1):

1 a hard nodule in one lobe of the prostate;
2 a craggy mass replacing the prostate and

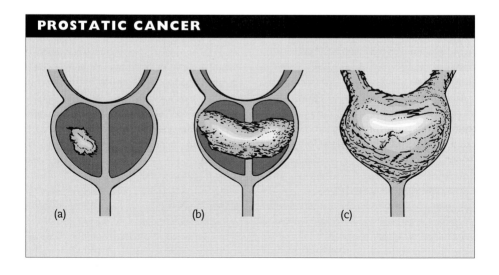

PROSTATIC CANCER

(a)   (b)   (c)

abolishing the normal sulcus between the two lateral lobes.

3 the same, together with infiltration of the tissues on either side of the prostate.

Special investigations

The same initial investigations are performed as for benign enlargement.

• *Prostate-specific antigen*, measured in the blood, is usually raised in the presence of prostate carcinoma.

• *Trans-rectal prostatic biopsy*, or prostatic chippings retrieved at trans-urethral resection, will confirm the diagnosis.

• *Trans-rectal ultrasound* gives good definition of the prostate. It can detect small tumours and can assess extracapsular spread.

• *Bone scan* will show the presence and extent of bony metastases.

Treatment

Localized disease

Occasionally, a tiny prostatic carcinoma is completely removable by prostatectomy; this fortunate occurrence happens most often by accident when an apparently benign prostate is removed and is found microscopically to contain a malignant focus. Small, well-differentiated tumours, which occupy less than 5% of the gland require no further treatment in the absence of metastatic disease.

Larger well-differentiated tumours, which are confined to the prostate, probably require no more than surveillance, although some would advocate radical therapy. More locally advanced, or poorly differentiated tumours have a greater tendency to spread and radiotherapy to the prostate is given. In the USA and increasingly in the UK, radical prostatectomy with pelvic lymphadenectomy is advocated, and is more appropriate for younger (under 70 years) patients.

Metastatic disease

Carcinoma of the prostate is more usually discovered at a stage when it has already spread beyond its capsule and may well have involved other organs, particularly the pelvic cellular tissues, bladder base and bone. The mainstay of treatment of this disease is androgen suppression or the use of specific androgen antagonists, which will produce symptomatic relief in disseminated prostatic cancer in about 75% of patients.

• *Castration* of patients with prostatic carcinoma often relieves their symptoms and sometimes produces dramatic remissions in the course of the disease.

• *Oestrogen administration*, e.g. stilboestrol, can produce similar results to castration, and is now used as primary therapy in the majority of cases. Stilboestrol may produce gynaecomastia, nipple and scrotal pigmentation and testicular atrophy. More importantly, it may result in fluid retention and precipitate congestive cardiac failure, so that in elderly patients with cardiovascular disease bilateral orchidectomy should be performed.

• *Cyproterone acetate*: a steroid androgen antagonist.

• *Aminoglutethimide*: which prevents suprarenal androgen secretion.

• *Gonadotrophin releasing hormone (GnRH) agonists*, e.g. buserilin and goserilin, which inhibit the release of luteinizing hormone (LH) from the anterior pituitary, with consequent reduction of testicular production of testosterone.

Palliation produced by hormonal treatment of prostatic cancer has completely changed the nature of this disease for many patients, a useful and happy life being preserved in some cases for many years. However, the results are not always so satisfactory. Radiotherapy may relieve the pain of bony deposits and can also be employed for local control to supplement hormonal therapy.

Urinary obstruction due to the prostatic carcinoma may resolve on stilboestrol therapy; if not, an endoscopic prostatectomy is indicated.

Prostatitis

Once commonly due to tuberculosis, bacterial infection of the prostate is now more commonly due to faecal organisms, particularly *Escherichia coli* and *Streptococcus faecalis*. Non-bacterial prostatitis may be due to *Chlamydia*, and occasionally patients may present with the symptoms of prostatitis in the absence of any inflammation (prostodynia).

Clinical features

Prostatitis may occur at any age in adult men. The patient will usually have symptoms of prostatism and urinary infection; he may present with acute retention. In addition, pain on ejaculation and blood in the semen (haematospermia) may be present. The patient is often pyrexial, and rectal examination reveals an enlarged exquisitely tender prostate, and occasionally an abscess may be palpable. Epididymitis is a common accompaniment, due to infection passing along the vas deferens. In chronic cases the prostate feels much firmer, and may resemble a carcinoma. Diagnosis may be helped by examination of a urine specimen taken immediately after prostatic massage. Urethroscopy and cystoscopy should be performed to exclude urethral stricture and prostatic or bladder tumours.

Treatment

If the disease is recognized early enough, treatment with the appropriate antibiotics (e.g. ciprofloxacin) may cause resolution. Long courses of 6–12 weeks are required. Untreated, an abscess may form and rupture spontaneously into the urethra.

Bladder neck obstruction

Bladder neck obstruction may be due to congenital valves in the region of the prostatic urethra and internal meatus, or fibrosis of the prostate.

Posterior urethral valves

Congenital valves which usually produce hydronephrosis and retention of urine in childhood. They may be difficult to diagnose because instruments may pass freely into the

bladder, although the valves obstruct micturition. Early treatment by surgical incision of the valves before renal failure occurs is important.

Prostatic fibrosis

Prostatic fibrosis produces the symptoms of prostatic hypertrophy but without enlargement of the prostate. The onset may be in childhood or early adult life. It may also result from scarring following instrumentation or prostatic resection.

Treatment

Endoscopic incision of the bladder neck is performed.

The management of urinary retention

Urinary retention may be either acute, chronic or acute on chronic. Acute retention presents with inability to pass urine, suprapubic pain and a suprapubic mass. The differential diagnosis that must always be considered is a ruptured abdominal aortic aneurysm, in which the mass may be pulsatile, the pain radiates into the back and the patient is shocked (causing anuria). Chronic urinary retention is a more insidious process with gradual enlargement of the bladder, dribbling incontinence and little or no pain.

The definite treatment of the urinary retention can only be decided upon after three essential steps have been carried out. These are:

1 diagnosis of the cause;
2 assessment of renal damage caused by the back pressure;
3 assessment of the general condition of the patient — is the patient fit for any surgical procedure that may be necessary?

Diagnosis of the cause

The diagnosis can be classified into the following.

1 *General causes* (no organic obstruction to urinary flow):

(a) post-operative;

(b) central nervous system (CNS) disease, e.g. tabes, multiple sclerosis, spinal tumour;

(c) drugs, e.g. anticholinergics, tricyclic antidepressants.

2 *Local causes:*

(a) in the lumen of the urethra, e.g. stone or blood clot;

(b) in the wall, e.g. stricture;

(c) outside the wall, e.g. prostatic enlargement (benign or malignant), faecal impaction, pelvic tumour, pregnant uterus.

General causes of retention of urine must always be borne in mind. The commonest cause of acute retention is indeed seen post-operatively. The patient is not used to passing urine lying in bed, is weak and often in pain. Usually the condition can be overcome by giving an injection of opiate and sitting the patient with his legs over the side of the bed within earshot of a running tap; if this does not succeed, catheterization may be required. The catheter can either be removed once the bladder has been emptied or, more commonly, may be left *in situ* until next morning. Sometimes a patient with an enlarged prostate is precipitated into retention of urine following some other surgical procedure and it may then be necessary to proceed to prostatectomy.

In every case the CNS must be carefully examined, as retention of urine may be due to interruption of the sacral nervous pathway. There is a tendency to think of retention of urine in an elderly man as being invariably due to prostatic disease, but every now and then one of these patients will be found to have a spinal tumour, tabes dorsalis or some other neurological condition.

The diagnosis of the cause of retention is made by the usual three steps:

History

This may reveal the typical progressive symptoms of prostatism, a story of urethral infection suggesting stricture, a preceding episode of ureteric colic suggesting stone, etc.

Examination

This includes a rectal examination to determine the size and nature of the prostate, palpation of the urethra for stone or stricture, inspection of the urethral meatus and examination of the CNS.

Special investigations

• *X-ray of the pelvis* may reveal a calculus at the bladder base or bony secondaries from prostatic carcinoma.

• *Prostate-specific antigen (PSA)* is estimated. A raised value is suggestive of carcinoma.

Assessment of the degree of renal damage

The patient with retention of urine may have damaged his kidneys by back pressure; obviously this is far more likely to occur in long-standing cases of chronic retention, but the possibility must be considered in every case. This assessment again is made under the three following headings.

History

Renal failure is suggested by headaches, anorexia, vomiting and mental disturbance.

Examination

Is the patient pale and drowsy with the dry, coated tongue of uraemia?

Special investigations

• *Urea and creatinine* are estimated: a blood urea over 7 mmol/L, and/or creatinine over 135 μmol/L suggest at least some degree of renal impairment.

Assessment of the general condition of the patient

The average patient with retention of urine admitted to hospital is an elderly man. Before proceeding to major surgery, his general condition must obviously be carefully investigated —again the three headings.

History

Exercise tolerance, the presence of cough and

sputum and a history of previous coronary episodes are enquired into.

Examination
Chest, cardiovascular system and blood pressure.

Special investigations
• *Chest X-ray and electrocardiogram* are performed if necessary.
• *The haemoglobin* level is checked.

Scheme of management of acute urinary retention
The three common causes for an emergency

Fig. 43.2   Treatment of acute retention.

surgical admission of a man with acute urinary retention are benign prostatic hypertrophy, malignant disease of the prostate and urethral stricture. The following scheme outlines the management of such cases (see Fig. 43.2). The patient is catheterized under full aseptic precautions.

Benign prostatic enlargement
Proceed to prostatectomy as soon as convenient if the renal function and general condition of the patient are satisfactory. If renal damage or general poor condition preclude operation, drainage by urethral catheter is continued until these can be improved. If the patient is in such poor health that operation is inappropriate, for example a bedridden cardiac cripple, then he is

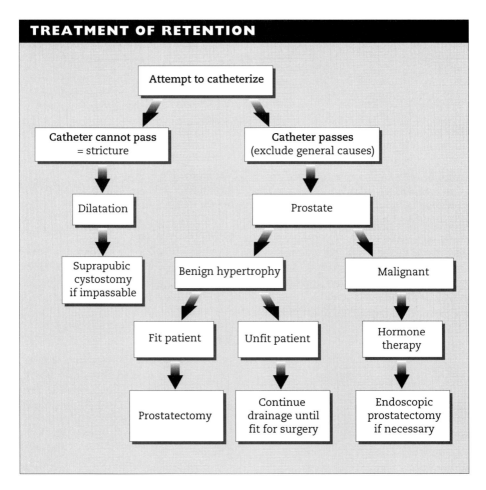

TREATMENT OF RETENTION

Attempt to catheterize

Catheter cannot pass = stricture

Catheter passes (exclude general causes)

Dilatation

Prostate

Suprapubic cystostomy if impassable

Benign hypertrophy

Malignant

Fit patient

Unfit patient

Hormone therapy

Prostatectomy

Continue drainage until fit for surgery

Endoscopic prostatectomy if necessary

best managed by permanent urethral drainage, the catheter being changed regularly and urinary antiseptics used if necessary should urinary infection occur. A self-retaining Foley catheter is far kinder to the patient than a leaky and smelly permanent suprapubic cystotomy tube.

Malignant disease of the prostate

In the presence of metastatic spread, hormone therapy is commenced. Endoscopic prostatectomy is required for localized tumours, or large tumours if symptoms persist on hormonal therapy.

Urethral stricture (see p. 349)

The catheter will not pass and the urethra must be gently dilated with bougies under local or general anaesthetic. Following this, it is possible to catheterize the patient and to continue with regular urethral dilatations or, preferably, to divide the stricture endoscopically with an optical urethrotome. Rarely, the stricture is impassable and the patient requires a temporary suprapubic cystotomy prior to urethrotomy. Occasionally, a plastic operation on the stricture is indicated but only rarely is permanent suprapubic drainage required.

Chronic urinary retention

If there is evidence of renal impairment, the patient is catheterized, and the catheter left in for a period to allow the renal function, and the general condition, to improve. Following relief of the hydronephrosis that accompanies chronic obstruction, there is a polyuric phase, and intravenous fluid replacement may be required to keep up with the fluid losses. Bleeding is common following decompression of a chronically distended bladder; there is no advantage in the intermittent catheter clamping that was once advocated when draining such bladders.

CHAPTER 44

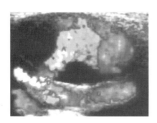

The Male Urethra

Congenital anomalies

Hypospadias

The male urethra is formed by the inrolling of the genital folds, which themselves form the corpus spongiosum. If the genital folds fail to develop or fuse completely, the tube is either short or absent. The urethra thus opens onto the ventral surface of the penis anywhere from the perineum up to the glans. Hypospadias is associated with an abnormal prepuce that is deficient ventrally, and so appears hooded. Proximal hypospadias is associated with a downward curvature of the penis on erection, termed *chordee*. Treatment involves plastic procedures utilizing the prepuce as a skin flap; circumcision before correction of the abnormality is therefore contraindicated.

Epispadias

The urethra opens dorsally on the penis. It is associated with other anterior abdominal wall defects including exstrophy of the bladder.

Posterior urethral valves (see also p. 344)

A valve-like membrane at the level of the verumontanum. This can obstruct the flow of urine, resulting in chronic retention of urine and uraemia in infants.

Injury to the urethra

These may be classified into rupture of (i) the bulbous urethra; (ii) the membranous urethra.

The bulbous urethra

This may be damaged by a direct blow, e.g. a fall astride a bar (e.g. a bicycle cross-bar), a kick in the perineum, or during forcible dilatation or cystoscopy. The patient will complain of severe pain in the perineum and usually bright-red blood will be seen dripping from the external meatus. There will be marked bruising in the region of the injury.

The membranous urethra

This is injured in pelvic fractures, especially those involving dislocation of a portion of the pelvis, it is torn at its junction with the prostatic urethra. As with extraperitoneal rupture of the bladder (p. 334), blood and urine are extravasated in the extraperitoneal space and produce a swelling dull to percussion above the pubis. If the urethra is torn from the bladder, the prostate is displaced and there will be a feeling of emptiness on rectal examination.

The attempted passage of a catheter in a patient with a pelvic fracture can be both misleading and dangerous; misleading in that the catheter may pass along a partially ruptured posterior urethra into the bladder so that the diagnosis is missed, and dangerous in that the catheter may complete the tear in a partially ruptured urethra or produce a false passage.

Management

Satisfactory management depends on a high index of suspicion leading to early diagnosis, as extravasation of urine is liable to lead to secondary infection, which will greatly complicate the condition. The presence of bleeding from the meatus, or a fracture of the pelvis, combined with urinary retention, should alert to the possibility.

Initial management

A *rectal examination* is performed to determine whether the prostate is palpable and in the normal position. An absent or high prostate implies a complete rupture of the membranous urethra, and urgent exploration is indicated.

A *urethrogram* is performed using water soluble contrast medium to identify any extravasation or loss of continuity, and localize the site of injury.

Membranous urethral injuries

Complete rupture. Where rectal examination confirms that the prostate (and therefore bladder) is floating out of the pelvis, urgent surgery is indicated. Primary anastomosis is rarely possible. Instead, the base of bladder and the urethra are approximated. The retropubic space is explored and haematoma evacuated. A urethral catheter is passed and railroaded into the bladder. The bladder is approximated to the ruptured urethra by means of sutures in the anterior prostatic capsule. The urethral catheter will remain *in situ* for 2 weeks; at the same time a suprapubic catheter is inserted into the bladder to drain the urine. The previous practice of inflating the urethral catheter and placing a weight on it has been abandoned because it could result in pressure necrosis of the bladder neck.

Incomplete rupture. If there is little extravasation, and continuity is preserved, a well-lubricated urethral catheter should be passed carefully, and left in place for 10 days.

Bulbous urethral injuries

Complete rupture. A complete laceration is an indication for urgent open repair, with suture of the tear and diversion of the urinary stream by suprapubic drainage.

Incomplete rupture. If there is little extravasation, and continuity is preserved, a well-lubricated urethral catheter may be passed carefully, and left in place for 10 days. Alternatively a suprapubic catheter can be inserted.

Complications

Stricture formation often occurs following injuries to the urethra due to scarring; subsequent repair may be necessary.

Impotence occurs in half the patients, either as a consequence of a pelvic injury involving the terminal branches of the internal iliac arteries, or injury to the nerves supplying the penis.

Urethral stricture

Aetiology
Congenital

For example meatal stenosis in hypospadias.

Acquired

1 *Trauma*:
   (a) urethral instrumentation including catheterization;
   (b) rupture of urethra;
   (c) previous urethral or prostatic surgery.
2 *Post-infection*:
   (a) gonococcal;
   (b) non-specific urethritis, e.g. *Chlamydia*.
3 Carcinoma of urethra (extremely rare).

Clinical features

The patient with a urethral stricture complains of difficulty in passing urine with a poor stream and states that only by straining can he empty his bladder. He is usually younger than 50 years (in contrast to prostatic disease), and may suffer urinary infection and acute retention as a consequence of the stricture.

Special investigations

• *Urethrogram* will demonstrate the location and length of the stricture.

• *Urinary flow rate*: the stricture limits the flow of urine, and measurement of the flow rate shows a flat plateau.

• *Urethroscopy* will visualize the stricture and facilitate treatment.

Treatment

In the elderly patient an established urethral stricture is treated conservatively by regular dilatation of the urethra by the passage of sounds. This can be carried out in the outpatient department and may be necessary once a month, or even more frequently.

In younger, fitter patients with short strictures, urethroscopy is performed and the stricture incised under direct vision (optical urethrotomy); this has a success rate up to 80%.

Recurrent strictures, or long strictures are treated by open surgery, either by simple resection of the stricture with end-to-end anastomosis of the ends, or interposition of a tube of perineal skin.

The management of acute retention due to urethral stricture is outlined on page 344.

CHAPTER 45

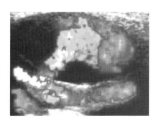

The Penis

Phimosis

Phimosis is gross narrowing of the preputial orifice. It occurs rarely as a congenital lesion, but may result from scarring following the trauma of forcible retraction of the prepuce (see below) or as a result of chronic balanitis.

Clinical features
On micturition, the prepuce is seen to balloon and the urinary stream is reduced to a dribble.

Treatment
Circumcision is performed. In some cases of chronic balanitis with considerable inflammation of the prepuce, a dorsal slit is an efficient, but less aesthetic, method of cure.

Paraphimosis

Paraphimosis results from pulling a tight foreskin proximally over the glans. The foreskin acts as a constricting band, interfering with venous return from the glans, which therefore swells painfully. Once swelling starts, it becomes more difficult to replace the foreskin.

Paraphimosis commonly occurs after an erection. It may also occur following urethral catheterization, when the foreskin is forcibly retracted over the glans to expose the meatus.

Once the catheter is inserted, the thickened scarred prepuce constricts the venous return, producing a paraphimosis. Hence it is important to always ensure that the patient's prepuce is pulled forward again after the insertion of an indwelling catheter — if not, paraphimosis may follow.

Treatment
Once a paraphimosis has become established it is difficult to reduce. There are three courses of action. Under a penile local anaesthetic block, the glans is squeezed for a few minutes to reduce the oedema, and enable the foreskin to be reduced. If squeezing fails to reduce the oedema, a hypodermic needle may be inserted into the glans and aspirated to relieve the congestion. Finally, the foreskin may be slit dorsally under general anaesthetic to release the constricting band.

Having once had a paraphimosis, the patient should be considered for a formal circumcision to prevent recurrence.

Non-retractile prepuce

Many male infants are presented to the doctor or nurse because the parents notice that the prepuce cannot be retracted. In fact, the foreskin is normally firmly adherent to the glans until 3 years of age. In the next 3 years the congenital adhesions between the glans and the foreskin lyse, progressively separating from the glans.

Forcible attempts to retract the foreskin traumatize the tissues, and the resultant scarring may lead to a true phimosis. Inability to retract the foreskin in the infant is no indication in itself for circumcision; indeed, in the 'nappy' stage the prepuce protects the delicate glans and the urethral orifice from the excoriation of ammoniacal dermatitis.

Circumcision

Circumcision is the resection of the foreskin, leaving the glans exposed. Indications for circumcision include:

- phimosis;
- paraphimosis;
- religious custom;
- non-retractile prepuce over 6 years.

Having the prepuce removed reduces the risk of carcinoma of the penis, probably because it prevents the accumulation of smegma, which is carcinogenic.

Ammoniacal dermatitis

This is a common cause of inflammation of the penis in children and is due to the presence of ammonia liberated by urea-splitting organisms. This is especially liable to occur if the child's nappies are infrequently changed and he is allowed to remain wet. The ammonia causes a painful, red, oedematous rash on the perineum, penis and foreskin.

Treatment

Treatment is to change the child's nappies frequently and to cover the skin with a protective barrier cream or zinc oxide and castor oil.

Circumcision should be avoided in the presence of ammoniacal dermatitis, as a meatal ulcer is likely to result.

Balanitis

Balanitis is an acute inflammation of the fore-skin and glans and it is usually due to the common pyogenic organisms, for instance coliform bacilli, staphylococci and streptococci. It may result in phimosis from scarring.

It is important to test the urine for sugar to exclude diabetes, which may predispose to the inflammation, in which case *Candida* may be the infecting organism.

Treatment

Treatment consists of administering the appropriate antibiotic after the organism has been cultured and its sensitivity has been determined. Local toilet with weak disinfectant solutions may give relief symptomatically.

Carcinoma

Pathology

This tumour usually affects elderly subjects. It is uncommon in the UK, although relatively frequently seen in Africa and the East. It is almost invariably associated with the presence of retained smegma and is virtually unknown among Jews, who are circumcised soon after birth.

The most frequent site of the tumour is in the sulcus between the glans and the prepuce.

Macroscopic appearance

Carcinoma of the penis may present either as a papillary growth on the glans or as an infiltrating ulcer; the latter is more common.

Microscopic appearance

The lesions are squamous carcinomas, which are usually well differentiated.

Spread

- *Local*: the tumour may fungate through the prepuce to present as an ulcerating lesion on the penile skin. Proximal spread along the shaft may destroy the substance of the penis.
- *Lymphatic*: the inguinal lymph nodes are frequently involved, often bilaterally.
- *Blood-borne* spread occurs late and is unusual.

Clinical features

The patient may report with an ulcer on the glans or because of a purulent or blood-stained discharge from below the non-retractile prepuce. He may wait until the tumour has ulcerated through the prepuce or until most of his penis has been destroyed by growth. Surprisingly enough, carcinoma of the penis never seems to occlude the urethra sufficiently to produce retention of urine.

Treatment

Diagnosis is achieved by biopsy, which often necessitates excision of the foreskin.

Early growths can be treated adequately by local radiotherapy using iridium wires, or by partial amputation of the penis if the urethra is encroached upon. Survival from early disease is good (near 100% at 5 years).

When the regional lymph nodes are involved, which is the case in 50% at presentation, treatment is more difficult. Radical surgery may effect a cure, and consists of total amputation of the penis and bilateral block dissections of the inguinal lymph nodes. This operation, although mutilating, does not interfere with micturition because both the internal and external sphincters are preserved. However, after a total amputation of the penis, the patient will need to micturate sitting down.

Inoperably fixed lymph nodes are treated by palliative irradiation.

In summary:
- urethra intact—radiotherapy;
- urethra involved—amputation;
- lymph nodes involved — block dissection if operable, radiotherapy as a palliative measure if matted together and fixed.

Impotence

Impotence is the inability to achieve, or sustain, an erection satisfactory to permit penetration for sexual intercourse.

Aetiology

The principal causes of erectile impotence are as follows:

Neurogenic

Erection is mediated via efferent parasympathetic fibres from S2, S3, S4. Reflex erection requires afferent signals via the pudendal nerve, while psychogenic erection requires out-flow from the brain via the spinal cord. Causes of neurogenic impotence include the following.
- Congenital: spinal bifida.
- Spinal causes: spinal cord injury, spinal cord tumour.
- Central causes: hypothalamic injury, cerebral infarction/tumour.
- Post-surgical causes, e.g. pelvic surgery such as anterior resection or abdomino-perineal resection.

Vascular

Erection requires increased arterial flow into the erectile tissue of the penis, together with some degree of venous out-flow inhibition. Arterial disease affecting flow in the internal iliac arteries, as may result from aorto-iliac disease, may result in impotence and buttock claudication (Leriche's syndrome*).

Hormonal
- Diabetes mellitus, the commonest hormonal cause, but probably acting via a diabetic neuropathy.
- Pituitary failure, primary testicular failure, hypothyroidism, and most other endocrine diseases may contribute to impotence.

Pharmacological

Some drugs, in particular anti-hypertensive agents, tranquillizers and oestrogens, may cause impotence. Alcohol is also a potent cause.

Psychogenic

Psychogenic impotence is usually of sudden onset, and the patient continues to have nocturnal erections and erections following masturbation, suggesting there is not a physical cause.

*René Leriche (1879–1955), Professor of Surgery successively in Strasbourg, Lyon and Paris.

Special investigations

• *Hormone screen*: abnormalities in the blood levels of testosterone, follicle-stimulating hormone, luteinizing hormone, prolactin and thyroxine should be excluded.

• *Penile brachial pressure index*: equivalent to the ankle–brachial index used in peripheral vascular disease, a small inflatable cuff may be placed around the penile shaft and the pressure measured at which a Doppler-detected systolic pulse returns; this is expressed as a ratio of the brachial pressure, an index of below 0.6 being suggestive of vascular disease.

• *Cavernosography*, to exclude a large venous leak.

• *Arteriography*, to identify arterial lesions and possibly to treat by balloon angioplasty.

Treatment

Hormonal disturbances are corrected where possible. Non-vascular causes may respond to intrapenile injections of vasodilators such as papaverine. Use of a vacuum condom, or an intrapenile inflatable prosthesis may be required.

CHAPTER 46

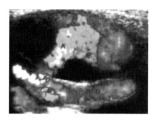

The Testis and Scrotum

Abnormalities of testicular descent

Embryology

The testis arises from the mesodermal germinal ridge in the posterior wall of the abdominal cavity. It links up with the epididymis and vas deferens, which develop from the mesonephric duct. As the testis enlarges, it undergoes caudal migration. By the third month of fetal life it is in the iliac fossa, by the seventh month it reaches the inguinal canal, by the eighth month it has reached the external inguinal ring and by the ninth month, at birth, it has descended into the scrotum. During this descent, a prolongation of peritoneum, called the processus vaginalis, projects into the fetal scrotum; the testis slides behind this and is thus covered in its front and sides by peritoneum. The processus vaginalis becomes obliterated at about the time of birth, leaving the testis covered by the tunica vaginalis. As expected from the embryology, abnormalities of descent are more common in premature infants (20% incidence) than full-term infants (2%).

Classification of maldescent

Testicular maldescent can be subdivided according to whether or not the testis followed the normal course of descent.

Ectopic testis (common)

A testis that has strayed from the normal line of descent is termed ectopic. The commonest position is in the superficial inguinal pouch, which lies anterior to the external oblique aponeurosis. The testis reached this site after migrating through the external inguinal ring and then leaves the normal track of descent to pass laterally. Other situations are the groin, the perineum, the root of the penis and the femoral triangle.

Undescended testis (relatively uncommon)

A testis that has followed the normal course of descent but has stopped short of the scrotum is termed an undescended, or more properly, an incompletely descended testis. It may lie anywhere from the abdominal cavity, along the inguinal canal, to the top of the scrotum. The vast majority are due to a local defect in development. The affected testis is always small and it is probable that this imperfect development impairs descent rather than that the imperfect descent impairs development. The incompletely descended testis is usually accompanied by persistent patency of the processus vaginalis, presenting as a congenital hernia. Unilateral undescended testes are four times as common as bilateral. The condition of bilateral undescended impalpable testes is termed cryptorchidism.

Most, if not all, testes that are going to descend do so within the first few months of life. If the testis is not in its normal scrotal position at puberty, it is very unlikely that it will be capable of spermatogenesis. However, the interstitial cells are functional, so that secondary sex characteristics develop normally.

Differential diagnosis: the retractile testis

The commonest mistake in diagnosis is to fail to differentiate a true maldescent from a retractile testis. The retractile testis is a normal testis with an excessively active cremasteric reflex resulting in the testis being drawn up to the external inguinal ring. It is a common condition and often the parents think that the testes have failed to descend; indeed, when the scrotum is palpated the testes may not be felt. However, careful examination will probably reveal the testis at the external inguinal ring or at the root of the scrotum and the testis can, by downward stroking or by gentle traction, be coaxed into the scrotum. A useful trick is to place the child in the squatting position for the examination; this often encourages a retractile testis to descend into the scrotum. It is also worth while asking the parents to examine the child when he is relaxed in a warm bath; again the retractile testis may now slip into its normal position.

If the testis is easily palpable in the groin and remains easy to feel when the child tenses his abdominal wall muscles, it is lying in the ectopic position and not in the inguinal canal—where it is usually impalpable or, at the most, in a thin boy, detected as a vague, tender bulge.

Treatment

The child with retractile testes is normal; reassurance of the parents is all that is required.

The ectopic or undescended testis must be placed in the scrotum if it is to function as a sperm-producing organ. The optimum age for surgery has been revised in recent times, and current recommendations are for surgery around the age of 3 years. After that age, definite changes in the testis can be seen on microscopy, which may lead to impaired spermatogenesis. The operation, termed orchidopexy, consists of mobilizing the testis and its cord, removing the coexisting hernial sac and fixing the testis in the scrotum without tension.

Complications of maldescent

• Defective spermatogenesis, sterility if bilateral.
• Increased risk of torsion.
• Increased risk of trauma.
• Increased risk of malignant disease, even if surgical correction is carried out.
• Inguinal hernia — persistence of the processus vaginalis.

Examination of swellings of the scrotum

When considering any swelling in the scrotum the following three questions should be considered in turn (Fig. 46.1).

1 *Can the examiner's fingers meet above the swelling?* If this is not possible, the swelling arises from the abdomen and is an inguino-scrotal hernia.

2 *If it is possible to palpate clearly the upper edge of the swelling, is the swelling cystic?* If it is cystic on transillumination and the testis is palpable separate from the swelling, the swelling is cyst of the epididymis. However, if the testis is not palpable because it lies within the cyst, it is a hydrocele.

3 *If the swelling is solid, the following must be considered:*

(a) the swelling is an abnormal testis, e.g. a tumour or (rarely) a gumma;

(b) the epididymis is involved — this is usually an inflammatory condition, either acute or chronic.

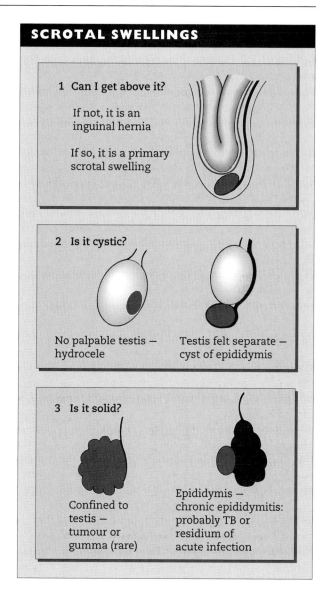

SCROTAL SWELLINGS

1 Can I get above it?

If not, it is an
inguinal hernia

If so, it is a primary
scrotal swelling

2 Is it cystic?

No palpable testis —
hydrocele

Testis felt separate —
cyst of epididymis

3 Is it solid?

Confined to
testis —
tumour or
gumma (rare)

Epididymis —
chronic epididymitis:
probably TB or
residium of
acute infection

Fig. 46.1 The differential
diagnosis of a scrotal swelling.

The latter is either tuberculous or the residual chronic thickening, which may persist for many months after an acute pyogenic infection that has been treated with an antibiotic.

Special investigation

• *Ultrasound of the swelling* is valuable in determining whether there is an underlying solid mass in relation to the presence of a scrotal cystic swelling, and may indicate its nature.

Cysts of the epididymis

Epididymal cysts arise as cystic degeneration of one of the epididymal or para-epididymal structures, and so are common in middle-aged and elderly men. They are often multiple, may be bilateral, and produce a fluctuant and usually highly translucent swelling in the scrotum. As they arise from the epididymis, the testis is palpable separately from, and in front of, the cyst. This is the main differentiating point from a hydrocele. The contained fluid may be water-clear or may be milky and contain sperm, hence the old term spermatocele. Clinically there is no way of differentiating between a cyst of the epididymis and a spermatocele and the latter term is best abandoned.

Large cysts of the epididymis may trouble the patient by getting in the way of his clothes and chafing his legs. If producing symptoms, cysts of the epididymis should be removed surgically. Aspiration is usually unsuccessful because it recurs.

Hydrocele

A hydrocele is an excessive collection of serous fluid in the processus vaginalis, usually the tunica. Hydroceles may be classified as follows.

Primary or idiopathic hydrocele (Fig. 46.2)
This is usually large and tense. There is no disease of the underlying testis. Hydroceles may be subdivided into the following.

Vaginal hydrocele. The vaginal hydrocele is the usual type of hydrocele surrounding the testis and separated from the peritoneal cavity. The patient presents with a cystic transilluminable swelling in the scrotum. On examination, the testis is difficult to feel and lies at the back of the swelling, which, due to the anatomy of the tunica, encompasses the anterior and lateral portions of the organ.

Congenital hydrocele. Congenital hydrocele is associated with a hernial sac, the still patent processus vaginalis. It opens into the peritoneal cavity through a narrow orifice. When elevated it gradually empties.

Infantile hydrocele. Infantile hydrocele extends from the testis to the internal inguinal ring but does not pass into the peritoneal cavity.

Hydrocele of the cord. Hydrocele of the cord is rare. It lies in, or just distal to, the inguinal canal, separate from the testis and the peritoneum, and represents a length of patent processus vaginalis in which upper and lower parts have closed. Diagnosis is confirmed by the simple test of downward traction on the testis, which pulls the hydrocele of the cord down with it. The equivalent in the female is a hydrocele of the round ligament within the

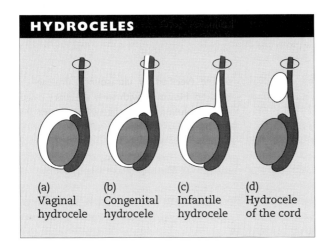

HYDROCELES

(a) Vaginal hydrocele   (b) Congenital hydrocele   (c) Infantile hydrocele   (d) Hydrocele of the cord

Fig. 46.2 The anatomical classification of hydroceles (the ring at the upper end of each diagram represents the internal inguinal ring).

inguinal canal, termed a *hydrocele of the canal of Nuck*.

Secondary hydrocele

A secondary hydrocele is usually smaller and lax and the testis is diseased. It is due to the serosal sac surrounding the testis becoming filled with an exudate secondary to tumour or inflammation of the underlying testis or epididymis.

Treatment

Infants

Hydroceles in infants should be left alone because most disappear spontaneously. If the hydrocele persists after the first year, operative treatment is advisable. The sac is identified, ligated and excised, care being taken not to damage any other structures in the cord.

Adults

In young adults the possibility of tumour should be borne in mind. Ultrasound examination will usually differentiate a normal from an abnormal testis in this situation.

The hydrocele can be treated by aspiration, the resultant fluid being straw coloured with flecks of cholesterol in it. Operative treatment is the treatment of choice in all but the very elderly, as hydroceles recur after aspiration.

Secondary hydroceles require treatment for the underlying condition.

Acute infections of the testis and epididymis

Acute infections usually arise as ascending infection via the vas deferens, spreading first to the epididymis and thence to the testis; occasionally, infection may be blood-borne.

Blood-borne infection

The commonest blood-borne agent to infect the testis is the mumps virus, the testicular manifestation of which usually follows within a week of the onset of parotid enlargement. Occasionally, it may occur in the absence of other manifestations. Diagnosis is confirmed clinically and by the rising level of mumps antibodies in the serum. Adults are particularly likely to be affected; there may be residual damage to the testis and if both sides are involved fertility may be impaired.

Ascending infection

Ascending infection is usually a consequence of a preceding urinary tract infection (e.g. with *Escherichia coli*) or a urethritis or prostatitis from a sexually transmitted organism such as gonorrhoea or *Chlamydia*, which result in epididymitis. Epididymitis may also follow urethral stricture where straining causes reflux of urine up the vas, or instrumentation of the urethra such as during prostatectomy.

Clinical features

The patient will have a very painful swelling of the epididymis, often with a secondary hydrocele and constitutional effects (pyrexia, headache and leucocytosis). There may be a history of dysuria suggesting a urinary tract infection, or urethral discharge suggesting a sexually transmitted organism. Examination of the urine may reveal the presence of organisms and pus cells, but the urine need not be abnormal. Rectal examination of the prostate may reveal coexistent prostatitis.

Treatment

Treatment is bed rest and the appropriate antibiotic given over a prolonged course (6 weeks); ciprofloxacin is a typical first-line agent with good specificity for the organisms most often encountered. If frank abscesses have formed (verified by ultrasound), drainage is required. However, with early adequate treatment resolution is more likely. The patient will often have residual swelling of the epididymis, which may be rather firm, and differentiation from the tuberculous epididymitis may be difficult unless the history of the previous acute attack is obtained.

Differential diagnosis

As with all acutely painful conditions of the

testis, torsion must be excluded. If the patient is in his teens, torsion is more likely; if he is in his twenties and sexually active, epididymitis is more likely. However, if doubt exists, urgent exploration is mandatory.

Chronic infections of the testis

Gumma

Although once common, syphilis of the testis is now a rarity. The testis is enlarged and is clinically difficult to distinguish from a carcinoma. On penicillin therapy, gummata of the testis melt away.

Tuberculosis

This often occurs in association with tuberculosis in other parts of the genito-urinary tract.

Clinical features

The patient usually presents with swelling of the epididymis. The vas deferens may be thickened and feel nodular. A cold abscess may develop in relation to the epididymis and rupture through the scrotum, usually posteriorly, resulting in a chronic sinus. The seminal vesicles may be enlarged and palpable on rectal examination.

Diagnosis depends on isolating tubercle bacilli from the urine or biopsy material, or evidence of tuberculosis elsewhere.

Treatment

This is the same as for tuberculosis in other situations. If a chronic sinus has developed, unilateral orchidectomy is probably the best form of treatment, as the testis is unlikely to be functional and is a continued source of infection and may lead to spread of the disease elsewhere.

Torsion of the testis

Aetiology

Usually this is a torsion of the spermatic cord in a congenitally abnormal testis, often malde-scended or hanging like a bell-clapper within a completely investing tunica vaginalis. Occasionally, true torsion of the testis occurs without involving the cord when there is an extensive mesorchium between the testis and epididymis. It is probably impossible for torsion to occur in an anatomically completely normal testis. Untreated, the testis undergoes irreversible infarction within a few hours and there is a typical transudation of blood-stained fluid into the tunica vaginalis. Torsion is more common in undescended and ectopic testes.

Clinical features

Torsion of the testis is a surgical emergency, which usually occurs in children or adolescents. There may be a history of mild trauma to the testis or of previous attacks of pain in the testis due to torsion and spontaneous untwisting, Cycling, straining, lifting and coitus are typical precipitants.

The history is of a sudden severe pain in the groin and lower abdomen, often accompanied by vomiting. The abdominal pain occurs because the nerve supply of the testis is mainly from T10 sympathetic pathway. Rarely, the pain is limited to the abdomen. Patients with torsion of the right testis have been operated on for acute appendicitis because the testis has not been examined with care, or more often not at all.

Examination of the scrotum reveals a swollen testis, painful to touch and lying high in the scrotum.

Differential diagnosis

The differential diagnosis is from acute epididymitis and torsion of a testicular appendage.

Epididymitis

The testis does not lie so high in the scrotum, there is a systemic reaction with pyrexia and leucocytosis, and there is usually a history of urinary infection with pus cells and organisms in the urine. A useful factor in differential diagnosis is the age of the patient, as torsion of the testis is unusual after the age of 20 years, whereas epididymitis is rare before that age.

Torsion of a testicular appendage

A number of embryological remnants exist around the testis, such as the appendix testis and appendix epididymis, which may themselves twist. They present in a similar fashion to testicular torsion, but on examination the testis does not lie high in the scrotum, and a dark-blue pea-like swelling may be visible through the scrotal skin.

Strangulated inguinal hernia

Torsion may also mimic a strangulated inguinal hernia.

Treatment

If there is any doubt as to the diagnosis, it is best to explore the testis as soon after admission as possible, because every hour increases the likelihood of irreversible damage to the testis. If still viable, the testis is untwisted and sutured to the tunica vaginalis. If infarcted, it is removed. In every case, fixation of the other testis should be performed at the same time, as any congenital anomaly is likely to be bilateral and torsion of the opposite testis may therefore occur.

Varicocele

This is a condition of varicosities of the pampiniform plexus of veins. It usually occurs on the left, and manifests first in adolescence. It is present in nearly 10% of males.

Its origin is due to the drainage of the left testicular vein at right angles into the left renal vein, unlike the right testicular vein, which drains obliquely into the inferior vena cava (IVC). Patients with varicoceles have absent or incompetent valves at the junction with the left renal vein.

Occasionally, a varicocele can be secondary to a tumour or other pathological process blocking the testicular vein. The best known example of this is a tumour of the kidney involving the renal vein and obstructing the drainage of the left testicular vein.

Clinical features

A varicocele may cause a dragging sensation in the scrotum. It is also associated with defective spermatogenesis, and patients with varicocele are often subfertile. On examination *in the standing position* the varicose veins within the scrotum feel like a 'bag of worms', but there may be little to feel when the patient lies down.

Treatment

Usually the condition requires no treatment apart from reassurance that the condition is not likely to give rise to any dangerous complications. If the weight of the varicocele and testis cause an ache, close-fitting underpants may help. If the patient demands treatment, and in cases of male infertility, the varicocele can be cured radiologically by embolizing the left testicular vein; it may also be treated surgically by ligating and dividing all the testicular veins as they traverse the inguinal canal.

Disorders of the scrotal skin

Idiopathic scrotal oedema

Characteristically affecting pre-pubescent boys, this inflammatory condition is characterized by an erythematous, oedematous swelling of the scrotal skin. It may involve both sides of the scrotum, and can extend into the groins. Unlike torsion it is painless, and the testicular apparatus is normal on examination. Spontaneous resolution within a few days is usual.

Fournier's gangrene

Fournier's gangrene,* or synergistic gangrene of the scrotum, is a result of synergistic infection with several species of bacteria, both aerobic and anaerobic; haemolytic streptococci, staphylococci and *Escherichia coli* are common isolates.

*Jean Alfred Fournier (1832–1914), Venereologist, Hôpital St Louis, Paris, France.

There may be a history of minor trauma, perianal abscess or surgery, although there is no obvious precipitating factor in half the cases. The patient develops sudden pain in the scrotum, and rapidly becomes profoundly toxic.

Treatment involves wide debridement of affected skin, often twice daily, and high-dose broad-spectrum antibiotics.

Carcinoma of the scrotum

Rare nowadays, this tumour is noteworthy as one of the first described industrial diseases. Percival Pott* (1779) noted an association with chimney sweeps, where chimney soot acted as a carcinogen when ingrained into the scrotal skin. Later, it was described in workers with mineral oils in whom the carcinogenic oils soak their trousers.

Presenting as an ulcerating growth, it is usually a squamous carcinoma and is treated by wide excision with block dissection of affected inguinal nodes.

Tumours of the testis

Testicular tumours are the commonest solid malignancy in young adult males, although they are relatively uncommon, representing around 2% of malignancies in the male.

Aetiology
Testicular tumours are associated with undescended and ectopic testis (sevenfold risk). There is also an increased incidence in patients who are infertile, and those who have had a previous contralateral testicular malignancy.

Pathology
There are two main forms of malignant tumours of the testis — seminoma and teratoma—although mixed forms also exist. Rare tumours include lymphoma, which affects an older age group.

*Sir Percival Pott (1714–88), Surgeon, St Bartholemew's Hospital, London.

Seminoma
The seminoma (60%) arises from cells of the seminiferous tubules, usually occurs between 30 and 40 years of age and is relatively slow growing. Macroscopically, the tumour is solid, appearing rather like a cut potato on section. Microsopically, cells vary from well-differentiated spermatocytes to undifferentiated round cells with clear cytoplasm. Some 10% arise in undescended testes.

Teratoma
Teratoma (40%) occurs in a younger age group, the peak incidence being 20–30 years. It is thought to arise from primitive totipotential germ cells. Macroscopically, it has a markedly cystic appearance and used to be called fibrocystic disease. The cut surface may appear like a colloid goitre, and areas of haemorrhage and infarction are common. Microscopically, the cells are very variable and the tumour may contain cartilage, bone, muscle, fat and other tissues.

Spread
• *Local*: the testis is progressively destroyed by the tumour. Spread through the capsule is unusual, but occasionally in an advanced case there may be ulceration of the scrotum.
• *Lymphatic*: to the para-aortic nodes via lymphatics accompanying the testicular vein. In advanced cases there may be enlargement of the supraclavicular nodes, especially on the left side.
• *Blood-borne*: spread from the teratoma occurs relatively early to the lungs and liver. In the seminoma this tends to be late in the disease.

Clinical presentations
• As a lump in the testis.
• As a hydrocele.
• Rarely as a painful rapidly enlarging swelling, which may be mistaken for orchitis.
• As secondaries, usually metastatic growths in the lung, as a mass in the abdomen due to involved abdominal lymph nodes or as a cervical lymphadenopathy.

Tumours of the testis usually present as a painless, swollen testicle, or lump on a testicle, which is hard and may be associated with an overlying secondary hydrocele, which sometimes contains blood-stained fluid. There is often a misleading history of recent trauma, and rarely it may present having undergone torsion.

Occasionally, gynaecomastia may be a presenting feature, due to the production of paraneoplastic hormones.

Special investigations

• *Scrotal ultrasound* may reveal a solid tumour in a hydrocele but a negative finding cannot exclude malignancy.

• *Tumour markers*: teratomas produce α-fetoprotein (AFP) and seminomas produce β human chorionic gonadotraophin (β-HCG). These are useful not only in making a diagnosis but in subsequent follow-up.

• *Chest X-ray and computed tomography (CT) of the abdomen* to seek secondary spread and so stage the disease.

Treatment

If it is suspected that the testicular swelling is due to a tumour, early exploration is mandatory. The spermatic cord is exposed through an inguinal incision, occluded by an atraumatic clamp and the testis delivered. The clamp prevents vascular dissemination of tumour cells. If the diagnosis is now obvious, immediate orchidectomy is performed. If the diagnosis is in doubt, a biopsy is taken and submitted to frozen section examination. Orchidectomy is performed if the diagnosis is now confirmed. Inguinal, rather than scrotal, exploration is performed to avoid exposure to the scrotal lymphatics, which drain to the inguinal nodes, unlike the spermatic cord, which drains to the internal iliac nodes.

Seminomas are highly radio-sensitive so that, following orchidectomy, radiotherapy is given to the ipsilateral iliac and para-aortic lymph nodes. For extensive disease, cytotoxic chemotherapy may also be given.

Teratomas are not as radio-sensitive and are best treated by combination cytotoxic therapy. As cytotoxic chemotherapy is likely to render the patient infertile, prior sperm banking is now offered.

Prognosis

Node-negative cases have an extremely good prognosis of nearly 100% 5-year survival. Even with early abdominal lymph node spread there is still a 95% 5-year survival and with disseminated disease long-term survivals are often achieved with chemotherapy.

Male infertility

The majority of couples who are trying for a pregnancy will be rewarded within 2 years. However, 1 in 10 couples suffer infertility, with the problem distributed evenly between each partner, with one-third of cases due to factors in both man and woman.

Aetiology
Congenital disorder

• *Chromosome abnormality*, e.g. Klinefelter's syndrome (XXY).

• *Developmental anomaly*, e.g. testicular maldescent, absent vas deferens.

Physical problems

• *Post-infection*, e.g. following mumps orchitis or epididymitis.

• *Trauma*, with subsequent atrophy.

• *Neurological*, e.g. spinal injury, producing erectile and ejaculatory dysfunction.

• *Temperature*, e.g. varicocele, tight-fitting underpants.

• *Iatrogenic*, e.g. vasectomy, damage during orchidopexy or hernia repair.

Hormonal

• *Pituitary insufficiency*, e.g. from a pituitary tumour or craniopharyngioma.

• *Liver failure*, causing increased circulating oestrogens.

Drugs
• *Chemotherapy and radiotherapy* for cancer, usually teratoma or seminoma — patients are offered sperm-bank facilities prior to treatment.

Clinical features

A full history and thorough examination are required to exclude obvious contributory pathology. Previous surgery or infection of the testicular apparatus is particularly important, especially as a child. Coexisting diabetes, renal or hepatic failure may contribute to infertility, as can smoking.

Examination should include assessment of hair distribution and general build for evidence of testicular failure (female distribution). Examination of the penis and scrotal contents is particularly important, verifying the course of the vas deferens on each side, the size of the testis and the presence of a varicocele (with the patient standing).

Special investigations

Before embarking on investigation, it should be ascertained that coitus is occurring regularly. Invasive tests are withheld until the infertile partner is identified.

• *Semen analysis.* This is produced following a period of 3 days' abstinence, and examined within 4 hours. A semen volume over 2 ml, with over 20 million sperm per millilitre, of which 50% are motile at 4 hours, and over 50% of normal morphology, is acceptable.

• *Hormone assays* in patients with no sperm (azoospermia), or few sperm. Raised prolactin is suggestive of a pituitary tumour. Raised follicle-stimulating hormone levels, with small testes, suggests primary testicular failure.

• *Seminal fructose levels*: fructose is produced by the seminal vesicles, and is absent in disease of the seminal vesicles and in congenital absence of the vasa deferentia.

• *Vasography and testicular biopsy*: obstruction of the vas may also cause azoospermia. Contrast radiography of the vas is performed under anaesthetic to identify obstruction. An obstruction may be bypassed, or an epididymo-vasostomy performed. If no obstruction is seen, a testicular biopsy is performed.

Treatment

Any underlying disease is treated. So, a varicocele is embolized or ligated, vasal obstruction bypassed, and hormone therapy administered as required. Non-specific measures, if no cause is found, includes wearing loose-fitting underpants, and cessation of smoking and excess alcohol intake.

Assisted conception techniques, including gamete intrafallopian tube transfer (GIFT), where ovum and sperm are transferred into the fallopian tubes directly, and *in vitro* fertilization, where fertilization of the ovum takes place outside the body, may be required.

Since the advent of contraceptive medication there has been an increase in the age of planned conception, with the result that more and more couples are having difficulty in conception, with fewer children available for adoption.

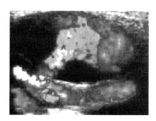

Transplantation Surgery

Historical background

Early attempts at organ transplantation were fraught with failure due to a lack of appreciation of the immune response that resulted in rapid destruction of the transplanted organ. It was not until the mid 1950s that successful replacement of a diseased organ with a transplanted organ occurred, when the immune response was bypassed by performing renal transplants between identical twins. By 1960, new immunosuppressive drugs appeared with which the immune response could be partly controlled, permitting longer useful function of organs from unrelated donors. In the subsequent decade regular haemodialysis also became increasingly available, able to support patients with renal failure while awaiting transplantation. In the 1980s more powerful immunosuppressants such as cyclosporin permitted a broader spectrum of organs to be transplanted successfully, such as hearts and lungs, together with an improvement in the results of kidney transplantation. With the advances in immunosuppression, better techniques of organ preservation and improved anaesthetic and intensive care management, the transplantation of replacement organs is now an accepted treatment for end-stage organ failure. It is also an important part of surgery, with results overall much better than those obtained with many common cancers.

Classification of grafts

• *Autograft*: transplant from one part of the body to another, e.g. skin graft.
• *Allograft*: between members of the same species, e.g. human to human.
• *Isograft*: between identical twins.
• *Xenograft*: between members of different species, e.g. pig to human.
• *Structural grafts*: act as a non-living scaffold. Can be of biological origin, e.g. arterial and heart-valve grafts, or synthetic, e.g. Dacron vascular prosthesis.

In addition to classifying a graft according to its source, grafts are also classified according to where they are implanted relative to the native organ.
• *Orthotopic*: the diseased organ is removed and replaced by the transplanted organ lying in

the normal anatomical position, e.g. heart, lung and liver transplants are usually orthotopic.

• *Heterotopic*: the transplanted organ is placed in a different position to the normal anatomical position, e.g. kidney and pancreas transplants. The diseased organ is not necessarily removed.

This chapter will discuss organ allografts for the functional replacement of diseased organs such as kidney, liver, heart, lungs and pancreas.

Organ donors

There are two potential sources of donor organs.

Living donors

Living donation applies mainly to kidney donation, where the donor can continue with adequate renal function with only one kidney and donate the other to a blood relative or, less commonly, their partner. There is a low (but definite) risk to the donor of post-operative events such as chest and wound infection, deep-vein thrombosis and pulmonary embolism. Donation of the left lateral segment of the liver to a child has been performed but with greater risk to the donor.

Cadaveric donors

Most organs for transplantation come from cadavers who have sustained a lethal brain-stem injury due to a head injury, intracranial haemorrhage or primary brain tumour, and who have been certified as 'brain-stem dead'. The organs are removed from the donor in the operating theatre after isolating their vascular pedicles and rapidly cooling and perfusing them with preservation solution while the heart is still beating.

Asystolic donation, in which the organs are removed from donor after cardiac standstill, is also used for renal donation. Up to 90 minutes of warm ischaemia between cessation of circulation and perfusion with cold preservation fluid can be tolerated by the kidney. In such cases the initial function of the kidney is inferior to that of a kidney from a 'heart-beating donor', but it is possible to support the renal

function with haemodialysis until recovery occurs, often 3 or more weeks later.

Exclusions to organ donation

There are three main reasons why a potential donor may be unsuitable.

1 *Potential transmission of infection*. The transplanted organ could carry with it infections such as the hepatitis B and C viruses, HIV and any bacterial infection that was disseminated in the donor.

2 *Malignancy*. Malignant disease in the donor can be transplanted into the recipient where it may become established in an immunosuppressed environment. Therefore, with the exception of primary brain tumours (which do not spread outside the central nervous system) and superficial non-melanoma skin tumours, malignancy is an exclusion for organ donation.

3 *Impaired function of donor organ*. If the function of the organ is impaired in the donor it is unsuitable for transplantation. For example, a heart with severe coronary artery disease is unsuitable, and a patient with polycystic kidneys who died from a subarachnoid haemorrhage from a berry aneurysm is an unsuitable renal donor.

Organ preservation

Once removed from the donor the organs must be maintained in their optimum state prior to transfusion. This is achieved by a combination of cooling the organ to approximately 4°C to reduce metabolic activity, and perfusing it with, and storing it in, a preservation solution that reduces intracellular fluid losses. One such solution is the University of Wisconsin (UW) solution. In this solution a kidney can be preserved for 36–40 hours, and a liver for up to 20 hours, although in both cases the shortest possible preservation period, or *cold ischaemia time* (the time between cessation of circulation in the donor, and implantation in the recipient) is desirable. No comparable preservation solution exists for the heart and lungs, and implantation must occur within 4–6 hours, as immediate life-sustaining function of these organs is necessary.

Organ recipients

Because no transplant operation is without risk, no-one should receive one until necessary, but they must still be fit enough to withstand the operative procedure. For renal transplantation, potential transplant recipients should be dialysis dependent. Liver transplant recipients have either chronic disease such as primary biliary cirrhosis, in which prognostic factors such as the degree of elevation of serum bilirubin concentration exist for working out the optimum time for transplantation, or acute liver failure in which elevation in prothrombin time is a more sensitive predictor of recovery of liver function without transplantation.

The immunology of organ transplantation

The major histocompatibility complex

When an organ is transplanted it is recognized as foreign by the host's immune system and the rejection response initiated. The recognition is mediated by an interaction between host T lymphocytes (T cells) and histocompatibility antigens on the surface of the allograft (the foreign organ). The major histocompatibility complex (MHC) is a group of genes that encode molecules (antigens) expressed on the surface of cells. The MHC molecules are of two principal sorts. MHC class I antigens are present on all nucleated cells. MHC class II antigens are present on certain cells (e.g. macrophages, monocytes and dendritic cells), and can be induced to appear on others by the presence of cytokines such as interferon-γ (IFN-γ).

The human leucocyte antigen system

The human leucocyte antigen (HLA) system describes the locus on chromosome 6 contain-

ing the genes encoding the MHC antigens. HLA-A, -B and -C loci encode class I molecules, while class II molecules are encoded by HLA-DP, -DQ and -DR loci. The considerable polymorphism at the loci, in particular the A and B loci, results in differences in the MHC antigens on allografts recognized by the host lymphocytes.

Organ matching

There are three levels of organ matching that can be performed, of which ABO matching is required for all transplants. Lymphocytotoxic cross-matching is required only in recipients who have previously been exposed to other HLA antigens following previous blood transfusions, transplants or in child birth. MHC matching is at present restricted to kidneys, where the availability of dialysis enables recipients to wait for an optimally matched kidney, and the better tolerance of cold ischaemia provides the necessary time required to tissue type the donor organ and move it between centres to the best matched recipient. This system requires central coordination of a large pool of recipients and donors which, in the UK, is based in Bristol.

ABO matching

Just like blood transfusions, the existence of pre-formed ABO antibodies means that the transplanted organs must be ABO compatible. Thus, while a group A recipient can have an organ from either a group A or group O donor, a group O recipient can only have a group O organ because of the presence of preformed antibodies to group A and B antigens. Crossing the ABO barrier with any other than liver transplants results in hyperacute rejection.

Lymphocytotoxic cross-match

To detect circulating antibodies in the recipient against donor antigens, a direct lymphocytotoxic cross-match is performed. This involves mixing donor cells (lymphocytes) from peripheral blood, lymph node or spleen, with recipient sera in the presence of complement and observing for cytolysis. Alternatively, the presence of anti-donor antibodies can be detected using flow cytometry. Presence of such antibodies results in hyperacute rejection.

MHC matching

In order to minimize the immune response to an organ allograft, the recipient's MHC antigens can be matched to the donor. The best matching, in fact perfect matching, comes from an identical twin. The inheritance of MHC antigens follows Mendelian genetics, and the antigens are codominantly expressed with a degree of linkage, so within a family there is a 1 in 4 chance that two sibs will share the same MHC antigens, a 1 in 2 chance of differing by a haplotype, and a 1 in 4 chance of inheriting a completely different set of antigens. One in four living related donors will thus offer a significant immunological advantage by complete HLA identity.

Unrelated donor–recipient pairs are also matched with a view to minimizing mismatching of MHC antigens. Three HLA loci, A and B (encoding class I antigens) and DR (encoding class II antigens) are specifically considered. The object of organ matching is to reduce the number of mismatched antigens out of the six possible MHC antigens encoded by the three loci. This strategy has been shown to be beneficial for renal transplantation. Retrospective analysis has also shown a benefit of matching for the survival of heart transplants, but the short preservation time prevents prospective matching.

Rejection

Hyperacute rejection

Where antibodies exist in the recipient to antigens expressed on the donor organ, either ABO antigens in incompatible grafts, or MHC antigens in recipients previously sensitized by child birth, blood transfusion or prior transplant, hyperacute rejection occurs. Antibody binds to the donor cells triggering graft destruction in minutes or hours.

Acute rejection

Acute rejection occurs when the initial dose of immunosuppression is inadequate to prevent the recipient's immune system attacking the graft. Clinically, acute rejection is characterized by a pyrexia, enlargement and tenderness over the transplanted organ, and biochemical dysfunction (a rise in creatinine in a renal transplant, elevated liver enzymes in a liver transplant). It is confirmed by biopsy of the organ. The commonest time for acute rejection is between 7 and 28 days after transplantation, and it usually responds to an increase in immunosuppression.

Chronic rejection

Chronic rejection is an insidious process of graft attrition, which generally results in graft loss. It is characterized by a progressive vasculopathy in the graft, the aetiology of which is related both to the immunosuppression and possibly also to infection of the graft by cytomegalovirus. While the vascular lesions are broadly similar in different organs, the time course is not. In liver transplantation, chronic rejection may occur as early as the first month, and has usually manifested with graft loss by the end of the first year, while in renal and heart transplantation it usually occurs after the first year.

Immunosuppression: principles of immunosuppressive therapy

Immunosuppressive therapy following organ transplantation is a balance between giving enough drug to prevent rejection, but not too much to cause infection. In addition, individual drugs have their own undesirable side-effects, which may be reduced by combining drugs with different modes of action and with different side-effect profiles, rather as is done with cancer chemotherapy regimens. A common protocol would be to combine prednisolone with an antinucleotide such as azathioprine and an inhibitor of T-cell activation such as cyclosporin, the so-called 'triple therapy'.

There are two other factors that influence immunosuppressive therapy. Some organs, such as intestine and lung, have an increased susceptibility to rejection, so higher doses of immunosuppression are required. Secondly, with most organs, after the initial few months the incidence of rejection is much less as the graft undergoes a degree of acceptance, so the total amount of immunosuppression may be reduced. This may be achieved either by reducing the dosage of the agents used, or by discontinuing one of the initial three agents.

Complications of transplantation

Following transplantation the complications can be divided into early (those occurring in hospital) and late.

Early complications

Early complications may be related to the four components of the transplant procedure.

1 *The surgical operation*, such as wound infections, anastomotic breakdowns, and vascular anastomotic thromboses.

2 *The quality of the organ*, dependent both on the donor organ and the quality of the preservation, in particular the ischaemia time. A donor organ with a long cold ischaemia time would be expected to perform less well initially.

3 *The immunological response* of the recipient to the donor (acute rejection).

4 *The effects of immunosuppression.* Initially, immunosuppression uses much higher doses than later in the life of the transplant, and it is in the early stages that the infective complications of over-immunosuppression are seen, in particular wound and chest infections, and that virus infections such as herpes simplex (cold sores) occur.

Late complications

The late complications of transplantation are either immunological, related to the immunosuppression, or due to recurrent disease.

Immunological complications include acute and chronic rejection.

Immunosuppressive complications reflect the difficulty in balancing adequate immunosuppression to stop rejection, but low enough to stop adverse effects. Such complications include:

- the side-effects of the drugs themselves;
- an increased risk of infection including opportunist infections such as *Pneumocystis carinii*;
- an increased risk of malignancy, in particular Epstein–Barr virus-related lymphomas and skin cancers such as squamous carcinomas (which may also have a viral aetiology).

Recurrent disease. In some cases, the original disease may recur in the transplanted organ. Common examples of glomerulonephropathies that may recur in the transplanted kidney include anti-glomerulobasement membrane (anti-GBM) disease, where antibodies attack the GBM, and IgA nephropathy. Transplantation of the liver to remove malignant tumours in the original liver commonly resulted in recurrent malignancy and death within 15 months, even where there was no evidence of spread beyond the liver at the time of transplantation. This indication has now been revised, and only patients with small hepatomas (less than 3 cm), on the background of cirrhosis, are considered.

Results in clinical organ transplantation

Kidney transplantation

Kidney transplantation has been a routine treatment for over 30 years, and there are several survivors with transplants functioning for that period. In the UK 1700 kidney transplants are performed annually, with over 5000 people on dialysis awaiting transplantation. The shortfall in supply is reflected worldwide, even in areas where living donation is more commonplace.

The kidney is transplanted heterotopically into the iliac fossa, with the donor renal vessels anastomosed to the external iliac vessels of the recipient, and the donor ureter anastomosed to the bladder directly to produce a new ureteric orifice. Unless the recipient's own kidneys are causing trouble (hypertension, source of infection) they are left *in situ*.

As with other organ transplants, results are usually quoted in terms of 1-year and 5-year graft survival, where the 1-year losses are higher and reflect the early complications, and the 5-year figures reflect the rate of chronic losses from recurrent disease or chronic rejection. One-year graft survival following renal transplantation is between 80 and 90%, and over 95% where the kidney resulted from an HLA-identical sibling donation. Thereafter, there is a gradual loss of around 3% per annum, giving a 5-year survival of 60–80% (better still for related grafts).

Liver transplantation

Liver transplantation is the treatment of choice for many forms of fatal liver disease. Patients are offered the operation before they become too sick for what is the most formidable of surgical assaults. The three main categories of patients are those with the complications of cirrhosis (recurrent variceal haemorrhage, intractable ascites and poor synthetic function), acute hepatic necrosis and metabolic disease (e.g. oxalosis, in which kidney grafting may also be required). Around 70–80% of liver-transplant recipients survive a year and the 5-year figure is over 60%, with a lower annual loss than renal transplants after the first year. The longest survivor is now alive and well over 25 years after operation.

Heart, lung and combined heart–lung transplantation

Heart transplantation is a relatively straightforward operative procedure in a unit where open heart surgery is performed. The indications are atherosclerotic coronary artery disease and cardiomyopathy. Solitary lung transplantation without the heart is now well established, either one or both lungs are grafted. when both lungs are transplanted *en bloc* with the heart, only three anastomoses are required, namely aortic, tracheal and right atrial. The indications for lung transplantation are primary pulmonary hypertension, chronic obstructive airways disease and cystic fibrosis. The survival of recipients of both heart and combined heart and lung grafts is approximately 80% at 1 year. The longest period of survival after heart grafting is 20 years and after combined heart–lung transplantation, 10 years.

Pancreas transplantation

It is likely that transplantation for the treatment of diabetes will eventually involve β-cells or islets, possibly with the help of genetic engineering, but although several hundred islet grafts have so far been attempted in humans, long-term results are poor. The only successful results have been with transplantation of the vascularized pancreas or a pancreatic segment. One of the complications of pancreas transplantation is leakage of pancreatic exocrine secretions containing all the digestive enzymes, which leads to severe surgical complications. The favoured technique is to place the pancreas in the iliac fossa vascularized from the iliac vessels, with the pancreas' exocrine drainage either into the bladder or into a Roux-en-Y enterostomy.

Pancreas transplantation is still in a developmental stage. The longest survivor with a functioning graft has lived more than 12 years. Approximately 70% of grafts are functioning after 1 year. It remains to be proved whether a pancreas graft will prevent the development and progression of the microangiopathy, which causes retinal and renal damage. Diabetic nephropathy has been the main indication for pancreas grafting and usually a kidney from the same donor has been transplanted simultaneously.

Index

Page numbers in *italics* refer to figures; those in **bold** refer to tables or boxes. Page numbers suffixed with an 'n' refer to footnotes.